Genetic Factors in Nutrition

Academic Press Rapid Manuscript Reproduction

Proceedings of an International Workshop
on Genetic Factors in Nutrition
Held in Teotihuacán, Mexico
August 4–8, 1982

Genetic Factors in Nutrition

Edited by

Antonio Velázquez

Department of Human Biochemical Genetics
National University of Mexico
Mexico City, Mexico

Héctor Bourges

Department of Nutritional Physiology and Food Technology
National Institute of Nutrition
Mexico City, Mexico

Editorial Assistant

Isabel Pérez Montfort

1984

ACADEMIC PRESS, INC.
(Harcourt Brace Jovanovich, Publishers)
Orlando   San Diego   New York   London
Toronto   Montreal   Sydney   Tokyo

ACADEMIC PRESS, INC.
Orlando, Florida 32887

United Kingdom Edition published by
ACADEMIC PRESS, INC. (LONDON) LTD.
24/28 Oval Road, London NW1 7DX

Library of Congress Cataloging in Publication Data

Main entry under title:

Genetic factors in nutrition.

    "Proceedings of an International Workshop on Genetic
Factors in Nutrition held in Teotihuacán, Mexico on August
4-8, 1982"--
    Includes index.
    1. Nutrition--Genetic aspects--Congresses.
I. Velázquez Arellano, Antonio. II. Bourges, Héctor.
III. International Workshop on Genetic Factors in
Nutrition (1982 : San Juan Teotihuacán, Mexico)
QP141.A1G46 1984   612.3   84-14473
ISBN 0-12-715950-9 (alk. paper)

PRINTED IN THE UNITED STATES OF AMERICA

84 85 86 87   9 8 7 6 5 4 3 2 1

Contents

III. Nutrient Requirements and Metabolism

IV. Energy Balance

V. Assessment of Nutritional Status

VI. Prospectives

Contributors

Numbers in parentheses indicate the pages on which the authors' contributions begin.

George H. Beaton (189), *Department of Nutritional Sciences, Faculty of Medicine, University of Toronto, Toronto, Ontario, Canada*

Margaret H. Beaver (211), *Department of Microbiology, Lobund Laboratory, University of Notre Dame, Notre Dame, Indiana 46556*

Henry Blackburn (105), *School of Public Health and Medical School, University of Minnesota, Minneapolis, Minnesota 55455*

George A. Bray (339), *Division of Diabetes and Clinical Nutrition, University of Southern California School of Medicine, Los Angeles, California 90007*

Luigi Cavalli-Sforza (423), *Department of Genetics, Stanford University Medical School, Stanford, California 94305*

Stephen D. Cederbaum (79), *University of California Mental Retardation Research Center, The Center for the Health Sciences, Los Angeles, California 90024*

Douglas L. Coleman (329), *The Jackson Laboratory, Bar Harbor, Maine 04609*

Sonja L. Connor (137), *Section of Clinical Nutrition and Lipid Metabolism, Department of Medicine, Oregon Health Sciences University, Portland, Oregon 97201*

William E. Connor (137), *Section of Clinical Nutrition and Lipid Metabolism, Department of Medicine, Oregon Health Sciences University, Portland, Oregon 97201*

Joaquín Cravioto (413), *Instituto Nacional de Ciencias y Tecnología para la Salud del Niño DIF, Mexico City, Mexico*

Janis S. Fisler (339), *Division of Diabetes and Clinical Nutrition, University of Southern California School of Medicine, Los Angeles, California 90007*

Lars Garby (319), *Department of Physiology, University of Odense, Odense, Denmark*

Alfred E. Harper (243), *Departments of Biochemistry and Nutritional Sciences, The University of Wisconsin–Madison, Madison, Wisconsin 53706*

Richard E. Hillman (199), *Division of Medical Genetics, Washington University Medical School, St. Louis, Missouri 63130*

Alan A. Jackson (297), *Tropical Metabolism Research Unit, University of the West Indies, Kingston, Jamaica*

Rubén Lisker (93), *Departamento de Genética, Instituto Nacional de la Nutrición Salvador Zubirán, Mexico City, Mexico*

Reynaldo Martorell (373), *Food Research Institute, Stanford University, Stanford, California 94305*

Arno G. Motulsky (157), *Division of Medical Genetics, University of Washington, Seattle, Washington 98195*

James V. Neel (3), *Department of Human Genetics, The University of Michigan Medical School, Ann Arbor, Michigan 48104*

M. C. Nesheim (417), *Division of Nutritional Sciences, Cornell University, Ithaca, New York 14853*

Philip R. Payne (177), *Department of Human Nutrition, London School of Hygiene and Tropical Medicine, London, England*

Rafael Ramos Galván (393), *Subjefatura de Investigación Clínica, Subdirección General Médica, Centro Médico Nacional, Mexico City, Mexico*

Rosa María Ramos Rodríguez (393), *Instituto de Investigaciones Antropológicas, Universidad Nacional Autónoma de Mexico, Mexico City, Mexico*

Leon E. Rosenberg (61), *Department of Human Genetics, Yale University School of Medicine, New Haven, Connecticut 06510*

William J. Schull (161), *Center for Demographic and Population Genetics, Graduate School of Biomedical Sciences, The University of Texas Health Science Center, Houston, Texas 77225*

Nevin S. Scrimshaw (17), *Department of Nutrition and Food Science, Massachusetts Institute of Technology, Cambridge, Massachusetts 02139*

Selma E. Snyderman (269), *Department of Pediatrics, New York University School of Medicine, New York, New York 10003*

Noel W. Solomons[1] (225), *Department of Nutrition and Food Science, Massachusetts Institute of Technology, Cambridge, Massachusetts 02139, and Instituto de Nutrición de Centro América and Panamá, Guatemala City, Guatemala*

Benjamin Torún (361), *División de Nutrición Humana y Biología, Instituto de Nutrición de Centro América y Panamá, Guatemala City, Guatemala*

Antonio Velázquez (57), *Unidad de Genética de la Nutrición, Instituto de Investigaciones Biomédicas, Universidad Nacional Autónoma de México, Mexico City, Mexico*

Richard H. Ward (37), *Department of Medical Genetics, University of British Columbia, Vancouver, British Columbia, Canada*

John C. Waterlow (279), *Department of Human Nutrition, London School of Hygiene and Tropical Medicine, London WC1E 7HT, England*

Bernard S. Wostmann (211), *Department of Microbiology, Lobund Laboratory, University of Notre Dame, Notre Dame, Indiana 46556*

[1]Present address: Divisíon de Nutrición Humana y Biológia, Instituto de Nutrición de Centro América y Panamá, Guatemala City, Guatemala.

Introduction

During the nineteenth century, one of the forefathers of human genetics, Francis Galton, used the terms "nature" and "nurture" to refer to biological heredity and to the environment, the two opposing forces which mold a living being and determine its phenotype. Although it is generally recognized that genes play a role in the use of nutrients, Galton's choice of words emphasizes the frequent perception of nutrition as a condition modulated essentially by the environment. The environmental aspects of nutrition have been amply studied, whereas studies on genetic factors are scarce.

For a long time now, scientists from both fields have recognized the enormous variation in all human populations. Genetic polymorphisms are widespread and essential for survival and evolution. On the other hand, nutritionists have been hindered by great individual variation in their subjects when establishing minimum nutritional requirements adequate for achieving optimal levels of health in various populations.

This great variability, seen both from the genetic and nutritional points of view, generates an enormous degree of individuality. But to what extent is nutritional individuality a consequence of genetic individuality? How do genes and food interact to determine nutritional state? How does this interaction influence health and disease? Why are some people obese without being gluttons or lazy, while others can eat almost limitless amounts without becoming obese? Why do some children fall victim to kwashiorkor or marasmus while others, seemingly equally undernourished, manage to adapt, survive, and reproduce? How in nutrition might we quantitatively interpret Ortega y Gasset's phrase "I am I and my circumstances?"

For many of these questions we lack even tentative responses. Finding the answers will depend on the joint interdisciplinary effort of nutritionists and geneticists. There have not been many such collaborations; geneticists and nutritionists have usually followed separate paths. For example, we know something about the importance of genotype in susceptibility to obesity, but we know nothing at all about the importance of genotype in predisposition to serious forms of malnutrition. We have the results of countless nutritional surveys carried out throughout almost the entire world. But students interested in the role of family factors will have a hard time finding anything useful because these factors are almost never considered in the questionnaires.

It is time for this situation to change. This book contains the proceedings of the International Workshop on Genetic Factors in Nutrition, sponsored by the National Autonomous University of Mexico and the National Institute of Nutrition "Salvador Zubirán" to promote the opening of communication between the two disciplines and to help develop a link between them. We aimed to define questions rather than answers, inventory methodological tools and strategies, and identify some of the most promising lines of interdisciplinary research.

The first papers establish the framework for consideration of genetic–nutritional interplay, utilizing the unifying perspective of biological evolution. Afterward, some examples of successful interaction between the two disciplines are reviewed. This is followed by a discussion of some aspects of nutrient requirements and utilization and consideration of methodological approaches to assess nutritional status, with emphasis on malnutrition. Finally the proceedings are summarized and genetic prospectives are presented. The discussions held by the participants during the meeting have been summarized by the chairmen of each session.

The editors were extremely fortunate in having the advice and support of the members of the program committee: Héctor Bourges, Stephen Cederbaum, Phillip P. Cohen, James V. Neel, Cecilia Salgado, Antonio Velázquez, and Richard Ward. They helped us plan the conference, define the approach, develop the program, and convince the participants, all of them very busy scientists, to temporarily set aside some of their obligations, prepare their manuscripts, and attend the meeting. This workshop on genetics and nutrition would never have come to fruition had it not been enthusiastically accepted and generously supported by the National University of Mexico's Coordinator de la Investigación Cientifica, Jaime Martuscelli; by the Director del Instituto de Investigaciones Biomédicas, Kaethe Willms; and by the Secretario Ejecutivo del Consejo de Estudios de Posgrado of the University, José Manuel Berruecos. We also want to acknowledge the valuable help of the Programa Universitario de Investigación Clínica, of the Dirección General de Asuntos de Personal Académico of the University, and the Consejo Nacional de Ciencia y Tecnología.

Special thanks go to Dr. P. P. Cohen and Cecilia Salgado, whose help and cooperation both before and during the workshop contributed greatly to its success, and to Paulina Rostín, whose constant and efficient work always made our job easier.

It is appropriate that this Workshop on Genetic Factors in Nutrition should be held in Mexico. For 40 years now, many excellent, internationally recognized nutritional research projects have been carried out here; the country has several mature groups of nutritionists.

The work sessions took place in Teotihuacán, near Mexico City. Two thousand years ago, the archeological site was the principal city on the American continent, a crucible in which the arts and sciences peacefully flourished. It is appropriate to point out that Teotihuacán was one of the few great metropolises never surrounded by defensive walls. Could there be a better place, then, for scientists from many countries to meet in harmony, as surely wise men of that ancient civilization often did, to work together for the advancement of knowledge?

A. VELÁZQUEZ
H. BOURGES

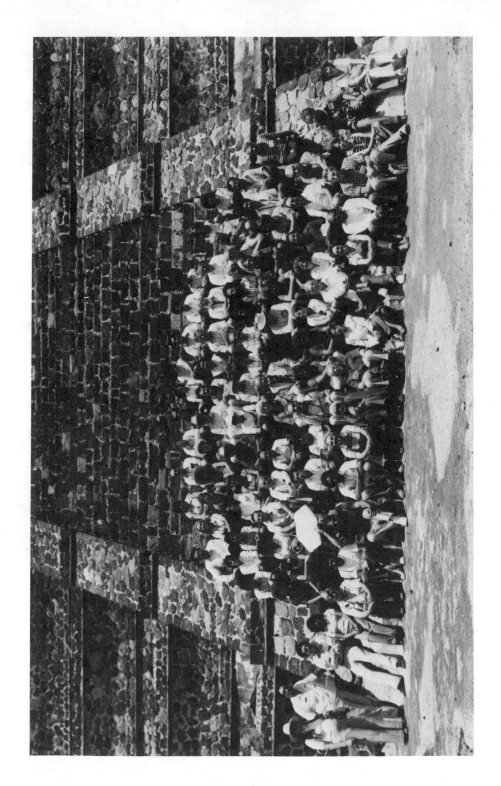

xiv

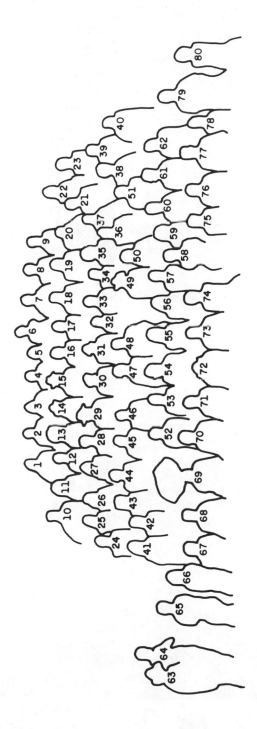

Participants of the International Workshop on Genetic Factors in Nutrition, held in Teotihuacán, México, on August 4-8, 1982. Key: 1. Mrs. Harper 2. A. Harper 3. P. Payne 4. A. González-Noriega 5. C. González-Noriega 7. Ignacio Méndez 8. Sergio Flores 9. Laura Moreno 10. Fabio Salamanca 11. Alessandra Carnevale 12. Miss Cavalli-Sforza 14. Mrs. Cavalli-Sforza 15. L. Cavalli-Sforza 16. L. Cavalli-Sforza Jr. 17. Reynaldo Martorell 18. M.C. Nesheim 19. G. Beaton 20. L. Garby 21. J. Waterlow 24. J. Miranda 27. S. Rodríguez 28. P. von Reisfeld 29. R. Hillman 31. L. Coleman 32. H. Bourges Jr. 33. H. Bourges 34. M. Bourges 35. Mrs. H. Bourges 36. H. Blackburn 39. R. Ortiz 40. W. Connor 41. M. Vázquez 42. C. Salgado 44. R. Garza-Chapa 45. S. Frenk 46. B. Torún 47. Mrs. J.V. Neel 48. J.V. Neel 49. G. Bray 51. R. Ward 52. C. de Céspedes 53. Mrs. A. Motulsky 54. A. Motulsky 55. B. Dahl 58. N.S. Scrimshaw 60. S. Cederbaum 61. R. Scott 62. B. Wostman 63. Mrs. R.E. Hillman 64. R. Chávez 65. R. Urzúa 67. J. Schull 68. Dr. Quintana 69. L. Rosenberg 70. Mr. Barbour 71. A. Velázquez 72. Mrs. P. Cohen 73. P.P. Cohen 74. S. Snyderman 75. Mrs. A. Velázquez 76. A. Jackson 77. A. Huberman 78. E. Casanueva 79. E. Jurado 80. S. Connor.

PART I

EVOLUTIONARY AND GENETIC FRAMEWORK

GENETICS AND NUTRITION:
AN EVOLUTIONARY PERSPECTIVE

James V. Neel

Department of Human Genetics
University of Michigan Medical School
Ann Arbor, Michigan

INTRODUCTION

The diet of our ancestors

Humans are exceedingly omnivorous animals. In the early stages of hominoid divergence from the other primates, we may presume the diet was very similar to that of present day chimpanzees. Our ancestors would have been scavengers, living on nuts, berries, fruits, roots, and an occasional small animal or egg, but, they posessed simple tools, and gathering was therefore much more efficient than in chimpanzees por example. As they began to develop hunting skills (as opposed to scavenging skills), perhaps 1,000,000 years ago, the amount of animal protein in the diet increased. Then came plant domestication, beginning some 20,000 years ago, and, even with early agricultural practices, a radical change in the diet occurred.

There are very few surviving human populations depending on pre-agriculture-type hunting-and-gathering for their livelihood, and such as there are - Australian aborigines - have usually been so displaced from their customary range that they do not project a very satisfactory picture of the nutritional balance of a hunting-gathering population. On the other hand, there still exist - or did until recently - relatively intact populations combining hunting-and-gathering with primitive agricultural practices. Two such groups are the Yanomama Amerindians, occupying the region drained by the Upper Orinoco and the two principal northern tributaries of the Amazon River, the Rio Branco and the Rio Negro, and the Xavante of the Brazilian Mato Grosso. In addition to our studies of these two groups, we have by now done field work among 10 other Amerindian tribes in various but more advanced stages of acculturation.

3

In this presentation, I shall tend to concentrate on findings among Amerindians, not only because this is the group with which I am most familiar but also because it seems especially appropriate to a meeting of this type in this hemisphere.

Although the studies of our group on the Xavante and Yanomama were never specifically dietary in nature, some aspects of their subsistence patterns were obvious. With respect to general nutritional status, we never encountered true obesity but an occasional young woman was 'pleasingly plump'. Neither, on the other hand, did we encounter the stigmata of chronic protein malnutrition. Although the Yanomama still are extensively engaged in hunting and gathering, the majority of their calories are derived from the cultivated cooking banana *(Musa paradisica)*. This is grown in gardens by the slash-and-burn technique, new gardens being started frequently. There may be periods of acute food shortages, when the old gardens are not yielding well and the new gardens are not yet mature, but I doubt if any undisturbed tribal population ever endured the chronic malnutrition which is a problem for so much of the world today. No group would voluntarily occupy an area that would not adequately support it.

In their efforts to achieve nutritional balance, the Xavante and Yanomama are most adaptable as to protein source. Although game - tapir, capybara, monkey, armadillo - are preferred, caterpillars, beatle larvae, turtle eggs in season, and small fish obtained by poisoning streams with rotenone, are quite acceptable.

In general, a child is breast fed for some 3 years, until the arrival of the next child. If an adult woman is not nursing her own child, she is nursing the child of some relative. The nutritional status of infants is by inspection usually excellent. The gamma-globulin levels of tribal populations are by the standards of civilized populations quite high; we have argued for a *relatively* smooth transition from passive to active immunity against the local pathogens [1]. By the time the child is weaned, its dentition enables it to cope with the local foods. It is our impression that the weanling diarrhea so characteristic of civilized tropical agrarian populations is a much less serious problem in a tribal group such as the Yanomama.

It is, in this connection, relevant that almost all primitive groups which have been adequately studied can be shown to have customs which sharply limit population growth. To what extent this results from a conscious effort to reconcile numbers with available resources is a much debated question among anthropologists. The prolonged lactation mentioned earlier may serve to suppress ovulation for some time following parturition; this can scarcely be seen as a conscious measure to limit population growth. An Indian mother will nurse her child several times an hour during the day, and several times in the course of the night. McNeilly [2] has argued that frequent nipple stimulation leads to regular prolactin surges and a suppression of estrogen and progesterone production, which is much more effective than the suppression induced by widely-spaced nursing.

In addition, however, there are conscious efforts to control the birth rate. There are often intercourse taboos for at least a year following the birth of a child. Further, abortion, induced by direct trauma to the abdomen, and infanticide are not uncommon among the Yanomama. Although precise figures are very difficult to obtain, we estimate, on the basis of anecdotal information plus the markedly unbalanced sex ratio among the very young, that approximately 30 percent of liverborn female infants and 5 percent of liverborn male infants are killed [3]. One stated reason for the abortion and infanticide is that the nursling is not yet ready to leave the breast. In addition, deformed children are customarily killed. The basis for the custom of such preferential female infanticide has no simple, compelling explanation.

Recently it has been argued that the apparent child-spacing among primitive populations may also be due to the fact that women below critical levels of fat storage do not conceive [4, 5, 6,]. This is a hypothesis that cannot-unfortunately-be pursued in many contemporary populations. As already suggested, the apparent nutritional level of the Yanomama and other relatively undisturbed tribes is such, that I doubt whether this is an important factor in Amerindian child spacing.

The ecology of disease is quite different in unacculturated Amerindians than in civilized communities [7, 8]. Of particular interest to us in the context of nutrition should be the parasitic and diarrheal diseases. I have already indicated the belief that weanling diarrhea is relatively uncommon among Amerindian infants. Our studies of parasites reveal a high prevalence of *Ascaris lumbricoides,* hookworm, *Trichuris trichiura, Strongyloides stercoralis, Entamoeba hartmanni, Entamoeba coli, Entamoeba histolytica, Iodamoeba buschlii, Giardia lamblia* and *Chilomastix mesnili,* plus several other less frequent parasites [9, 10]. But despite the high prevalences, the parasitizations, as judged from very limited stool samples, were not heavy. In the instance of hookworm, the custom of changing the village site every 3 or 4 years plus lack of a fixed place for defecation undoubtedly prevented the super-infection characteristic of many rural agricultural populations. The vicious combination of recurrent diarrhea, intense parasitization, and chronic malnutrition seen among the caboclos and campesinos of Central and South America is much less apt to occur amongst unacculturated Amerindians. On the other hand, in some areas parasitization by microfilaria of *Mansonella ozzardi* is very heavy [11, 12]; it has never ceased to amaze me how the tissues (at least as judged by the skin) can so swarm with these worms with so little apparent medical consequence.

The result of all this is for the Yanomama a life curve rather different from those encountered in civilized populations (Fig. 1) [3]. We estimate that, aside from death due to infanticide, some 22% of liveborn males and 13% of liveborn female infants die during infancy. This is high by the standards of developed countries, but well below the situation in most peasant populations until rather recently. The continuing mortality during the childhood and adult years has a large traumatic component. Approximately 10% of liveborn infants can expect to reach age 60. An analysis of skeletal material from Indian burial mounds suggests prehistoric mortality patterns very similar to those of the Yanomama [13, 14, 15]. We suggest that with this population structure, the natural rate of population

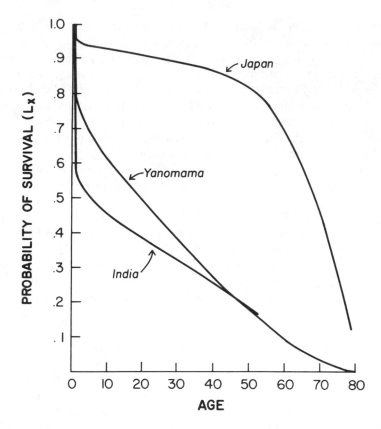

Figure 1. Life curve of the Yanomama compared to other populations.

increase per year is 0.5 -1.0% per year. Howell [16] reports similar findings among the contemporary !Kung San. We believe that because of the decimation of their neighbors plus the relatively recent acquisition of steel tools, the Yanomama are expanding more rapidly than characterized Indian tribes during prehistory. Even lower rates of increase - say 0.3% - were presumably periodically offset by a variety of disasters - the most important probably being intervillage warfare -otherwise given 20,000 years and even a very small founding population, the total numbers of Indians at the time of first contacts [estimated at 20,000,000 for South America [17]] would have been larger.

Our altered nutritional circumstances

I hardly need dwell on how dramatically the nutritional circumstances of modern man depart from those of his ancestors. The most obvious differences are, on the one hand, the emergence, all over the world, of groups who are chronically malnourished, but, on the other hand, a striking frequency of over-nutrition, some 15% of the U.S. population, for instance, is classified as obese, the precise figure, of course, depending on rather arbitrary standards. In those areas where malnutrition is rampant, the children, of course, suffer disproportionately, in no small measure because of a relatively high birth rate, with the inevitable concomitant of less time on the breast for any specific infant.

In addition to this very obvious development, there are of course many much more subtle changes in dietary patterns. Let me mention only three, to whose possible genetic implications we can return later. The first of these is a major change in the bulk of the diet. Primitive people did not have access to refined foods. Intestinal transit time was more rapid [18]. The various products of protein putrefaction could not accumulate in the feces to the same extent. As one who has handled a fair number of stool samples from both civilized and remote Amerindian populations, I can testify that to the extent the olfactory sense can be trusted, the indoles and skatoles - hallmarks of protein putrefaction - are a much less prominent component of Amerindian stools. Efforts to type the strains of *E. coli in* Yanomama stools led to the identification of 13 new 0 serotypes before we gave up (19). We have no idea whether these result from the persistence of chance mutations in an isolated population or have adaptive significance.

The second change is the introduction with civilization of a wide variety of chemicals into the diet, usually as food preservatives, coloring agents, or texturing agents, but sometimes inadvertently. This is not to present the world of primitive man as free of what might broadly be termed pollutants. For instance, in a survey designed to yield baselines from which to appreciate the added body burden with civilization of a number of chemicals of potential toxic significance, we were surprised to find, in two very remote Yanomama villages, blood mercury levels in males significantly higher than those in comparable Ann Arbor males (Red Cross blood donors). By contrast, lead and cadmium levels were lower, and copper very similar (20). We presume the mercury is derived from some natural constituent of the diet, presumably plant-life growing in a mercury-rich environment, but have no real evidence to that effect. At any rate, dietary chemical contamination was not unknown in such populations, but presumably less common than among civilized groups.

The third striking change is in the mineral content of the diet. The Yanomama do not add salt to their diet. The collection of 24-hour urine samples from males who have no understanding of why one would wish to do such a foolish thing (and even give a gift in return) presents a few problems not encountered on a metabolic ward; our best estimate of the 24-hour excretion of Na+ in adult males, adequacy of the sample judged by creatinine content, is 1.02 ± 1.51 mEq/liter (21). Spot urine samples confirm the 24-hour findings. The large standard deviation is due to a few 'outliers' whom we suspect helped the expedition's cook dispose of excess food; without them the mean would be well below 1 mEq/liter/24 hours. This is roughly 1% of the amount recovered in the urine of the average European or North American male.

The genetic significance of changing dietary patterns

Against this brief background, let us now begin a consideration of genetic factors in relation to nutritional requirements and excesses. It is an article of genetic faith that every species has evolved genetic adaptations to its diet, some obviously structural, like teeth, but others more subtle, such as the enzymatic armentarium. The intestinal tract of herbivores is adapted to plant material and of carnivores, to meat. Presumably, despite the fact that we are omnivores, and very adaptable ones at that, we too have evolved certain genetic adaptations and limitations with respect to our customary diet, adaptations now being challenged by the many dietary changes upon which I have commented so briefly [cf. 22].

Human populations represent storehouses of genetic variability, greater than appreciated until recently. From the genetic studies on blood groups, serum proteins, and erythrocyte enzymes, it has been estimated that electrophoretically - identified variants occur at a level greater than 2% (i.e., as genetic polymorphisms) at 20-25% of all human genetic loci so far examined, and that the average individual is heterozygous at 6% of his loci for such variants [23]. Since electrophoresis only identifies charge-change variants, the true amount of genetic variation is appreciably higher. Recent studies employing 2-dimensional polyacrylamide gel electrophoresis are revealing lower levels of variation, but to what extent; this is due to technical reasons is not yet clear [24]. On the other hand, analysis of variation at sites of action for the DNA restriction endonucleases is suggesting an unexpectedly high frequency of genetic polymorphisms of DNA [31-35]. Some of these must relate to translated DNA sequences and potentially significant genetic differences between individuals. While, then, we cannot exactly evaluate the pool of genetic variability in human populations, clearly it is considerable.

When nutritional patterns - or, for that matter, any other aspect of the environment - change dramatically, these changes will thus impact on a genetically highly heterogeneous population. Because of individual genetic differences, it may be anticipated that some individuals will respond quite differently to the change from others and this difference in response will be transmitted. Otherwise stated, individual differences which might otherwise go unnoticed can be thrown into high relief by a significant change in the environment - in this case, diet. For this reason, it is a propitious time for the geneticist concerned with understanding inherited nutritional differences between individuals.

In this context it is important to draw a distinction between two different classes of genetically-influenced nutritional diseases. There are, on the one hand, nutritional inadequacies determined by single genes. As currently known, these inadequacies are usually severe, often life-threatening. Examples include phenylketonuria, the glycogen storage and urea cycle disorders, and abnormalities of branched chain amino acid metabolism. We believe that the genes responsible for these diseases are largely maintained by the pressure of mutation. Although there are no reliable historical data, such rare diseases have probably been part of the human scene for millenia.

On the other hand, there is an important group of diseases which appear to be multigenic in origin with considerable genetic heterogeneity, behind the symptomatology which brings them to medical attention. Some of these diseases, such as maturity-onset-type diabetes mellitus and essential hypertension, are relatively common. Their apparent rarity in primitive populations, but emergence in civilization, suggests that the altered environment - especially its nutritional aspects - is uncovering genetic predispositions not previously expressed in this way. These predispositions have not simply been accumulating waiting to be uncovered - presumably the genes involved have legitimate functions in the bodily economy, but the altered nutritional environment has resulted in new phenotypic expressions for these genes.

Although at this meeting we are concentrating on nutritional disorders, we must recognize, even if we do not discuss, how other aspects of our life style, such as the pattern of physical activity, are also changing. It is by no means clear how the patterns of exercise and diet interdigitate, but the influence of exercise on insulin requirements is just one small example that they do.

The monogenic disorders in a changing nutritional environment

The monogenic nutritional disorders are the 'classical' inborn errors of metabolism, now amounting to several hundred. The dietary shifts I have mentioned are not apt to alter their basic expression appreciably, although the concomitant improvement in understanding and medical care will increase the likelihood of survival, and even reproduction. These disorders, caused by enzyme or receptor defects, are unremittingly present from birth onwards, qualitative impairments of a magnitude incompatible with normal functioning.

Every sweeping generalization has its exceptions, including the foregoing. About 1 in 500 Caucasoids exhibits hypercholesterolemia because of a genetically determined defect in cellular surface receptors for low density lipoprotein (LDL), a cholesterol complex [36]. Individuals heterozygous for the allele(s) in question on the 'typical' diet of Western Civilization tend to exhibit cholesterol levels in the 300 to 550 mgm % range and a 2.5 fold elevation in the plasma level of low-density lipoprotein. Myocardial infarctions between the ages of 35 and 55 are common. The homozygotes for this allele-about 1 per 1,000,000 persons - show a much more extreme picture, with cholesterol levels of 650 to 1000 mgm % and death from myocardial infarction in the second decade quite common. These manifestations of the disease are against a dietary background such that the average young adult has a cholesterol level of 200 to 250 mgm %. Among the Xavante of the Brazilian Mato Grosso the serum cholesterol level was (M $\pm$ σ) 127.1 $\pm$ 29.5 mgm % in young males and 164.9 $\pm$ 47.2 mgm %

in young females at the Sao Domingos village and even lower at the villages of Simoes Lopes and Sao Marcos [1, 9]. Similar low values have been reported for other tribal populations [refs. in 1]. Since the hypercholesterolemia of the heterozygote for the receptor defect is seen as a compensatory elevation of substrate in the presence of the receptor defect, one can speculate that the manifestation of the trait should be altered in "low cholesterol" cultures, but there are in fact no pertinent data.

The multigenic disorders in a changing nutritional environment

We turn now to what I will term for present puposes the 'emerging multigenic nutritional disorders'. Time permits brief mention of only three examples, genetic responses to a changing environment. Two of these examples - maturity - onset-type diabetes mellitus and essential hypertension -will come as no surprise, but the third, carcinoma of the colon, is one not usually viewed in this light.

Although the kind of data one really wants on the incidence of maturity-onset-type diabetes mellitus is simply not available for relatively undisturbed Amerindians, the impression is of an uncommon disorder. By contrast, diabetes mellitus is rampant among North American Indians, in whom obesity is also extremely common, the Pima and Papago being especially well-studied in this respect [37-43]. The disease is also emerging as a major problem among other recently acculturated groups [44-47]. A recent small study of the response of unacculturated male Yanomama and Panoan Marubo to a standard glucose load revealed plasma blood sugar, insulin, pancreatic polypeptide, and growth hormone levels which in the context of a multivariate analysis were significantly different from those of an age-and sex-matched control assembled in Ann Arbor [48]. The differences were not, however, characteristic of a higher frequency of incipient diabetes among the Indians. The 2-hour glucose level of the Marubo [5.9 ± 1.4 μmol/l], although somewhat higher than that of Caucasian controls, was much less elevated than would be the case for a similar sample of Pima [estimated 7.8 ± 5.6 μmol/l], it may thus be presumed that the diabetes so characteristic of the North American Indian has emerged with acculturation.

The familial nature of maturity onset diabetes in civilized populations is well established, but the precise mechanism(s) for what is very likely a heterogeneous collection of diseases remains unclear [49]. The failure in genetic studies to find a clear distinction between diabetics and non-diabetics within the family argues in the general case for multigenic control [50, 51]. On several occasions I have suggested that the disease may result from a perversion of the 'normal' genetically controlled physiological system for sugar metabolism, a perversion due to excessive stimulation of that system by refined carbohydrate [52, 53]. This excessive stimulation in time results in responses which impair sugar metabolism. I have suggested a number of precise mechanisms, which we cannot stop to consider now. My colleagues and I have shown that in the statistical sense, the disease is very gradual in onset, minor impairments of the glucose tolerance test being present in some instances 20 years before the onset of clinical disease [50, 54]. Given the ameliorative (and possibly 'curative') effect of a properly disciplined diet in the very early stages of the disease, it seems proper to term this a nutritional disease.

Along with changes in the protein-calorie content of the diet with acculturation, there have in some instances been striking changes in the mineral content of the diet. Salt is a good case in point. Earlier we documented the low salt intake of the Yanomama. We have encountered only one case of (borderline) hypertension among the Xavante and Yanomama [55, 21], and the disease is well known to be rare among primitive populations, usually on relatively low salt diets [1]. The conservation of sodium under these conditions requires levels of renin and aldosterone encountered in the United States only in the presence of an adrenal adenoma or renal artery stenosis [21, 56]. Hypertension can be controlled by an extremely low salt diet. The familial nature of the disease is well established. As for maturity-onset-type diabetes mellitus, hypertension is a major cause of illness among recently acculturated populations, including Amerindians [57, 45]. It seems a reasonable hypothesis that salt at the levels injested by most civilized populations, while not directly causative of hypertension, permits the expression of a still poorly understood genetic predisposition, a 'predisposition' serving a different genetic purpose under 'no salt' conditions.

A final example of a dietary change may result in the expression of previously inapparent genetic differences between individuals pertains to the decreasing bulk content in our diet. Carcinoma of the colon is now the second most common cause of cancer mortality; this malignancy appears to be very uncommon amongst primitives. One hypothesis suggests that the relative intestinal stasis of civilized man permits the formation of mutagenic protein decomposition products [18] -much as charring meat results in the formation of mutagens [58, 59]. Even after the exclusion of such clear genetic predispositions to carcinoma of the colon as multiple polyposis of the colon and Gardener's syndrome, carcinoma of the colon has a 'familial predisposition', first degree relatives of patients exhibiting a 3-fold elevation in risk over controls [60, 61, 62]. Although it has not been excluded that this familial predisposition stems from familial dietary patterns, it is also a reasonable postulate that there are a variety of inherited differences between individuals in the ability to detoxify potential carcinogens formed in the large bowel, which differences find this particular mode of expression only as the diet changes.

The special case of chronic malnutrition

As I have stated earlier, I believe the condition of chronic protein - calorie malnutrition was extremely uncommon in primitive man. It would be an article of genetic faith that as food conditions deteriorate, individual differences in the ability to adjust would emerge. Such differences will certainly be influenced by acquired attributes, such as the nature of the intestinal flora and the degree to which, prior to the onset of malnutrition, antibodies to some of the intestinal pathogens had been acquired. On the other hand, one can easily visualize innate factors which would influence the adjustment. Within the euthyroid state there is a considerable range in the basal metabolic rate. Let us assume that the precise setting to the normal thermostat is to some extent under control. A case can be made for the individual whose setting is on the low side, and who consequently has lower requirements for metabolic balance, adapting to malnutrition better than the individual with the higher requirements.

This is a problem one would prefer not to have the opportunity to study. I regard the challenge of reconciling the numbers of people on the earth with the earth's capacity for sustained food production as equal in importance only by the task of bringing the nuclear armaments race under control, and would prefer that malnutrition disappear long before the geneticist got organized for proper studies. Unfortunately, this will not be the case.

There is a considerable range in obligatory urinary and fecal nitrogen losses in young Caucasian males, and the position of an individual in the spectrum is quite reproducible [63]. To what extent this is genetic and to what extent acquired is unclear. Likewise, the pattern of obligatory urinary and fecal nitrogen loss of young Chinese males differs from that observed in the previously referenced studies on Caucasians [64]. The genetic significance, if any, of these differences is unknown. There is at least the presumption, however, of differences that might influence the response to malnutrition, and in a world where local protein deficiencies are common, understanding the nature of these differences - be they inherited or acquired - is of potential practical value.

There are some difficult ethnical problems in the study of how genetic differences may influence the response to malnutrition. There are observations which one would like to make upon severely malnourished children who, however, so require treatment that it is difficult to justify any delay in therapy, valuable though the data to be gained might be.

Some philosophical issues in the prevention and treatment of genetically influenced nutritional disease

In closing, I would like to devote a few minutes to a consideration of some philosophical issues in the prevention and treatment of genetically - conditioned nutritional disease. Once nutritional genetic disease is apparent - be it of the monogenic or multigenic type - there is no ethical alternative to the fullest treatment possible. But the strategy of prevention is quite different for the two genetic types of nutritional disease. For the monogenic, it is genetic counseling and prenatal diagnosis through amniocentesis, the latter followed by elective abortion if the fetus has the defect in question and if abortion is compatible with the law of the land and the beliefs of the parents. For the multigenic, however, the strategy is quite different. One can identify high risk families and recommend stringent precautionary measure within these families -rigid weight control or extreme salt restriction. But there is an alternative -promulgate measures for the general population which will decrease the likelihood of disease among the susceptibles within the population. Although you might expect the geneticist to favor the former aproach, I have become convinced that with limited resources for medical care, the latter will be much more cost - effective. And if, with a general educational push towards avoiding obesity and excessive salt intake, plus regular exercise, it is suggested that those who have a particular family history of diabetes mellitus, hypertension, or gout should in particular observe these measures, so much the better.

REFERENCES

1. Neel, J.V., Salzano, F.M., Junqueira, P.C., Keiter, F., and Maybury-Lewis, D. Studies on the Xavante Indians of the Brazilian Mato Grosso. *Am J. Hum. Genet.* 16:52, 1964.
2. McNeilly, A.S. Effects of lactation on fertility. *Brit. Med. Bull.* 35:151, 1979.
3. Neel, J.V., and Weiss, K.M. The genetic structure of a tribal population, the Yanomama Indians. XII. biodemographic studies. *Am. J. Phys. Anthrop.* 42:25, 1975.
4. Frisch, R.E. Population, food intake, and fertility. *Science* 199:22, 1978.
5. Cohen, M.N. Speculations on the evolution of density measurement and population regulation in *Homo sapiens*. *In* "Biosocial Mechanisms of Population Regulation" (M.N. Cohen, R.S. Malpass, and H.G. Klein, eds.), pp. 275-304. Yale University Press, New Haven. 1980.
6. Huss-Ashmore. Fat and fertility: demographic implications of differential fat storage. *Yearbook of Phys. Anthrop.* 23:65, 1980.
7. Neel, J.V. Genetic aspects of the ecology of disease in the American Indian. *In* "The Ongoing Evolution of Latin American Populations" (F.M. Salzano, ed.), pp. 561-590. C.C. Thomas, Springfield, 1971.
8. Neel, J.V. Health and disease in unacculturated Amerindian populations. *In* "Health and Disease in Tribal Societies. Ciba Foundation Symposium 49" pp. 155-177. Elsevier-North Holland Inc., Amsterdam, 1977.
9. Neel, J.V., Mikkelsen, W.M., Rucknagel, D.L., Weinstein, E.D., Goyer, R.A. and Abadie, S.H. Further studies on the Xavante Indians. VIII. Some observations on blood, urine, and stool specimens. *Am. J. Trop. Med.* 17:474, 1968.
10. Lawrence, D.N., J.V., Abadie, S.H., Moore, L.L., Adams, L.J., Healy, G.R., and Kagan, I.G. Epidemiologic studies among Amerindian populations of Amazonia. III. Intestinal parasitoses in newly contacted and acculturating villages. *Am. J. Trop. Med. Hyg.* 29:530, 1980.
11. Beaver, P.C., Neel, J.V., and Orihel, T.C. *Dipetalonema perstans* and *mansonella ozzardi* in Indians of Southern Venezuela. *Am. J. Trop. Med. Hyg.* 25:263, 1976.
12. Lawrence, D.N., Erdtmann, B., Peet, J.W., Nunes de Mello, J.A., Healy, G.R., Neel, J.V., and Salzano, F.M. Epidemiologic studies among Amerindian populations of Amazonia. II. Prevalence of *Mansonella ozzardi*. *Am. J. Trop. Med. Hyg.* 28:991, 1979.
13. Blakely, R.L. Comparison of the mortality profiles of Archaic, Middle Woodland, and Middle Mississipian skeletal populations. *Am. J. Phys. Anthrop.* 34:43, 1971.
14. Blakely, R.L. Sociocultural implications of demographic data from Etowah, Georgia. *In* "Biocultural Adaptation in Prehistoric America" (R. L. Blakely, ed.), pp. 45-66. University of Georgia Press, Athens.
15. Lovejoy, C.O. Paleodemography of the Libben Site, Ottowa County, Ohio. *Science* 198:291, 1977.

16. Howell, N. "Demography of the Dobe !Kung." New York, Academic press, 1979.
17. Denevan, W.M. (ed.) "The Native Population of the Americas in 1492." University of Wisconsin Press, Madison, 1976.
18. Burkitt, D.P. Epidemiology of cancer of the colon and rectum. *Cancer* 28:3, 1971.
19. Eveland, W.C., Oliver, W.J., Neel, J.V. Characteristics of *Escherichia coli* serotypes in the Yanomama, a primitive Indian tribe of South America. *Infect. Immun.* 4:753, 1971.
20. Hecker, L.H., Allen, H.E., Dinman, B.D., and Neel, J.V. Heavy metal levels in acculturated and unacculturated populations. *Arch. Env. Hlth.* 29:181, 1974.
21. Oliver, W.J., Cohen, E.L., and Neel, J.V. Blood pressure, sodium intake, and sodium related hormones in the Yanomama Indians, a "no-salt" culture. *Circulation* 52:146, 1975.
22. Neel, J.V. The study of natural selection in primitive and civilized human populations. *Hum. Biol.* 30:43, 1958.
23. Harris, H., "The Principles of Human Biochemical Genetics" 3rd revised ed., 554 pp. Elsevier/North-Holland Biomedical Press, Amsterdam, 1980.
24. Leigh Brown, A.J., and Langley, C.H. Reevaluation of genic heterozygosity in natural populations of *Drosophila melanogaster* by two-dimensional electro-phoresis. *Proc. Nat. Acad. Sci. USA* 76:2381, 1979.
25. Comings, D.E. Pc 1 Duarte, a common polymorphism of a human brain protein, and its relationship to depressive disease and multiple sclerosis. *Nature* 277:28, 1970.
26. McConkey, E.H., Taylor, B.J, and Phan, D. Human heterozygosity: A new estimate. *Proc. Nat. Acad. Sci. USA* 76:6500, 1979.
27. Walton, K.E., Styer, D., and Guenstein, E.I. Genetic polymorphism in normal human fibroblasts as analyzed by two-dimensional polyacrylamide gel electrophoresis. *J. Biol. Chem.* 254:7951, 1979.
28. Racine, R.R., and Langley, C.H. Genetic heterozygosity in a natural population of musculus assessed using two-dimensional electrophoresis. *Nature* 283:855, 1980.
29. Smith, C.R., Racine, R.R., and Langley, C.H. Lack of genic variation in the abundant proteins of human kidney. *Genetics* 96:967, 1981.
30. Hamaguchi, H., Ohta, A., Mukai, R., and Yamada, M. Genetic analysis of human lymphocyte proteins by two-dimensional gel electrophoresis: 1. Detection of genetic variant polypeptides in PHA-stimulated peripheral blood lymphocytes. *Hum. Genet.* 59:215, 1981.
31. Kan, Y.W., and Dozy, A.M. Polymorphism of DNA sequence adjacent to human β-globin structural gene: relationship to sickle mutation. *Proc. Nat. Acad. Sci. USA* 75:5631, 1978.
32. Avise, J.C., Lansman, R.A., and Shade, R.O. The use of restriction endonucleases to measure mitochrondrial DNA sequence relatedness in natural populations. I. Population structure and evolution in the gene *Peromyscus. Genetics* 92:279, 1979.
33. Brown, W.M., George, M., and Wilson, A.C. Rapid evolution of animal mitochondrial DNA. *Proc. Nat. Acad. Sci. USA* 76:1967, 1979.
34. Jeffreys, A.J. DNA sequence variants in the G_γ-, A_γ-, δ-and β-globin genes of man. *Cell* 18:1, 1979.
35. Brown, W.M. Polymorphism in mitochondrial DNA of humans as revealed by restriction endonuclease analysis. *Proc. Nat. Acad. Sci. USA* 77:3605, 1980.
36. Brown, M.S., and Goldstein, J.L. Familial hypercholesterolemia: model for genetic receptor disease. *Harvey Lectures* 73:163, 1979.
37. Johnson, J.E., and McNutt, C.W. Diabetes mellitus in an American Indian population isolate. *Tex. Rep. Biol. Med.* 22:110, 1964.
38. Doeblin, T.D., Evans, K., Ingall, G.B., Dowling, K., Chilcote, M.E., Elsea, W., and Bannerman, R.M. Diabetes and hyperglycemia in Seneca Indians. *Hum. Hered.* 19:613, 1969.
39. Henry R.E., Burch, T.A., Bennett, P.H., and Miller, M. Diabetes in the Cocopah Indians. *Diabetes* 18:33, 1969.
40. Elston, R.C., Namboodiri, K.K., Nino, H.V., and Pollitzer, W.S. Studies on blood and urine glucose in Seminole Indians: Indications for segregation of a major gene. *Am. J. Hum. Genet.* 26:13, 1974.

41. Stein, J.H., West, K.M., Robey, J.M., Tirador, D.F., and McDonald, G.W. The high prevalence of abnormal glucose tolerance in the Cherokee Indians of North Carolina. *Arch. Intern. Med.* 116:842, 1965.

42. Bennett, P.H., Rushforth, N.B., Miller, M., and LeCompte, P.M. Epidemiologic studies of diabetes in the Pima Indians. *In* "Recent Progress in Hormone Research 32" pp. 333-376. Academic Press, New York, 1976.

43. Bennett, P.H., Knowler, W.C., Rushforth, N.B., Hamman, R.F., and Savage, P.J. The role of obesity in the development of diabetes in the Pima Indians. *In* "Diabetes and Obesity" (J. Vague, and P.H. Vague, eds.), pp. 117-126, 1979.

44. Prior, I.A.M., Rose, B.S., Harvey, H.P.B., and Davidson, F. Hyperuricaemia, gout and diabetic abnormality in Polynesian people. *Lancet* I:333, 1966.

45. Bassett, D.R., Rosenblatt, G., Moellering, R.C., Jr., and Hartweell, A.S. Cardiovascular disease, diabetes mellitus, and anthropometric evaluation of Polynesian males on the Island of Niihau-1963. *Circulation* 34:1088, 1966.

46. Zimmet, P., Taft, P., Guinea, A., Guthrie, W., and Thoma, K. The high prevalence of diabetes mellitus on a Central Pacific island. *Diabetologia* 13:111, 1977.

47. Zimmet, P., Faaiuso, S., Ainuu, J., Whitehouse, S., Milne, B., and DeBoer, W. The prevalence of diabetes in the renal and urban Polynesian population of western Samoa. *Diabetes* 30:45, 1981.

48. Spielman, R.S., Fajans, S.S., Neel, J.V., Pek, S., Floyd, J.C., and Oliver, W.J. Glucose tolerance in two unacculturated Indian tribes of Brazil. *Diabetologia,* in press.

49. Creutzfeldt, W., Köbberling, J., and Neel, J.V. (eds). "The Genetics of Diabetes Mellitus," 248 pp. Springer Verlag, Berlin, 1976.

50. Neel, J.V., Fajans, S.S., Conn, J.W., and Davidson, R. Diabetes mellitus. *In* "Genetics and the Epidemiology of Chronic Diseases" (J.V. Neel, M.W. Shaw, and W.J. Schull, eds), pp. 105-132. Public Health Service Publication #1163, Government Printing Office, Washington, D.C, 1965.

51. Neel, J.V. Diabetes mellitus-a geneticist's nightmare. *In* "The Genetics of Diabetes Mellitus" (W. Creutzfeldt, J. Köbberling, and J.V. Neel, eds.) pp. 1-11, Springer Verlag, Heidelberg, 1976.

52. Neel, J.V. Diabetes mellitus: a "thrifty" genotype rendered detrimental by "progress." *Am. J. Hum. Genet.* 14:353, 1962.

53. Neel, J.V. The thrifty genotype revisited. *In* "The Genetics of Diabetes Mellitus" (J. Köbberling, and R. Tattersall, eds.). Academic Press, Amsterdam, in press.

54. Beatty, T.H., Neel, J.V., and Fajans, S.S. Identifying risk factors for diabetes in first degree relatives of non-insulin dependent diabetic patients. *Am. J. Epid.* 115:380, 1982.

55. Weinstein, E.D., Neel, J.V., and Salzano, F.M. Further studies on the Xavanté Indians. VI. The physical status of the Xavantes of Simöes Lopes. *Am. J. Hum. Genet.* 19:532, 1967.

56. Oliver, W.J., Neel, J.V., Grekin, R.J. and Cohen, E.L. Hormonal adaptation to the stresses imposed upon sodium balance by pregnancy and lactation in the Yanomama Indians, a culture without salt. *Circulation* 63:110, 1981.

57. Bennett, C.G., Tokuyama, G.H., and McBride, T.C. Cardiovascular-renal mortality in Hawaii. *Am. J. Publ. Hlth.* 52:1418, 1962.

58. Sugimura, T., Nagao, M., Kawachi, T., Honda, M., Yahagi, T., Seino, Y., Sato, S., Matsukura, N., Matsushima, T., Shira, A., Sawamura, M., and Matsumoto, H. Mutagen-carcinogens in food, with special reference to highly mutagenic pyrolytic products in broiled foods. *In* "Origins of Human Cancer" (H.H. Hiatt, J.D. Watson, and J.A. Winsten, eds.), pp. 1561-1577. Cold Spring Harbor Labs, Cold Spring Harbor, 1977.

59. Powrie, W.D., Wu, C.H., Rosin, M.P., and Stich, H.F. Mutagens and carcinogens in food. *In:* "Chemical Mutagenesis, Human Population Monitoring and Genetic Risk Assessment" (K.C. Bora, G.R. Douglas, and E.R. Nestman, eds.) pp. 187-199. Elsevier/North-Holland Biomedical Press, Amsterdam, 1982.

60. Woolf, C.M. A genetic study of carcinoma of the large intestine. *Am. J. Hum. Genet.* 10:42, 1958.
61. Macklin, M.T. Inheritance of cancer of the stomach and large intestine in man. *J. Nat. Cancer Inst.* 24:551, 1960.
62. Burdette, W.J. Heritable cancer of the colorectum. *In* "Carcinoma of the Colon and Antecedent Epithelium" (W.J. Burdette, ed.), pp. 78-102. C.C. Thomas, Springfield, 1970.
63. Scrimshaw, N.S., Hussein, M.A., Murray, E., Rand, W.M., and Young, V.R. Protein requirements of man: variations in obligatory urinary and fecal nitrogen losses in young men. *J. Nutr.* 102:1595, 1972.
64. Huang, P.C., Chong, H.E., and Rand, W.M. Obligatory urinary and fecal nitrogen losses in young Chinese men. *J. Nutr.* 102:1605, 1972.

EVOLUTION, MAN, AND FOOD: A NUTRITIONIST'S VIEW

Nevin S. Scrimshaw

Massachusetts Institute of Technology
Cambridge, Massachusetts

INTRODUCTION

The Importance of Man's Omnivorous Heritage

Early humans emerged from the trees as omnivores with the capability of digesting and obtaining adequate sustenance from a wide variety of foods of plant and animal origin. Those hunting and gathering societies that have maintained their way of life more or less intact into the current century still survive in this manner. For example, Australian Aborigines live in harsh desert conditions and must exploit a wide variety of food in their environment, including vegetable seeds, yams, root fruits such as onion grass, bush fruits, honey from bees and ants, birds' eggs, insects, a number of small desert marsupials, birds, lizards, leaves and nectar flowers, ant hill clay, to give just a sampling of the extraordinary variety of foods utilized [32, 46]. The African bushman is familiar with at least 85 species of edible plants, and 223 local species of animals are known and named by bushmen [28].

This remarkable ability to obtain nutrients from such a variety of foods is quite different from the specificity of the food supply of most animal species. It made it possible for humankind to adapt to a wide range of environments offering heterogeneous mixes of foods, ranging from those of the rain forest to arid zones even deserts, highlands at many different latitudes, and the Arctic. This adaptability includes not only the ability to obtain nutrients from many different food sources, but also the ability to adapt metabolically to enormous variations in the kind and timing of dietary energy supply.

The traditional Eskimo thrived on a diet in which up to 45% of his food energy came from fat, and most of the remainder from protein. Conversely, the lower income populations of many tropical developing countries have diets with no recognizable fat. The corn and bean diet of Mexico and Guatemala

17

may supply less than 10% of calories as fat, and the root and tuber diets of eastern Nigeria only 5%. However, there is no indication that *genetic* variation is a significant factor in this adaptation. Stefansson and the members of his expedition to the Arctic adapted well to the traditional Eskimo diet [45, 19]. Today one can find populations such as the Masai in East Africa whose diet consists chiefly of raw milk and blood, living in the same region as the Akikuyu, who eat almost exclusively cereals, roots, and fruits. Had it not been possible for humankind to give up a diet with liberal amounts of animal protein and subsist primarily on cereals and other foods of vegetable origin, the transition to dependence on agriculture and the progressive growth of world population could not have occurred.

Physiological Adaptability to Dietary Differences

(a) Protein. If populations that were forced by environmental circumstances, including social as well as physical and biological factors, to subsist on a high intake of maize, wheat, or rice were better able to digest and absorb nutrients from that kind of a diet, they would have an advantage. Table I shows that, in fact, when a Guatemalan diet of corn and beans was given to Berkeley, California students, their absorption of protein from that diet proved to be significantly less than that of Guatemalans who were accustomed to it [8].

As Figure 1 illustrates, the differences in absorption of good quality protein by children recovering from malnutrition and healthy MIT students are even more striking and in the opposite direction. Most Americans and Europeans

TABLE I. % Absorption of nitrogen and calories from diets of varying fiber content by Guatemalan and U.S. males fed 0.6 gm protein/kg body weight

		Guatemalan black bean	Corn-diet	Egg formula fiber-free-diet	Egg formula diet with oat bran
13 Rural Guatemalan males after 30-23 mos. Military service	N^1		85 ± 5	—	—
	Energy²		92 ± 2	—	—
6 U.S. male university students	N^1		69 ± 2	91 ± 3	86 ± 4
	Energy²		89 ± 2	97 ± 1	94 ± 2

[1]*Apparent protein digestibility, % dietary N - fecal N/ dietary N × 100.*
[2]*Digestible energy, % = dietary kcal (bomb) - fecal kcal (bomb) / dietary kcal (bomb) × 100.*
Source: Reference 8.

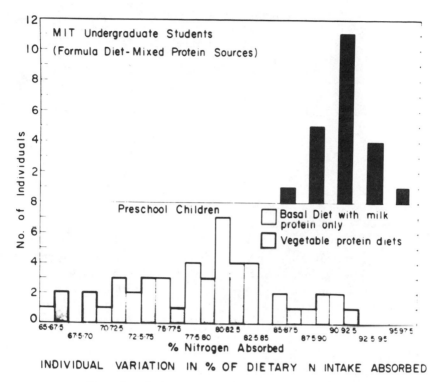

INDIVIDUAL VARIATION IN % OF DIETARY N INTAKE ABSORBED

Figure 1. Individual variation in % of dietary N intake absorbed.

find themselves generally unable to consume the quantities of rice that are commonplace for Asians. However, these and similar patterns of adjustment to various kinds of diets are phenotypic and not genotypic.

At one time, we thought we *had* discovered a possible genetic adaptation to a predominantly rice diet. Individuals consuming a diet with little or no protein reduce their urinary nitrogen excretion. When we placed 100 MIT students on a nitrogen-free diet to measure the minimum urinary loss under these conditions, the six Asians all fell below the mean of the distribution [42]. This stimulated Po Chao Huang, who had observed the MIT study, to repeat it with 50 Taiwanese students [25]. As shown in Table II, he found the mean and distribution of the obligatory nitrogen losses of these individuals to be significantly below those of the Cambridge, Massachusetts sample. Unfortunately for our hypothesis, he repeated the study in a hotter season of the year and found still lower obligatory nitrogen losses, a change that was just sufficient to compensate for the higher losses of nitrogen measured in sweat. Moreover, when obligatory urinary *and* fecal losses were combined, they were the same for the two groups.

TABLE II. Obligatory Urine and
Fecal N Losses in Two Populations of
Young Adult Men

Parameter	M.I.T.[1]	Taiwan[2]
Urine		
mg N/kg	37.2 ± 5.5	33.2 ± 4.2
mg N/kcal	1.7 ± 0.30	1.3 ± 0.2
Fecal		
mg N/kg	8.8 ± 2.1	13.1 ± 2.5

[1]Source: reference 42.
[2]Source: reference 25.

This ability of individuals experiencing increased losses of nitrogen in *sweat* to compensate by decreased *urinary* nitrogen excretion was confirmed by Hector Bourges with MIT students subjected to two hours daily of treadmill exercise at 4 miles per hour and a 10% grade. After adaptation, the measured nitrogen losses in sweat before and after the two hours of exercise were approximately equal to the decrease in urinary nitrogen excretion. Unpublished data from the work of T.R. Davis (1964) shows that there is also adaptation by a decrease in the nitrogen content of the sweat lost with prolonged high temperatures with a proportionately greater conservation of essential than non-essential amino acid N. Adaptation has also been described in Jamaican sugar cane cutters [2].

More recently, the United Nations University has sponsored studies in Bangladesh, Brazil, Chile, China, Colombia, Egypt, Guatemala, India, Korea, Mexico, Nigeria, the Philippines, and Turkey for comparison with those in the United States, Japan, and the USSR [47, 34]. For the ten of these populations for which obligatory nitrogen data are available, no significant differences in obligatory nitrogen loss emerged.

In each of the locations, the amount of protein in the usual diets necessary for nitrogen equilibrium was determined, taking into acount the *measured* obligatory urine and fecal nitrogen losses and the *estimated* integumental and miscellaneous losses. The amounts of protein per kg of body weight required for nitrogen balance were remarkably similar for diets as diverse as those based primarily on rice, corn, wheat, or cassava as the main staple, and ranged from those with little or no animal protein to relatively generous amounts.

It was apparent that the amino acid patterns of foods in the mixed diets complement each other sufficiently that the essential amino acid compositions is *not* the limiting factor in most diets when they are consumed to supply protein at requirement levels. Instead, the observed variation in protein requirement could largely be accounted for by inherent differences in the *digestibility* of the diets, due mainly to their varying fiber content. The studies in rural Mexico of Bourges [4] that might have been expected to show an adaptation to centuries of a maize diet whose protein is of relatively poor quality fell into the *middle* of the range.

In order to calculate the amount of protein required to cover the needs of nearly all of the populations, by definition the mean plus two standard deviations, a pooled standard deviation of all of the studies was used to avoid the exaggeration associated with the calculation of variance from a very small sample. It was reasoned that if the average protein requirement were fed to a number of individuals, there should be aproximately equal numbers in negative and positive nitrogen balance during the observation period. On the other hand, if an amount equivalent to the average plus two standard deviations were fed, individuals in negative nitrogen balance should be exceedingly rare.

Studies were completed in Chile by Uauy [34], Mexico by Bourges [5], and Turkey by Ozalp [34]. A pooled standard deviation of 18% was used. The average zero nitrogen balance intercept in each case was that observed in an earlier study at multiple intake levels [47], and a pooled standard deviation from all of the studies was used. In the Turkish study the average requirement was fed. The results with the 12 subjects conformed well with expectations: 5 negative, 4 positive, and 3 close to zero N balance.

In the other two studies, the calculated safe allowance was fed. Of the 53 Chilean and 20 Mexican young men, 97.5% of them should have been in positive nitrogen balance, but 15 of 33 and 9 of 20, respectively, were observed to be in negative nitrogen balance for the ten days. This was true despite the fact that the coefficient of variation was taken to be 18%, whereas for reasons to be explained shortly, a figure of 12.5% will be used in future calculations of this sort. Clearly, environmental or other factors were acting to raise requirements of some of these individuals.

(b) *Energy*. Although international tables boldly present mean caloric requirements for every age and sex group, the "requirement" for dietary energy can vary over an extraordinarily wide range among populations, individuals, and, over time, for the same individual. When observed dietary energy intakes in some developing country populations are only 90 or even 80% or less of the 1973 FAO/WHO [13] estimated mean requirement for energy, only one of two explanations is possible. Either the apparently "deficient individuals" are wasting away and dying, or they have adapted in some manner to energy intakes well below estimated requirements. In fact, it is the latter that occurs to bring the individuals in such a population into zero energy balance.

Since no more than about 15% of this adaptation can come from metabolic adjustement [15], the remainder must come from a reduction in physical activity. The first reduction is in those "discretionary activities" that are so important for social development, and then in the amount of energy available for work. Viteri has documented the extent to which Guatemalan plantation workers are limited by their food intake in the amount of work they can do and then virtually collapse for the remainder of the day, with little further activity [48, 49]. When additional food is provided to them, their consumption and activity both increase.

This reduction in activity when less food is available is true for children as well as adults. Stimulation is essential to normal mental development. The reduced interaction of undernourished children with their environment, including with parents and siblings, is probably a critical factor in the poor cognitive performance of such children, as suggested by the work of Chávez and Martínez in Mexico [9]. They particularly noted the increase in their interactions with the environment and with other persons as a result of giving supplementary food to under-nourished preschool children. This reduced stimulus to poorly growing children helps to explain the observation of another pioneer Mexican nutritionist, Joaquin Cravioto [10], who, in the 1960s, demonstrated and impairment in intersensory coordination of children in the lowest quartiles of weight-for-age compared with those in the upper ones among *lower* socioeconomic group children in both Mexico and Guatemala. In the upper socioeconomic groups in which differences in growth performance were not so influenced by diet and infectious disease, no such relationship was found.

Reduced physical growth is, of course, another adaptation to low food intake, and the smaller final body size leads to a population with lower *per capita* food requirements. This may appear to be a successful and innocuous adaptation, but it is not. The degree of malnutrition sufficient to retard growth is also associated with decreased resistance to infection and increased morbidity and mortality from infectious disease. In young children, the relationship between retardation in weight-for-age and cognitive perfomance is usually not made up. Finally, agricultural and other physical work output has been clearly demonstrated to be related to body size [1].

In comparisons of energy intake among populations, cultural patterns are important determinants of the adequancy of *per capita* calorie intake. An intake of 80% of the 1973 estimated FAO/WHO mean requirement may severely restrict the desired discretionary and work activities of a developing country population, and yet be associated with obesity in a privileged population living a very sedentary existence, dependent on automobiles, elevators, and air conditioning. It is probable that some *social* patterns, such as the long siesta common to many societies, are adaptations to chronically low food intakes.

(c) *Thermogenesis.* The issue of energy requirements is greatly complicated by thermogenesis. The first FAO Expert Committee on Calories Requirements in 1950 [17] provided a 5% increase or decrease for every ten degree change from a mean environmental temperature of 10°C. The second Committee Report in 1957 [18] reduced this correction to 3% for each ten degrees *below* 10°C on the grounds that individuals were partly protected from the major effects of such change by clothing, but retained the 5% decrease for every 10°C *above* the reference temperature. The 1973 Joint FAO/WHO Expert Committee Report [13] abolished the adjustment altogether because the macro-environment reflects the micro-environment of individual to such a limited degree. Eskimos in igloos in the Arctic are found to be at environmental temperatures permitting the transmission of tropical parasites [21], and when outdoors are extremely well protected from the cold. On the other hand, the early visitors to Tierra del Fuego found the natives sleeping naked on frozen ground noted by Magellan, and there is abundant evidence that individuals habitually exposed to the cold develop considerable tolerance [11, 12].

Part of the explanation lies in non-shivering thermogenesis, which enables the body to increases its metabolic rate and hence internal heat production when exposed to seasonal or continuos cold, and yet to decrease it promptly when entering a warm environment. Experimentally, it takes several months of exposure to cold to develop non-shivering thermogenesis to a maximum capacity, and it is slowly lost when it is not called into play. However, basal metabolic rate does not change, and heat and cold adaptation are not mutually exclusive.

The heat produced by thermogenesis must, of course, come from food energy, and any metabolism of food produces an energy loss that must be made up by the energy value of the food ingested. It has long been known that the heat of internal combustion, the so-called specific dynamic effect, varies with the nature of the dietary energy source, being greater for protein than for carbohydrates and fat. It is now realized that variations in thermogenesis also enable the body to dispose of excessive calories without becoming obese, or, put another way, to maintain body weight over a wide range of dietary energy intakes and the same average energy expenditure. Some individuals can apparently overeat without becoming obese, and others have such limited capacity for increased dietary thermogenesis that they put on weight easily and at energy intakes well below those that would be considered normal for their body composition and level of activity. Most recently it has been suggested that these differences are associated with the proportion of brown fat in the body [24, 37], a factor that may well vary systematically or adaptively among populations, although there are no data available.

The variation in calories intake of normal, healthy adults is extraordinary. In our metabolic balance studies at MIT from 1966 to 1982, we have estimated the usual dietary intake of more than 600 student volunteers and then determined whether this estimate was, in fact, adequate for weight maintenance. The range is from 36 to 56 kcals per kg of body weight. Much of this, but not all of it, can be accounted for by differences in life-style, from the very sedentary to the individuals preparing for marathons, training for crew, long-distance swimming meets, and the like. However, there are also significant differences among individuals whose activity patterns appear similar.

It has long been recognized that physical activity has an anabolic effect on protein utilization [57]. Although not yet confirmed by rigid analysis of sufficient data, there is evidence from some of our metabolic studies that high levels of physical activity lead, not only to a more efficient utilization of protein, but also to lower requirements for protein per kg of body weight.

The Significance of Within-Population Variation

(a) *Normal variation*. Nutritionists, in attempting to assess nutrient requirements, pay a great deal of attention to the variation of nutrient requirement within populations. The distribution in obligatory nitrogen losses found among 83 Caucasian young men in the study referred to earlier [42] is as follows: for urinary loss, the mean is 37.2 g per kg with a coefficient of variation of 18%, but including fecal losses, it is 16%. The pooled coefficient of variation in the amount required for zero nitrogen balance in the multicountry UNU studies was also 18%.

These figures for variation have two components: inter-individual variations and intra-individual variation. The recent joint FAO/WHO/UNU Expert Consultation on Protein-Energy Requirements [15] concluded that these components were probably more or less equally represented in this pooled variant figure. If this is the case, then the coefficient of variation attributable to inter-individual variation would be 12.5% i.e. ($\sqrt{S^2}$ intra-individual + S^2 within-individual).

Variations for the requirement of other essential nutrients in normal individuals appear to be in this same range. Thus, if all the world were "normal", and average requirement figures were available, the needs of nearly all of the population would be met by a figure approximately 25% higher than the mean. In theory, this would allow for the needs of 97.5% of the population on a one-tailed distribution. To meet the needs of 99% of the population would require the mean plus 3 standard deviations, or, in this example, about 37% above the mean. The probability of any particular intake figure's being adequate or inadequate for individuals can be given, assuming that they are free of disease [56].

In the case of protein, MIT and ONU multi-level short-term studies indicated the average requirement for young adults to be 0.64 grams of egg, milk, meat, or soy protein per kg of body weight [34]. Thus, a safe allowance for the majority of the population would be 25% more, or approximately 0.8 grams of protein per kg of body weight. Unfortunately, the issue is far more complicated. This figure needs to be confirmed by long-term studies. Furthermore, it is for single protein sources that are highly digestible and essentially completely utilized. For ordinary mixed diets, this figure must be corrected for digestibility if the needs of the great majority of the population are to be safely met.

Such a correction applied to the 0.8 gm per kg figure would bring the allowance for protein in ordinary mixed diets back near to the 1 gram of protein per kg body weight of the 1935 League of Nations and the early U.S. Food and Nutrition Board recommendations. It cannot, of course, be stated that individuals consuming less than the safe allowance are receiving insufficient protein. In fact, under such circumstances, by definition the great majority should be receiving more protein than they require. It should always be remembered that estimated requirements and allowances are merely probability statements, as indicated in Table III [14].

It would be convenient if I could end my discussion of variation in protein requirements at this point, but the issue is far more complicated. Still limiting the discussion to individuals considered to be normal, we have the intriguing problem, already mentioned above, of the outliers that turn up in almost every metabolic study. Even in metabolic balance studies with groups of subjects as small as 6 or 8, there is usually one individual whose digestion or retention of a given dietary protein diverges markedly from that of the remainder of the group. At first it was assumed that these were the result of breaks in the rigid requirement for standardization of dietary intake and complete collection of all urine and fecal samples. Since most of these studies were part of the research of students for doctorate degrees, they were embarrassing to the investigators and generally discarded in the final analysis and discussion. Also, since each set of studies covered a limited time plan, there was rarely an opportunity to repeat the same study in an individual to confirm whether or not it was a characterictic of the individual or an artifact of the study. We still have very few repeat observations on individuals showing apparently aberrant results, but have come to believe that such such outliers are part of the variation in human populations, and must not be discarded.

b). *Effects of infections and other stress.* Even more significant, in interpreting "safe allowances" for protein, however, is the fact that there is no assurance that even probability figures are applicable to a given individual or population because of the frequency with which pathological factors supervene to increase requirements.

It is estimated that preschool children in the lower socio-economic groups of developing countries have diarrheal, respiratory, or other infections from

TABLE III.

Intake Vs. Requirement	Proportion of Individuals Inadequate
25% above average	2.5
12.5% above average	33
Average	50
12.5% below average	67
25% below average	97.5

(1 S.D. = 12.5%)

20 to 40% of the time between the ages of 6 and 36 months and a serious but lesser burden of infection before and after this critical period [30]. Each episode of infection, no matter how mild or subclinical, adversely influences nutritional status [38].

Food intake decreases because of anorexia; the quality of the diet is decreased by the tendency to remove solid food and substitute watery gruels; the stress response results in the increased loss of essential nutrients in the urine; the immune response diverts nutrients from normal synthetic pathways, and if the gastrointestinal tract is affected, absorption of nutrients is decreased.

The so-called catabolic period associated with any infection, even subclinical, depletes the body of nutrients than must be replaced when the acute episode is over. Trauma induces a similar response. Unless the diet is adequate to provide more than "normal" nutrient requirements, this replacement may occur slowly or not at all, and repeated episodes of infection progressively deplete the individual and may precipitate clinical nutritional deficiency desease. The symptoms will depend on the nutrients most limiting in the individual's diet and the differential effects of disease.

The majority of the population in the rural areas of developing countries suffer from multiple intestinal parasites that, when, severe, can contribute to decreased absorption of nutrients. The frequent intestinal infections associated with an unsanitary environment and poor personal hygiene also produce changes in the morphology of the villi and micro-villi of the small intestine known as tropical jejunitis [36] that are more significant in their effect on protein absorption than the usual parasitic infection. Even U.S. Peace Corps. volunteers working in rural villages in developing countries experience these same changes, and it takes many months after return to the U.S. for them to disappear.

c) *Variations in child growth.* Another example of the tendency to minimize protein requirement estimates is the past approach to the needs of growing children by FAO/WHO committee, and national bodies followed their example. These requirements have been estimated by taking the average daily change and the calculating the additional protein and energy that would be required for that amount of daily weight gain. These amounts are then added to the maintenance requirement and amount to approximately 2% of the total for energy and 12% for protein.

Only recently has it been recognized by nutritionists that even normal children do not grow in this way [50]. Instead, there are some periods of little or no growth followed by periods of growth up to two to four times the average daily rate. Moreover, when normal children experience one of the common communicable diseases of childhood, or other infection, the episode is followed by a period of more rapid catch-up growth if the diet is sufficient to permit this. Since the dietary protein intakes of European and American children and those of upper income groups in all parts of the world are usually well above the 1973 and earlier FAO/WHO allowances, and because such children experience relatively infrequent episodes of infection, the matter was and is of merely academic interest to privileged populations.

It has been mistakenly ussumed that when dietary protein intake appears adequate for normal growth, defined as above, it cannot be a limiting factor. However, analysis of the factors limiting the growth of low-income children in Peru [22] and Guatemala [52] indicates that protein rather than caloric intake is responsible. This fits the preceding discussion and is exceedingly important because retardation in growth and development is almost universal in developing countries. It also offers an explanation for the secular trends seen in the U.S. and Europe and most recently in Japan toward taller children and adults. More liberal protein diets with increasing affluence would allow for all growth spurts and optimum catch-up growth after episodes of infection.

For populations of developing countries, even when diets appear to meet normal protein requirements for young children, the intakes may not be sufficient for appropriate recovery from the frequent episodes of infection or to allow for decreased protein absorption from the gastrointestinal tract of individuals with frequent diarrhea and intestinal parasites. In such a case, using the 1973 FAO/WHO estimates, the 10% additional *energy* required for a catch-up rate of six times the daily average of a normal child would be much easier to achieve than the 60% additional *protein* that simple extrapolation would indicated to be needed. Increase efficiency of utilization of protein under these circumstances would help a little, but far less than needed.

Even if a 10% increase in energy intake is not available when the child's appetite increases during the recovery period, the difference *could* be made up by reduced activity. Viteri and co-workers (personal communication) demonstrated that experiment reduction of dietary energy intake to 92% did not affect the growth of Guatemalan preschool children recovering from malnutrition as long as protein intake continued at 2 gm per kg. The children promptly came into zero energy balance by reducing their activity. At 83%, however, both activity and growth were reduced.

(d) *Myth of the daily requirement.* Although it is convenient to express human nutrient needs in terms of a mean *daily* requirement and safe allowance, and, in the case of growing children, also estimate the nutrient needs for an average daily growth rate, this has led to a great deal of misunderstanding and misuse. Individuals will have no adverse consequences from even zero intakes for a number of days, weeks, or months, depending on the nutrient and on the circumstances as long as the diet provides a safe intake of that nutrient over a longer interval.

In the case of a normal adult, there are few objective signs and symptoms in the first 30 days of a complete fast other than weight loss and ketosis because the body has the capacity to use fat as a major energy source and canabalize its lean body mass for the amino acids required for normal gluconeogenesis and protein synthesis [6]. Once adequate food intake is resumed, the lean body mass is rapidly replenished. The latter also serves as a reserve for fluctuations in protein intake within each 24-hour period and over periods of several days or weeks. Humans have evolved not only with a capacity to subsist on a very wide range of habitual foods and diets, but also to tolerate considerable variation in their daily availability.

It is when situations arise in the modern world that are unlikely to have been common during the early period of human evolution that problems come. When starch gruel or sugar water is given to young children, the mobilization of amino acids from skeletal muscle for gluconeogenesis is blocked and the amino acids thus are not available for protein synthesis. It is only under these circumstances of a deficiency of protein relative to calories that signs and symptoms of protein deficiency and, in children, kwashiorkor develop [40]. Similarly, sustained over-eating combined with a sedentary existence is in the same category —the limits of adaptation are surpassed.

In the case of vitamin A, liver stores built up during the seasonal availability of fruits and vegetables rich in vitamin A are adequate to sustain individuals for many months of low or even zero intake of vitamin A. While body stores of the water-soluble vitamins are more limited, it still requires many weeks of a deficient diet for clinical symptoms to develop in a previously well-nourished subject, although the time can be sharply reduced by superimposed infection or trauma.

The point is that the human ability to consume a wide range of foods and to tolerate variation in their availability gives leeway for adaptation to new foods and new environments through cultural rather than genetic mutation. Thus it is that large numbers of new foods have been introduced in recent years with few problems in tolerance. Moverover, novel sources of protein and energy, such as from bacteria and yeast grown on methanol, and even synthetic energy sources are feasible. The synthetic compound, 1-3 butanediol, does not occur in nature. It has a caloric density of 6 calories per gram, and yet is metabolized through normal carbohydrate pathways with no evidence of toxicity in animal and human feeding trials [33, 26]. It is yet another example of the broad spectrum human adaptability to exotic foods.

Evidence of the Limits of Physiological Adaptability

It must be noted that all of the above phenotypic adaptations provided for in the normal human genotype are useful for the maintenance of health under conditions confronting the hunter-gatherer and would be expected to facilitate adaptation to either a primarily hunting or primarily agricultural existence. However, biological evolution simply did not occur under the conditions of modern societies, such as a very sedentary existence combined with an abundance of calorie-dense food leading to sustained over-eating and diets consistently high in refined carbohydrates or in the consumption of large amounts of salts. It is not surprising that the limits of adaptatility are passed for many individuals in such societies, with a consequent increase in diabetes, hypertension, and ischemic heart disease.

(a) *Atherosclerosis and coronary heart disease.* I am well aware of the controversy over the relationship between diet and coronary heart disease and the claims that the data are inadequate to justify a conclusion. Such objections, however, are based primarily on the inconclusive results often observed in intervention studies and lack of an appreciation of the results of comparisons among natural populations.

An Inter-American Atherosclerosis Study conducted from 1959 to 1963 [31] collected aortas and coronary vessels from consecutive autopsies in a general hospital in the cities of Bogotá, Cali, Caracas, Guatemala, Kingston, Lima, Manila, San José (Costa Rica), San Juan (Puerto Rico), Sao Paulo, Santiago, Oslo, and New Orleans. All vessels were stained in a standard manner and evaluated separately by four different pathologists unaware of the origin of any particular specimen. In the developing countries, even though the samples came from city hospital necropsies, the study indicated that atherosclerosis increased slowly throughout life, but usually did not become sufficiently severe to be likely to be associated with either coronary or cerebrovascular disease.

In the U.S. and Norway in this period, arteriosclerotic heart disease accounted for about one-fourth of the deaths in males 10 to 69 years of age compared with 6% in Guatemala and Costa Rica. For example, for men 55 to 64 in New Orleans dying of all causes, 46% had narrowing of one more coronary arteries. The populations of Costa Rica and Guatemala also showed decreasing standard weight-for-age, which meant that they became leaner, whereas the populations of the United States and Europe showed a shift in body composition with age to a higher proportion of fat.

When we examined the cholesterol and lower density lipoprotein in blood serum of the kinds of populations in Guatemala and Costa Rica from which the autopsy sample were drawn, we found them to be so much lower than those of upper income populations in the same countries and normal values for the United States that there was virtually no overlap of the distributions. The average serum cholesterol among 251 Mayan Indians aged 10 to 80 years was 135 ± 31 mg/dl [29, 43].

Similar differences in serum cholesterol were also seen in children. There was virtually no overlap in the values for serum cholesterol in Guatemalan children from low-income, rural families of 121 ± 23 mg/dl, low-income urban families of 143 ± 29 mg/dl, and from middle-and upper-income urban populations of 187 ± 27 mg/dl. Corresponding percentages of dietary calories from fat were 8, 15, and 37. Animal protein intake was estimated to be 35 mg per day for the urban upper-income group, 10 gm for the urban low-income children, and only 6 gm for the rural children from low-income families [39].

We attempted to relate the findings to the known dietary intakes of the various populations and found the best correlation to be with the percentage of calories from fat. This in turn correlated with protein intake, but presumably as a secondary correlation. The Costa Rica sample from a population obtaining 20 to 40% of its calories from crude brown sugar [16] had no higher levels of cholesterol and low density lipoproteins than the population sample from Guatemala for whom only 8 to 9% of the calories came from sugar.

These results indicate that the dramatic differences in aortic atherosclerosis and coronary heart disease and in related serum levels of cholesterol and lower density lipoproteins are certainly of environmental origin. Moreover, the principal environmental factor appears to be the nature of the diet. These population differences in serum lipoproteins, atherosclerosis, and coronary heart disease are clearly not genetic, although just as clearly, within populations there are major genetic differences in tendency to hyperlipidemia and heart disease, as is discussed elsewhere in this volume.

(b) *Essential hypertension.* For the large differences in the distribution of essential hypertension among populations, a similar situation exists. Where they have been carefully investigated with good epidemiological techniques, the differences appear to be due to environmental rather than genetic factors. For example, the higher frequency of hypertension and cerebrovascular accidents of Japanese in Japan appears to be associated with the high salt content of the diet, and they are now decreasing as consumption of the traditional salty foods becomes less a percentage of the total diet.

Tea plantations in Bangladesh where the people use salt instead of sugar in their tea have a much higher incidence of hypertension beginning at early ages than other populations in Bangladesh in which this condition is rare. The higher frequency of hypertension in Negroes and Caucasian populations living in the same areas [3] was easy to attribute to racial differences until comparative studies showed that the frequency of hypertension in Black populations depended largely on environmental circumstances, although it appears that the factors in this case are more ones of psychological than dietary stress [41].

(c) *Diabetes.* For diabetes, the situation is not nearly as clear, but certainly clinical diabetes is relatively rare among populations whose food supply is limited, and increases greatly in prevalence when those same populations have sudden access to much larger amounts of food, particularly refined carbohydrates, and to become obese. Of course, once the food increase occurs, the variation in genetic predisposition to diabetes is one of the factors determining its within-population distribution.

(d) *Endemic goiter.* Endemic goiter due to iodine deficiency is another disease that depends primarily on environmental differences, even though within-population genetic factors are responsible for both hypo- and hyperthyroidism. In the endemic disorder the enlargement of the thyroid gland represents a generally successful adaptation in that it is rare to find a reduced basal metabolic rate in individuals with endemic goiter. The hypertrophy of the gland improves the efficiency of trapping iodine from the blood stream and protects against metabolic dysfunction. It is really only under the extraordinary demands of pregnancy that the consequences of iodine deficiency of which endemic goiter is an indicator are manifest, and then not in the women themselves, but in their offspring. The result is an increase in the frequency of feeble-mindedness, deafmutism, and the occasional occurrence of a cretin.

(e) *Gout.* Primary gout is a form of hyperuricemia with recurrent attacks of acute arthritis that is associated with a number of different inborn errors of metabolism. In some individuals, the defect is excessive uric acid production by one of several different mechanisms, and in others there is a reduction in renal urate clearance. The result of a sustained elevation of serum urate levels is the development of recurrent attacks of acute arthritis and sometimes urate tophae in tissues, or urate renal stones. Since uric acid is the end-point of the purine part of the nucleic acid molecule, diets that are high in sources of nucleic acid, such as organ meats and single-cell protein, are more likely to precipitate attacks of gout in susceptible individuals. The wide differences in the occurrence of clinical gout among different populations has been attributed to differences in dietary nucleic acid content, alcohol ingestion, surface area, and body weight. It virtually disappeared in Europe and Japan during World War II and has become common in these areas once again. The evidence for the influence of social class is strong. While there is no evidence for genetic differences in age- and sex-matched uric acid levels, this should be explored more systematically.

Genetic Variations Capable of Influencing Nutrient Requirements

(a) *Differences among populations.* Lactase deficiency, a genetically determined characteristic that causes differences in the metabolic effect of diet among populations, is the gradual loss soon after the weaning period of the intestinal enzyme, lactase, responsible for the digestion of lactose, the principal carbohydrate in both human and animal milk. This topic is discussed in more detail elsewhere in this volume. It is worth pointing out here, though, that this is one of the few clear-cut examples of a genetically determined metabolic factor that does influence the nutritional effects of diet among populations.

It is apparently normal to lose intestinal lactase once the period of breast-feeding is over. This is not an example of loss of enzyme activity because of lack of substrate; i.e., lactase does not appear to be an inducible enzyme. Instead, the loss is genetically determined. However, the importances of the loss of intestinal lactase has been greatly exaggerated, since even individuals with little or no intestinal lactase activity can ingest a single glass of milk without intestinal discomfort. Protein absorption is not affected [7], and the loss of energy caused by inability to split lactose in the small intestine is negligible. Even in the elderly, we found no one unable to tolerate a glass of milk regardless of their lactase status [35].

It could, however be an advantage for northern Europeans as older children and adults to be able to derive a substantial amount of energy as well as protein from animal milk. It was long assumed that the Masai, who depend heavily on animal milk for their sustenance, must be an exception among Africans and that they somehow retained their intestinal lactase while it was lost in other Negro and Negroid groups. It appears, however, that the adaptation is different —simply the development of tolerance to relatively large amounts of dietary lactose, even though the lactose continues to pass largely undigested into the large intestine [27].

b) *Alcohol sensitivity.* Individual and racial differences in alcohol intoxication have been reported by many investigators. Alcohol-sensitive persons exhibit rapid facial flushing, elevation of skin temperature, and an increase in pulse rate when they drink more than 0.2 ml of alcohol per kg of body weight. Such sensitivity is far more commonly observed in individuals of Oriental origin, such as the Japanese, Korean, and American Indian than in Caucasians. According to Wolff, more than 80% of Orientals are alcohol-sensitive, while only 5% of Caucasians respond abnormally after alcohol administration [53, 54].

One of the major alcohol dehydrogenase isoenzymes is structurally different in Causasians and Oriental [23]. Liver aldehyde dehydrogenase components also differ between Caucasians and Orientals [55]. It might be predicted that alcoholism would be less prevalent among Orientals than Caucasians, and a comparison of Japanese, Chinese, and Koreans with North American and Europeans would suggest that this is indeed the case. The powerful effect of social factors, however, is indicated once again in the paradox that American Indians are of Mongoloid origin and have a frequency of alcohol sensitivity equally as high as that of Orientals in Asia, and yet alcoholism is a particulary serious social problem among them.

c) *Taste and smell.* While a functional basis for the origin of a difference in alcohol sensitivity among populations is not immediately apparent, it is one more interesting example of the interplay of genetic and social environmental factors. Another kind of genetic variation for which it might be possible to discern a nutritional influence is difference in the ability to taste or smell certain substances. There are, for example, marked differences among populations in the ability to taste phenolthio-carbamide (PTC). Inability to taste PTC is a simple recessive, but with wide differences in penetrance. Indians and Orientals are usually able to identify PTC readily, whereas about one-third of Caucasians, Negroes, and inhabitants of the Middle East are non-tasters [20]. Similar variations are found for a number of other chemical compounds, and as a non-taster who perceives the artificial sweetener used in diet beverages as metallic and non-sweet, I am curious to know whether these differences originally conferred selective advantage in one direction or another. Could they have been of assitance in enabling individuals to avoid toxic plants in a region? To my knowledge, this has never been demonstrated.

Inborn Errors of Metabolism

No topic is more fascinating than the seemingly infinite number of inborn errors of metabolism that have consequences varyin from the trivial to the lethal, and whose study has been so instrumental in advancing our knowledge of normal metabolism and of the functional role of various enzymes and substrates. Indeed, this book considers such disorders as: lactase deficiency, phenylketonuria, the hyperlipidemias, and inborn errors of metabolism as an epidemiological tool. Not considered in detail are the large array of other known metabolic defects.

These include such additional disorders of carbohydrate metabolism as diabetes, pentosuria, functosuria and intolerance; glycogen deposition diseases, galactosemia, and primary hyperoxaluria and oxalosis. The additional diseases of amino acid metabolism include tyrosinosis, alcaptonuria, albuminuria, the hyperglycinuria, branched chain ketonuria, histidemia, cystathioninuria, homocystinuria, and disorders of proline and hydroxyproline and the urea cycle. In addition to the lipoproteinemias covered in the conference are lipid abnormalities such as Tay-Sachs disease, Niemann-Pick disease, Fabry's disease, etc. This does not even begin to include the disorders of steroid metabolism deficiencies of circulating enzymes and protein, Wilson's disease and hemochromatosis, and diseases manifested primarily in blood and blood-forming tissues, connective tissue, muscle and bone [44].

It is reasonable to ask what the relationship of these disorders may be to the variation in nutrient requirements in a normal population, or to the ability of populations to survive stress and environmental change.I would suggest that the answer does not lie in attempting to find a utility for these particular metabolic disorders, which may be considered Nature's failed experiments, but rather in considering them the tip of a vast underseas mountain of metabolic variations of varying degrees of severity, some of which may account for outliers or be responsible for obscure ill health. Thousands of less serious inborn errors must occur without being either detected or perpetuated. Some of them may, however, have subtle effects on the health of individuals without necessarily affecting that of populations. Roger Williams has gone to great lengths to stress biochemical individuality [51], and although I do not agree with him in all particulars, believe he is right in doing so. He argues that many human disorders of obscure etiology, wich strike certain individuals and leave others untouched, have roots in the failure of affected individuals to receive continuously, or at crucial times, adequate nutrition in terms of their own peculiar needs.

Given the large number of essential nutrients and the still larger number of enzymes associated with their utilization, it would indeed be surprising if *every* individual did not have one or more genetic traits or mutations sufficient to make the individual differ from the general population in regard to metabolism or requirement for a specific nutrient. In some cases this would be expected to render a seemingly adequated diet insufficient for that individual.

Nutritionists must be aware of "wild card" in all of their metabolic experiments and calculations. Differences in the frequency of such metabolic variants should continue to be sought in population studies as well. Because of the influence of environmental factors, it is a mistake, when dealing with free-living populations, to view requirements in rigid terms of "normal" needs, even allowing for "normal" variation. Nutritionists should also be less dogmatic in asserting that a given diet must be adequate for *specific* individuals because it meets the "safe allowance" calculated by a committee for a *normal population*. The combination of genetic and environmental factors influencing nutrient requirements calls for larger margins of safety than expert committees have commonly seen fit to allow.

REFERENCES

1. Arteaga, L. The Nutritional status of Latin American adults. *In* "Nutrition and Agricultural Development", 500 pp. (N.S. Scrimshaw and M. Béhar, eds.), pp. 67-76. Plenum Fress, New York and London, 1976.
2. Ashworth, A. and Harrower, A.D.B. Protein requirements in tropical countries: Nitrogen losses in sweat and their relation to nitrogen balance. *Brit. J. Nutr.* 21:833, 1967.
3. Bays, R.P. and Scrimshaw, N.S. Facts and fallacies regarding the blood pressure of difference regional and racial groups. *Circulation* 8:655, 1953.
4. Bourges, H. Nitrogen balance response of young male adults fed predicted requirement levels of a Mexican rural diet. *In* "Protein-Energy Requirements of Developing Countries: Results of International Research" (W.R. Rand, R. Uauy, and N.S. Scrimshaw, eds.), in press. The United Nations University Publications on Food and Nutrition, Supplement, Tokyo, Japan.
5. Bourges, H. and Lopez-Castro, B.R. Protein requirements of young male adults with a rural Mexican diet. *In* "Protein-Energy Requirements of Developing Countries: Evaluation of New Data" (B. Torún, V.R. Young, and W.R. Rand, eds.), pp. 71-76. The United Nations University Publications on Food and Nutrition, Supplement No. 5, Tokyo, Japan. 1981.
6. Cahill, G.F., Jr. Starvation in man. *New Engl. J. Med.* 282:668, 1970.
7. Calloway, D.H. and Chenoweth, W.L. Utilization of nutrients in milk and wheat-based diets by men with adequate and reduced abilities to absorb lactose. 1. Energy and nitrogen. *Am. J. Clin. Nutr.* 26:939, 1973.
8. Calloway, D.H. and Kretsch, M.J. Protein and energy utilization in men given a rural Guatemalan diet and egg formulas with and without added oat bran. *Am. Clin. Nutr.* 31:1118, 1978.
9. Chávez, A. and Martínez, C. "Growing Up in a Developing Country," 155 pp. (This English version has been published by the Institute of Nutrition of Central America and Panama [INCAP], 1982, and is a United Nations University translation of the book, "Nutrición y Desarrollo Infantil" originally published by the Nueva Editorial Interamericana, S.A. de C.V., Mexico, 1979).

10. Cravioto, J. and De Licardie, E.R. Intersensory development of schoolage children. *In* "Malnutrition, Learning, and Behavior" (N.S. Scrimshaw and J.E. Gordon, eds.), pp. 252-269. MIT Press, Cambridge, Massachusetts and London, England, 1968.
11. Davis, T.R. Chamber cold acclimatization in man. *J. Appl. Physiol.* 16:1011, 1961.
12. Davis, T.R. and Joy, R.J. Natural and artificial cold acclimatization. *In* "Biometeorology" (S.W. Tromp, ed.), pp. 286-303. Pergamon Press, Oxford, London, New York, Paris, 1962.
13. "Energy and Protein Requirements." Report of a Joint FAO/WHO *Ad Hoc* Expert Committee. WHO Tech. Rep. Ser. 522, WHO, Geneva, 1973.
14. "Energy and Protein Requirements." Recommendations by a Joint FAO/WHO Informal Gathering of Experts. *Food Nutr.* (FAO) 1:11, 1975.
15. "Energy and Protein Requirements." Report of a Joint FAO/WHO/UNU Expert Consultation, Rome 5-17 October, 1981. WHO, Geneva, in press.
16. Flores, M. Nutritional studies in Central America and Panama. *In* "The Ongoing Evolution of Latin American Populations" Part III (F.M. Salzano, ed.), pp. 311-331. Charles C Thomas, Springfield, Illinois, 1971.
17. Food and Agriculture Organization Nutritional Studies No. 5, "Calorie Requirements" Report of the Committee on Calorie Requirements, FAO, Rome, 1950.
18. Food and Agriculture Organization Nutritional Studies No. 15, "Calorie Requirements." Report of the Second Committee on Calories Requirements, FAO, Rome, 1957.
19. Freuchen, P. "Book of the Eskimos." Bramhall House, New York, 1961.
20. Gates, R.R. "Human Genetics," Vol. II, pp. 1066-1072. MacMillan Co., New York, 1946.
21. Gordon, J.E., Freundt, E.A., Brown, E.W., Jr., and Babbott, F.L., Jr. Endemic and epidemic diarrheal disease in Arctic Greenland. *Am. J. Med. Sci.* 242:374, 1961.
22. Graham, G.C., Creed, H.M., MacLean, W.C., Jr., Kallman, C.H. Rabold, J., and Mellits, E.D. Determinants of growth among poor children: Nutrient intake-achieved growth relationships. *Am. J. Clin. Nutr.* 34:539, 1981.
23. Harada, S., Agarwal, D.P., and Goedde, H.W. Isozyme variaons in acetaldehyde dehydrogenase (E.C.1.2.1.3) in human tissues. *Hum. Genet.* 44:181, 1978.
24. Himms-Hagen, J. Determinants of human obesity. *Clin. Nutr.* 1:4, 1982.
25. Huang, P.C., Chong, H.E., and Rand, W.M. Obligatory urinary and fecal nitrogen losses in young Chinese men. *J. Nutr.* 102:1605, 1972.
26. Kies, C., Robin, R.B., Fox, H.M., and Mehlman, M.A. Utilization of 1,3-butanediol and non-specific nitrogen in human adults. *J. Nutr.* 103:1155, 1973.
27. Kretchmer, N. Lactose and lactase - a historical perspective. *Gastroenterology* 61:805, 1971.
28. Lee, R.B. and Devore I. (eds.), "Man the Hunter." Aldine Press, Chicago, 1 68.
29. Mann, G.V. Muñoz, J.A., and Scrimshaw, N.S. The serum lipoprotein and cholesterol concentrations of Central and North Americans with different dietary habits. *Am. J. Med.* 19:25, 1955.
30. Mata, L.J. "The Children of Santa Maria Cauqué," 395 pp. MIT Press, Cambridge, Massachusetts and London, England, 1978.
31. McGill, H.C., Jr. (ed.) The Geographic Pathology of Atherosclerosis. *Lab. Invest.* 18:463-653, 1968 (Special Issue).
32. Meggitt, M.J. Notes of vegetable foods of the Walbiri. *Oceania* 28:143, 1957.
33. Miller, S.A. and Dymsza, H.A. Utilization by the rat of 1,3-butanediol as a synthetic source of dietary energy. *J. Nutr.* 91:79, 1967.
34. Rand, W.R., Uauy, R., and Scrimshaw, N.S. (eds.) "Protein-Energy Requirements of Developing Countries: Results of International Research," in press. The United National University Publications on Food and Nutrition, Supplement, Tokyo, Japan.
35. Rorick, M.H. and Scrimshaw, N.S. Comparative tolerance of elderly from differing ethnic backgrounds to lactose-containing and lactose-free dairy drinks: A double-blind study. *J. Gerontol.* 34:191, 1979.
36. Rosenberg, I.H. and Scrimshaw, N.S. (eds.), Malabsorption and Nutrition. *Am. J. Clin. Nutr.* 25: Part I:1046; Part II:1226, 1972.

37. Rothwell, N.J. and Stock, M.S. A role for brown adipose tissue in dietinduced thermogenesis. *Nature* 281:31, 1979.
38. Scrimshaw, N.S. Effect of infection on nutrient requirements. *Am. J. Clin. Nutr.* 30:1536, 1977.
39. Scrimshaw, N.S., Balsam, A., and Arroyave, G. Serum cholesterol levels in school children from three socio-economic groups. *Am. J. Clin. Nutr.* 5:629, 1957.
40. Scrimshaw, N.S. and Béhar, M. Protein malnutrition in young children. *Science* 133:2039, 1961.
41. Scrimshaw, N.S., Culver, G.A., and Stevenson, R.A. Toxic complications of pregnancy in Gorgas Hospital, Panama Canal Zone, 1931-1945. *Am. J. Obstet. Gynec.* 54:428, 1947.
42. Scrimshaw, N.S., Hussein, M.A., Murray, E., Rand, W.M., and Young, V.R. Protein requirements of man: Variations in Obligatory Urinary and fecal nitrogen losses in young men. *J. Nutr.* 102:1595, 1972.
43. Scrimshaw, N.S., Trulson, M., Tejada, C., Hegsted, D.M., and Stare, F.J. Serum lipoprotein and cholesterol concentrations. Comparison of rural Costa Rican, Guatemalan, and United States Populations. *Circulation* 15:805, 1957.
44. Stanbury, J.B., Wyngaarden, J.B. Fredrickson, D.S., Goldstein, J.L., and Brown, M.S. (eds.) "The Metabolic Basis of Inherited Disease," McGraw Hill Book Co., 1982.
45. Stefansson, V. "The Fat of the Land," McMillan and Co., New York, 1956.
46. Sweeney, G. Food supplies of a desert tribe. *Oceania* 17:239, 1947.
47. Torún, B. Young, V.R., and Rand, W.M. (eds.), "Protein-Energy Requirements of Developing Countries: Evaluation of New Data," 268 pp. The United Nations University Food and Nutrition Bulletin, Supplement No. 5, Tokyo, Japan, 1981.
48. Viteri, F.E. Definition of the nutrition problem in the labor force. *In* "Nutrition and Agricultural Development—Significance and Potential for the Tropics" (N.S. Scrimshaw and M. Béhar, eds.), pp. 87-98. Plenum Press, New York, 1976.
49. Viteri, F.E. Nutrition and work performance. *In* "Nutrition Policy Implementation—Issues and Experience" (N.S. Scrimshaw and M.B. Wallerstein, eds.), pp. 3-13. Plenum Press, New York, 1982.
50. Viteri, F.E., Whitehead, R.G., and Young, V.R. (eds.), "Protein-Energy Requirements under Conditions Prevailing in Developing Countries: Current Knowledge and Research Needs, "The United Nations University Food and Nutrition Bulletin Supplement No. 1, 73 pp., Tokyo, Japan, 1979.
51. Williams, R.J. "Physician's Handbook of Nutritional Science," Charles C. Thomas, Springfield, Illinois, 1975.
52. Wilson, A.B. Longitudinal analysis of diet, physical growth, verbal development, and school performance. *In* "Malnourieshed Children of the Rural Poor (J.B. Balderston, A.B. Wilson, M.E. Freire, and M.S. Simonen, eds.), pp. 39-81. Auburn House Publishing Co., Boston, Massachusetts, 1981.
53. Wolff, P.H. Ethnic differences in alcohol sensitivity. *Science* 175: 449, 1972.
54. Wolff, P.H. Vasomotor sensitivity to alcohol in diverse mongoloid populations. *Am. J. Hum. Genet.* 25: 193, 1973.
55. Yoshida, A. Genetic differences in alcohol metabolism between Caucasians and Orientals. City of Hope Quarterly 11 (3):5, 1982.
56. Young, V.R. and Scrimshaw, N.S. Genetic and biological variability in human nutrient requirements. *Am. J. Clin. Nutr.* 32:486, 1979.
57. Young, V.R. and Torún, B. Physical activity: Impact on protein and amino acid metabolism and implications for nutritional requirements. *In* "Nutrition in Health and Disease and International Development." Symposia from the XIIth International Congress of Nutrition (A.E. Harper and G.K. Davis, eds.), pp. 57-85. Alan R. Liss, Inc., New York, 1981.

GENETIC EPIDEMIOLOGY AS A POTENTIAL TOOL IN NUTRITIONAL RESEARCH

R.H. Ward

Department of Medical Genetics
University of British Columbia
Vancouver, British Columbia
Canada

INTRODUCTION

Before discussing the statistical methodology and study design that the genetic epidemiologist might usefully bring to bear upon the problem of determining causation in malnutrition, it will be helpful to adopt an evolutionary perspective. This will help define which etiological models are most likely to be realistic for our understanding of "malnutrition". As indicated below, selection of an appropriate study design, along with a set of statistical methods, is conditional on our assumptions of underlying causation.

Throughout the symposium the influence of the interaction between biological and cultural components of evolution, on the distribution and consequences of malnutrition has been emphasized. The following general conclusion obtains. First, today's nutritional environment for our species is substantially different from the nutritional environment with which our species contendend for most of the past four million years. Second, the change in our nutritional environment occurred extremely recently on an evolutionary time scale. Hence for many populations today, there is a considerable imbalance between the actual nutritional environment and the optimal nutritional environment for which our genome evolved. As Blackburn indicates [3], this imbalance results in an appreciable proportion of the total burden of morbidity and mortality in many modern populations.

The nutritional adequacy of an environment is a consequence of the efficiency with which the environment is utilised. Early in Man's history, when food was obtained almost exclusively by biological strategies, such as foraging, this efficiency was low relative to later periods. However, for the majority of individuals in the population, the nutritional adequacy of the environment was commensurate with their requirements. For a small minority, utilisation of the

37

environment would have been a limiting factor, resulting in an overall selection for increased efficiency of utilisation of scarce resources [43]. In general, the selection pressure would have been slight, since nutritional requirements were not likely to be substantially greater than could be obtained in the average environment. As cultural evolution proceeded, there would have been an overall increase in the efficiency of environmental utilisation. This would have resulted in a slight relaxation of selective pressure, so that genetically defined nutritional requirements would have also increased over time, tracking just behind the nutritional potential of that cultural stage. Selection of the type envisioned by Neel twenty years ago [43] would still have ocurred, though occasional saltations in cultural evolution would have resulted in a temporal disappearance of any selective pressure. Examples of a cultural saltation would be the inovation of a radically new tool, or the development of a novel strategy to utilise a formerly limiting resource.

This essentially steady state situation changed dramatically about 10,000 years ago with the development of domestication. Suddenly the degree of nutritional abundance in the environment far exceeded the genetically defined requirements of the population. For the first time, limitations on nutritional intake were due to cultural factors influencing the distribution of relatively abundant resources, rather than the limitations imposed by scarce environments. As the culturally based potential to exploit the environment increased exponentially, the degree to which socio-political factors dictated the distribution of food also increased. This eventually lead to excessive heterogeneity in the distribution of food, so that some individuals had a definite overabundance of food, while others suffered from minimal or inappropriate nutrition. Following domestication the inevitable development of empires and consequent colonial expansion, lead to increasing heterogeneity in the distribution of food. Today there is a tendency for individuals to exist either in a state of feast, or in a state of famine largely because of their cultural an sociopolitical environment. Thus the major nutritional problems that confront us today are of quite recent origin and are inherently unlikely to be caused solely by faulty genotypes.

The Likelihood of Genetic Etiology in Nutritional Problems

If the above synopsis represents a reasonably close approximation to the manner in which the biological and cultural aspects of man's species have interacted, the genetic epidemiologist has a difficult task. Whereas genetic lesions that determine malnutrition are unlikely to be prominent in the human genome, specific environmental "insults", or deficiencies, are much more likely to play a dominant role. This conclusion does not exclude the possibility that genetically-defined susceptibilities to certain deleterious environments may play a critical role in influencing the distribution of "malnutrition" within, and between populations. This is the area in which the genetic epidemiologist is likely to make the greatest contribution. However, while the variable response to a specific environmental factor may be due to genetically determined sensitivity, the final outcome will depend on the presence, or absence, of an environmental variable.

Few examples exist where a specific genetic lesion interacts with the nutritional environment to cause disease. Despite twenty years of hard work, type II diabetes still gives little evidence of a single major gene causing disease [61]. One striking example is afforded by the series of genetic lesions which collectively cause significant defects in cholesterol metabolism [15, 21, 26, 42, 46, 59]. As the seminal work of Goldstein and Brown [22] shows, individuals possessing mutant forms of the cell surface receptor for cholesterol will exhibit a substantial aberration of cholesterol metabolism, irrespective of cholesterol intake. These, and closely related genetic lesions, are an example of a presumably rare class of genes in which the deleterious outcome appears independent of nutritional intake, or other aspects of the environment. However, it seems apparent that, despite the dramatic effects of these genes, they contribute only a small proportion of the total burden of cardiovascular mortality. Also more comparative data from populations of different backgrounds, and existing under different nutritional regimes, are required before the possibility of environmental interaction can be excluded. As noted in this conference, investigating the presumptive genetic basis of lactose intolerance in western European populations has lead to similar cautions.

At this point it should be noted that genetic sensitivity to inadequate nutritional environment may be manifested in other ways than frank malnutrition. The recent intriguing findings from Britain suggesting that recurrence of neural tube defects in high risk women may be prevented by high doses of vitamins, especially folic acid, or even better dietary habits (Laurence, pers. comm.) is such an example. In this case it appears that certain genotypes may be particulary susceptible to inadequate nutrition and both factors must occur to produce the deleterious outcome with high frequency. Thus there is a wide range of opportunity for the genetic epidemiologist interested in the interface between genetics and nutrition, especially if the concept of genetic susceptibility to nutritional inadequacy is brought to bear on such related areas as pregnancy outcomes and the consequences of impeded growth and development. For example the genetic epidemiology of neurological defects might well benefit from a nutritional component.

The essence of epidemiology is a preoccupation with the patterns of morbidity and mortality in order that causation may be deduced from the correlated distribution of putative risk factors. For our purposes, concepts of causation can be conceived in terms of a basic dichotomy between environmental cause and genetic cause. Whatever else, genetic epidemiology may be preoccupied with [40], it is certainly concerned with identifying the relative role of genotypic factors and environmental factors as they contribute to the etiology of complex disease. Hence, it will be helpful to consider how traits may be conceptualised in terms of the orthogonal relationship between genetic and environmental cause. Until about a decade ago, human geneticists and epidemiologists contended with four main classes of etiological cause.

a) The underlying etiology is essentially random.

This category includes instances of morbidity and mortality which exhibit no readily definable pattern in their temporal or spacial distribution, apart from rather broad trends which are of little help in partitioning risk within a population. The general characteristic of this class is that afflicted individuals do not have any identifiable characteristic, or any set of genetic or environmental attributes that allow reliable prediction of risk. Certain classes of accidents fall into this category, as well as conditions associated with natural, or man-made catastrophes.

In our own time, such factors have been important in determining malnutrition, since the extensive distribution of famine in many areas of Africa and south east Asia, results from a combination of natural, and manmade disasters. In such situations, neither classical epidemiology nor genetic epidemiology, has much to offer in terms of estimating components of risk. While such generalised disasters may be thought a recent phenomena, the archeological and historical record indicates this is not so. One of the consequences of domestication and the subsequent occurrence of large, concentrated, urbanised populations, has been an increasing ecological instability, so that large scale disasters have probably affected our species for at least the last 12,000 years.

b) The underlying etiology is essentially environmental.

These are the conditions that occupy the attention of the classical epidemiologist. The environmental factors which underlie the condition of interest, tend to have characteristic distribution in space and time and these in turn result in a non-random occurrence of disease. Since the time of John Snow, epidemiology has been at pains to define ways of identifying clusters of disease in space and time and thus identify specific factors which, by virtue of their similar distribution, may be viewed as prime candidates for the underlying etiology. The great success of epidemiology, first with infectious disease and, more latterly, with chronic disease, has occurred by applying these procedures. The continuation of this approach to study problems of malnutrition is likely to be extremely profitable since environmental components play a dominant role in many instances. Of some methodological interest is the fact that the most popular statistical procedures for assigning relative risk to categorical data [19] have obvious extensions to the definition of genetic risk [8,58] so that epidemiologists and geneticists may be utilizing the same analytic strategies, though directed to different ends.

c) The underlying etiology is Mendelian in nature.

These conditions, loosely known by the term "genetic traits", arise as the consequence of the action of a specific gene product. As in the case of the environmental diseases, genetic traits also display a markedly non-random distribution in the population. In this case, the clustering, which occurs within family units, is due to the classical patterns of segregation as dictated by the Mendelian laws of heredity. While such conditions may be relatively rare in terms of their contribution to their total burden of malnutrition, they can be of considerable importance to certain segments of the population. In addition, as the presentations of Cederbaum (this volume) and Lisker (this volume) have indicated, the intensive study of such conditions may be extremely instructive in identifying physiological modes of action that have a more general importance for our understanding of metabolism of malnutrition.

d) The underlying etiology is "multifactorial", both genotype and environment playing a role.

The fourth group, encompasses features of both the two previous classes and stretches between them. In this category, the etiological contribution to disease may best be regarded as a linear model, where the total variance can be regarded as the sum of a genetic component plus an environmental component. The total variance may represent the variance of a measurable trait or the variability in the unmeasurable liability of disease.

There are two important features of the multifactorial model as been traditionally applied to human diseases, that need to be mentioned. First, the genetic contribution to the overall variance is deemed to be polygenic in nature. Instead of the genetic contribution to variability arising form the segregation of one, or a few, alleles, at a single locus, variability is the consequence of the accumulative effect of many alleles at many loci. Hence, instead of the discrete distributions characteristic of the binomial (or multinomial) consequences of Mendelian segregation, liability is a continuously distributed variable, with affection lying in the tail of the distribution. When the variable in question is itself continuous, such as lipoprotein levels, or blood pressure, the concept of a continuous distribution poses little problem. However, when the trait is discontinuous, then it is necessary to assume that affection status is a consequence of individuals distributed beyond a given threshold which defines the categorically different tail of the liability distribution [18, 49].

Second, in this model, genetic factors are considered to be independently distributed from the distribution of environmental factors. Hence, the probability of two individuals sharing a vector of environmental variables is uncorrelated with the probability of their possessing identical genotypic vectors. Both these restrictions on the multifactorial model are somewhat unrealistic and result from the difficulty of deriving appropriate statistical measures for evaluating human disorders. Since experimental situations are virtually non existen for human populations environmental or genetic manipulation, is not possible. The freedom with which plant and animal geneticists are able to elaborate their model of causation is denied the genetic epidemiologist.

The multifactorial model is of prime importance in evaluating a great many conditions associated with "malnutrition" in the broadest sense. There is considerable evidence that suggests that lipid abnormalities such as hypercholesterolemia, are essentially multifactorial in nature rather than being monogenic [27, 31, 37, 42, 44, 48, 52, 59]. Similar conclusions obtain for diabetes [61] and related disorders. While the evidence for conditions due to undernutrition still needs to be collected, it seems reasonable that a classical multifactorial model will also prove instructive in this case.

Further Etiological Models

The past ten years have witnessed some progress in removing the restrictions from the multifactorial model which had made it less than appropriate for the analysis of complex problems. As a consequence, some of the gaps in the "etiological space", have now been filled. Essentially, two main developments have occurred.

e) Multifactorial model with major gene effects (the "mixed model").

This model bridges the gap between etiological models dependent on a classical Mendelian model involving a single locus, and the traditional multifactorial model which relies on a polygenic component to describe genetic diversity, plus a randomly varying environmental component. The "mixed model" combines both these concepts and thus adds the last link to the general bridge between these two areas first established by Fisher [20]. The resulting model incorporates fixed effects due to the influence of the alleles at the major locus (each genotype having a distinctive expected value), as well as a random component due to polygenic and environmental variables. Each genotype has a normally distributed set of values around its expected value, though the resulting displacement of genotype means may make the overall distribution significantly non-normal. This model, encompassing a mixture of normal distributions, has analogies with the "mixed model" concept in analysis of variance [50], since the underlying factors of the model include both constants (the fixed genotypic effects of major locus) and random variables (the random variability about each genotypic mean caused by the polygenic and environmental components of variance).

This concept was first introduced explicitly into formal analysis for human genetics by Elston and Stewart [14], and then was more extensively defined for the nuclear family situation by Morton and MacLean [41]. From this initial beginning, a great deal of effort has been expended in making this somewhat complex model applicable to general pedigree structures [23, 24, 45] as well as to nuclear families which have been ascertained by affected individuals elsewhere in the pedigree [34].

f) Genotype-environmental interaction

Although this concept is likely to be of paramount importance in our understanding of common disease, the development of analytic strategies and research designs for such situation are still in an elementary stage. Traits falling into this category have a very different relationship between causal components than do the other categories. The correlated interaction of genotype and environmental components of etiology lead to considerable difficulties of estimation in situations where direct experimentation is not possible. Kempthorne [32] has commented on the overall problem of inferring causation from studies that are merely observational, for even simple linear models. When genotype-environmental interactions also need to be incorporated into the model, the problems of making valid inferences about causation increase by an order of magnitude.

However, some progress has been made. One approach has been to recognise the non-random distribution of environments within human pedigrees. While this is an old problem, statistical procedures now exist to incorporate the concept of a shared common environment in sibships [37, 44, 45, 52] genotype-environmental interactions, it does at least give an approach to tackling the important problem of the correlated distribution of environments and genes in human pedigrees.

Another approach has been to take the concept of correlated response as this is used by animal breeders and utilise this as a way of defining interactions. Using Falconer's concept that the measurement of the same variable in two distinct environments is tantamount to measuring two traits in the same environment, the elements of statistical methodology now exist for estimating such interactions. At least two developments have occurred along these lines in recent years. Lathrop et al. [35] have devised a method of incorporating physiological interactions in a path analysis approach, while Hanis (pers. comm.) has considered interactions from the point of view of correlated response. While much work needs to be done in this area, these developments represent a promising beginning to a conceptually difficult and statistically daunting task.

Relative Risk

The estimation and assignment of relative risk is one of the basic objectives in epidemiology. While specification of relative risk to a vector of environmental factors cannot be equated with identification of causal factors, it provides a sharply defined set of possible etiologies. In genetic epidemiology, the concept of relative risk is equally useful. Here, the major axes along which relative risk estimates can be defined are either genetic or environmental in type. Ideally, one would be able to identify a vector of relative risks associated with a specific, and measurable, genotype analogous to the assignment of relative risks to specific environmental categories. The clearest example of the assignment of relative risks to specific genotypes by epidemiological techniques, is the identification of very high relative risks for the development of reactive arthritis (Ankylosing spondilitis, Reiter's disease, etc.) with the HLA B27 antigen. Similar assignments of relative risks have been made for other HLA haplotypes, and antigens, for a variety of autoimmune and related diseases. Unfortunately, our ability to assign relative risks to identifiable genotypes is severely limited by the fact that only a small fraction of the human genome can be unambiguously identified. Thus, apart from these relatively few genetic polymorphisms, calculation of relative risks associated with genetic traits is not possible to do in the standard epidemiological manner.

The alternative strategy is to estimate relative risk in terms of the coefficient of kinship which defines the probability that a relative shares an allele identical by descent with one of the alleles of the affected proband. This leads to a continuous distribution of relative risks, whith specific relatives forming arbitrary discontinuities. The same concept can be applied to the definition of relative risk for environmental variables. Rather than directly measuring a specific set of environmental variables, relative risk can be estimated along an axis which specifies the probability that two individuals share environments. This is sometimes explicitly done in epidemiology when the putative risk factor cannot be directly measured, but a surrogate measure is utilised instead. The concept of defining relative risk along a shared environmental axis, without directly measuring the environment, is also implicit in the definition of a sibship environment by the genetic epidemiologists. This is now routinely used in specifying linear models that attempt to identify relative influences of genetic and non-genetic causes without having to explicitly specify the constitution of the environment.

Strategies

The different etiological models will tend to require distinct kinds of research strategies in order to elucidate the underlying causal component. In genetic epidemiology there is a graded series of strategies that can be employed. Depending on the strategy used, the degree of inference concerning genetic etiology will vary from being suggestive, as in the case of familial aggregation, to conclusive as in the case of genetic linkage.

Defining familial aggregation

This can be regarded as the preliminary step in any attempt to determine whether genes play any significant role in the distribution of the trait. If the trait being analysed does not cluster within families, then it is unlikely that genetic factors play a major role in influencing the distribution of the trait in the population. However, the converse does not apply. A variety of factors, other than genetic etiology, can result in familial aggregation. Among them are the familial clustering of relevant environments, which have been shown to be important in the distribution of cholesterol levels [37, 52]. A striking example of the importance of familial environments in nutrition is given by Cravioto and DeLicardie [12] who found that the existence of severe malnutrition in infants was to a large extent a function of the social and behavioural environment created by the mother. Cultural transmission is also a phenomenon which can cause aggregation of a trait in biologically related individuals. This is likely to be an especially important issue in studies of nutrition and malnutrition, since food habits and methods of food preparation are cultural traits that tend to be transmitted along the maternal line.

Identifying genetic associations

Estimating the association of a trait with a specific genetic marker is analagous to the estimation of relative risk associated with an environmental variable. The same class of statistics tend to be used in both instances-usually contingency chi-square analysis or extensions thereof. The same cautions apply, in that causation cannot be infered from a relative risk estimate. Although the association of a disease with a known genetic trait is suggestive of some underlying genetic involvement in causation, there are three potential problems. First there are the statistical issues of correctly identifying the "associated" allele, or haplotype. This is especially critical for complex systems like HLA, where linkage disequilibrium amongst four highly variable loci provides a daunting number of possible interpretations. In such situations, it is best to first test for a general non-random distribution of the trait amongst the allelic, or genotypic, classes [53] and if this is significant, proceed to identify the relevant alleles in a hierachical fashion. It is also important to partition the allelic classes properly so that estimates of relative risk do not involve mixtures of high and low risk classes. Also the standard chi-square proceedure can lead to a biased estimate of relative risk, with the percentage bias being approximately equal to the expected number of individuals in a given class. Hence for rare alleles, or haplotypes, large samples will be needed to reduce both standard error and bias.

Second, confounding can lead to biassed estimates of relative risk. Potential causes of confounding when estimating genetic associations are excessive heterogeneity in the case population, or inappropriate selection of a comparison population. The first problem can be avoided by ensuring that the population of cases is as homogeneous as possible. A valid relative risk estimate requires that the population of controls represent the genetic background of the cases as closely as possible. Matching for ethnic background of grandparents, or, for parental community of origin is a fairly simple proceedure that would ensure comparability, though this is rarely done.

Third, genetic associations are often overinterpreted. It is unwise to assume that association with a genetic marker is the inevitable consequence of a linked gene, since this can lead to contradictions which are difficult to resolve.

Analysis of transmission

Under this heading are grouped the strategies and analytic proceedures that are directed towards a specific test of hypothesis. Familial aggregation is assumed and the pertinent issue is whether the distribution of the trait in defined sets of relatives is consistent with a specific transmission model. Traditionally, the only models given serious consideration were genetic models of Mendelian segregation. Classical segregation analysis, as first proposed by Weinberg [57] and then subsequently elaborated upon, was the method used to test the hypothesis for a given Mendelian model. Many of the formal analysis for segregation can now be carried out on complex pedigrees [2, 15, 23, 24] by use of a recursive probability functions [5]. However, care has to be taken in the ascertainment of such pedigrees [3, 55], and even for simple situations, the power to discriminate between competing genetic models may not be great [1]. The stronger the inference, the higher the likelihood of genetic causation. As Lalouel et al [33] have recently pointed out, a critical evaluation of complex segregation analysis should incorporate the "mixed model" [41] and requires testing the transmission parameters of the model [16, 17, 33].

Recently, Cavalli-Sforza and Feldman [6], among others, have elaborated models of cultural transmission which are equally worthy of testing. While the most efficient study designs and statistical analyses have yet to be developed for such models, this is an especially important concept to be considered in the nutritional area. Once the appropriate tests are formulated, it will be possible to make strong inference about traits that exhibit familial clustering because of cultural factors, as opposed to Mendelian segregation.

Genetic linkage studies

This strategy represents the most specific test of hypothesis in terms of defining genetic etiology. Formulating a research design to identify linkage relationships implicitly assumes that the trait being studied segregates as a Mendelian character. Like the strategies concerned with the mode of transmission, the success for outcome of a linkage study results in a clearcut assignment of genetic etiology. Since the genetic locus involved becomes positioned on the human genome as a consequence of a linkage study, this last strategy gives the most precise information of any of the strategies so far discussed. However, the instances where this strategy will be useful in the nutritional area are likely to be confined to the relatively few traits which involve single gene products.

Evaluating Familial Aggregation

In the majority of instances the first step in the investigation of a trait thought to have an underlying genetic component is to define the nature and extent of familial aggregation. This can be thought of as a preliminary descriptive exercise with the analytic proceedures employed considered as "Exploratory Data Analysis" in Tukey's original sense. Exceptions to this general principle would occur when there is already good evidence to indicate that the trait in question is influenced by a major gene. In such cases it is more appropriate to proceed to the stategies involving more formal tests of hypothesis outlined in the preceding section. When dealing with a complex field such as malnutrition, analysis of familial aggregation will be frequently called for.

Irrespective of whether the focus is on a clinical feature such as kwashiokor, or on the distribution of the kinetic properties of ATPase, it is essential to specify how the trait is distributed in families. The results of such analysis will determine which is the most appropriate next step in the investigation. A variety of relatively straightforward proceedures exist whereby familial aggregation can be defined. In general they can be considered as falling into two analytic strategies: correlational analysis, and cluster analysis.

Correlational Analysis. The objective of this strategy is to estimate the correlation coefficient of a trait amongst pairs of relatives. The primary objective of such an analysis is to determine if the correlations between defined sets of relatives are significantly different from zero, since this indicates familial aggregation. An advantage of correlational analysis is that the resulting correlations can be used to provide crude estimates of the contribution of presumptive genetic factors to the overall variance of the trait in the population. Such analyses which build on Fisher's original results [20] attempt to discern if the *pattern* of correlations amongst various sets of relatives varies systematically with the genetic coefficient of kinship.

While estimates from individual sets of relatives can be used for this purpose, a more structured analysis such as path analysis [39, 40, 60] is preferable. Path analysis gives the opportunity to construct environmental indices and in this way the importance of cultural transmission can be guaged [10,11]. The path analysis strategy is also quite suitable for the modelling of genotype environmental interactions [10,35] and can also handle qualitative data, such as clinical status [47]. Thus, there is much to recommend the estimation of simple correlations, since they are readily understood and, if estimated from an epidemiologically sound sampling design, can be informative regarding the nature of familial aggregation in the population.

However, there are some cautions which should be mentioned. First, the individuals are presumed to be a random sample from the population and, second, the different pairs of relatives in the sample are presumed to be independent of each other. Frequently both these conditions are difficult to meet. Random sampling is costly when the trait is rare and in communities, it may be difficult to find independent sets of relatives. The first difficulty can be overcome by explicitly selecting affected individuals and estimating the relative risk of affection in relatives which is equivalent to estimating familial correlations in genetic liability for a threshold trait [18]. With the extension of this concept to multiple thresholds [11,49], a potentially useful strategy arises for evaluating familial aggregation of graded series of malnutrition.

However, the problem of non-independent sets of relatives still remains, as does the potentially more serious problem of non-random distribution of relevant environmental variables. Both issues can be successfully circumvented by the use of the fixed cluster sampling design first promulgated by Schull in the guise of the "family set" method [51]. In this study design, a relationship cluster which is deemed to be most useful for a given problem is defined and this then forms the sampling unit, rather than individuals. A number of different kinds of relationship sets have been defined, such as nuclear family; extended nuclear family; sibs and cousins; extended sets of cousins, etc, and their properties examined [9,38]. Multivariate analysis results in the joint estimation of all relevent correlations simultaneously, thereby maximising the amount of information in the sample. Even more importantly the fixed clusters can be selected on the basis of a properly defined epidemiologically protocol [13]. By randomising environments across clusters, or by stratifying clusters within defined environments, the influence of environmental variables on familial aggregation can be estimated and controlled. In the complex and largely unknown area of nutrition, this type of sampling strategy and study design shows a great deal of promise.

Cluster Analysis. Methods of investigating the clustering of traits in groups of relatives form an alternative strategy for defining familial aggregation. The essence of this approach, which is ideally suited for clinical traits, is to investigate whether the occurence of a condition (e.g. marasmus) in a group of relatives is more concentrated than would be expected by chance. Two techniques have been recently suggested.

The first method, which requires the development of extensive pedigrees for a community or population, considers a group of cases and compares their mean coefficient of kinship with the mean coefficient of kinship for a group of appropriately selected controls. Higher coefficients of kinship amongst the cases, indicate familial aggregation. This implies that common descent from an ancestor has influenced the distribution of disease. This model which has been used to gauge familial aggregation of cancer [25] has the advantage that controls and cases can be matched for relevant concomitant variables, but has the disadvantage that the demographic structure of the population and the resulting pedigree is often ignored [56]. Other methods which requiere less extensive pedigrees [76], or which take demographic structure into account [56] have also been proposed. Although they have promise in certain areas they are unlikely to be useful in the area of nutrition because of their dependence on extensive pedigrees. By and large, the majority of populations that exhibit severe nutritional problems do not lend themselves to the construction of multi-generational pedigrees. This, plus the formidable problem of ensuring that cases and controls come from equivalent environments suggests such techniques will not be useful.

The second method is the converse of the first in the sense that a group of relatives are initially selected and then the frequency of occurrence of a trait in the group is compared with the expected frequency based on population distributions. Following the development of a general test for aggregation [54], a statistic has been developed for an arbitrary set of relatives [7]. This strategy which is formally related to the calculation of relative risk, is still in the stage of being formulated but shows considerable promise. Originally developed for general pedigree structures, the model could be extended to incorporate the concept of fixed cluster designs mentioned earlier. Since the model already allows for the incorporation of age specific incidence rates, other attributes influencing the probability of affection status could also be added in conjunction with an epidemiologically sound sampling strategy. Whether this would be more useful than the multivariate analysis of fixed clusters is a moot point, but for exploratory analysis of clinical data the strategy appears promising.

EPILOGUE

This brief presentation summarises some of the research strategies that are available in the area of genetic epidemiology and which might be applied to the area of nutrition. Overall, it seems premature to expend a great deal of energy on the sophisicated statistical techniques that formally embody the Mendelian and polygenic models. Once the field has been defined and well formulated hypotheses can be set up for specific issues in nutrition, the rigour of estimating transmission parameters will be appropriate. At that time, there will be sufficient information to ensure the collection of sample units in such a way that ascertainment bias does not skew the conclusions. For the present, it seems best to emphasize the somewhat more prosaic strategy of defining familial aggregation for specific clinical and biochemical variables that influence, or indicate, nutritional status. Even in this exercise, the problems are sufficiently daunting to satisfy even the most ambitious genetic epidemiologist.

REFERENCES

1. Beaty, T.H. Discriminating among single locus models using small pedigrees. *Am. J. Med. Genet.* 6:229-240, 1980.
2. Bishop, D.T. The analysis of pedigree information. *In* "The Genetics and heterogeneity of Common Gastrointestinal Disorders" (J.I. Rotter, I.M. Samloff, and D.L. Rimoin, eds), pp. 453-475. Academic Press, New York, 1980.
3. Blackburn, H (manuscript)
4. Cannings, C.m and Thompson, E.A. Ascertainment in the sequential sampling of pedigrees. *Clin. Genet.* 12:208-212, 1977.

5. Cannings, C., Thompson, E.A., and Skolnick, M. Probability functions on complex pedigrees. *Adv. Appl. Probab.* 10:26-61, 1978.

7. Chakraborty, R., Weiss, K.M., Majumder, P.P., Strong, L.C. and Herson, J. The detection of excessrisk of disease in family or other structured data based on individual outcomes. (Manuscript).

8. Chakraborty, R., Weiss, K.M. and Ward, R.H. Evaluation of relative risks from the correlation between relatives: A Theoretical approach, *Med. Anthropol.* 4:395-414, 1980.

9. Chakraborty, R. and Schull, W.J. Fixed cluster designs in human genetic studies: Interpretations and usefulness. In "Genetic analysis of Common Diseases: Applications to Predictive factors in Coronary Disease" (C.F. Sing and M. Skolnick). Alan R. Liss Inc., New York, 1979.

10. Cloninger, C.R. Interpretation of intrinsic and extrinsic structural relations by path analysis: Theory and applications to assortative mating. *Genet. Res.* 36:133-145, 1980.

11. Cloninger, C.R., Lewis, C.E., Rice, J., and Reich, T. Strategies for resolution of biological and cultural inheritance. In "Genetic Research Strategies in Psychobiology and Psychiatry" (E.S. Gershon, S. Matthysse, X.O. Breakefield, and R.D. Ciaranello). Boxwood Press, Pacific Grove, Calif, 1981.

12. Cravioto, J., and DeLicardie, E. La desnutricion infantil y el ambiente social. *Ciencia y Desarrollo* 13:63-72, 1977.

13. Donner, A., Birket, N. and Buck, C. Randomization by cluster. Sample size requirements and analysis. *Am. J. Epi.* 114:906-914, 1981.

14. Elston, R.C., and Stewart, J. A general model for the genetic analysis of pedigree data. *Hum. Hered.* 21:253-542, 1971.

15. Elston, R.C., Namboodiri, K.K., Glueck, C.J., Fallat, R., Tsang, R., and Leuba, V. Study of the genetic transmission of hypercholesterolemia and hypertriglyceridemia in a 195-member kindred, *Ann. Hum. Genet.* 39:67-87, 1975.

16. Elston, R.C., and Rao, D.C. Statistical modeling and analysis in human genetics. *Ann. Rev. Biophys. Bioeng.* 7:253-286, 1978.

17. Elston, R.C. Segregation Analysis. In "Advances in Human Genetics" 13:62-121, 1981.

18. Falconer, D.S. The inheritance of liability to certain diseases estimated from the incidence among relatives. *Ann. Hum. Genet.* 29:51-76, 1965.

19. Fienberg, S.E. "The Analysis of Cross-Classified Categorical Data," MIT Press, Mass, 1977.

20. Fisher, R.A. The correlation between relatives on the supposition of Mendelian inhereitance. *Trans. R. Soc. (Edinburgh).* 52:399-433, 1918.

21. Goldstein, J.L., Schrott, H.G., Hazzard, W.R., Bierman, E.L., and Motulsky, A.G. Hyperlipidemia in coronary beart disease. II. Genetic analysis of lipid levels in 176 families and delineation of a new inherited disorder, combined hyperlipidemia. *J. Clin. Invest.* 52:1544-1568, 1973.

22. Goldstein, J.L., and Brown, M.S. The LDL receptor locus and the genetics of familial hypercholesterolemia. *Ann. Rev. Genet.* 13:259-289, 1979.

23. Hasstedt, S.J., and Cartwright, P. PAP: Pedigree Analysis Package. Technical Report 13, Department of Medical Biophysics and Computing. University of Utah, 1979.

24. Hasstedt, S.J. Genetic models. In "The Genetics and heterogeneity of Common Gastrointestinal Disorders" (J.I. Rotter, I.M. Samloff, and D.L. Rimoin, eds), pp. 475-487. Academic Press, New York, 1980.

25. Hill, J.R. A survey of Cancer sites by kinship in the Utah Mormon population. In 'Branbury Report: Cancer incidence in defined populations' (J. Cairns, J. L. Lyon and M. Skolnick eds.) Cold Spring Harbor Lab, 1980.

26. Iselius, L. A major locus for Hyper-beta lipoproteinemia with xanthomatosis. *Clin. Genet.* 15:530-533, 1979.

27. Iselius, L. Complex segregation analysis of hypertriglyceridemia. *Hum. Hered.* 31:222-226, 1981.

28. Joreskog, K. The analysis of covariance structures. In "Multivariate Analysis III" (P.R. Krishaigh, ed). Academic Press, New York, 1973.

29. Karlin, S., Carmelli, D., and Williams, R. Index measures for assessing the mode of inheritance of continuously distributed traits. I. Theory and justifications. *Theor. Pop. Biol.* 16:81-106, 1979.

30. Karlin, S., Williams, P.T., and Carmelli, D. Structured exploratory data analysis (SEDA) for determining mode of inheritance of quantitative traits. I. Simulation studies on the effect of background distributions, *Am. J. Hum. Genet.* 33:262-281, 1981.

31. Karlin, S., Williams, P. T., Haskell, W. L., and Wood, P.D. Genetic analysis of the Stanford LRC family study data. II. Structured exploratory data analysis of lipids and lipoproteins. *Am. J. Epidemiol.* 113:307-323, 1981.

32. Kempthorne, O. Logical epistemiological and statistical aspects of nature nurture data interpretation. *Biometrics.* 34: 1-23, 1978.

33. Lalouel, J.M., Rao, D.C., Morton, N.E. and Elston, R.C. A Unified model for complex segregation analysis. (Manuscript).

34. Lalouel, J.M. and Morton, N.E. Complex segregation analysis with pointers. *Hum. Hered.* 31:312-321, 1981.

35. Lathrop, G.M., Lalouel, J.M. and Jaquard, A. Path analysis of family resemblance and gene-environment interactions. (Manuscript)

36. MacLean, C.J., Morton, N.E., and Lew, R. Analysis of family resemblance. IV. Operational characteristics of segregation analysis. *Am. J. Hum. Genet.* 27:365-384, 1975.

37. Moll, P.P., Powsner, R., and Sing, C.F. Analysis of genetic and environmental sources of variation in serum cholesterol in Tecumseh, Michigan. V. Variance components estimated from pedigrees. *Ann. Hum. Genet.* 42:343-354, 1979.

38 Moll, P.P., and Sing, C.F. Sampling strategies for the analysis of quantitative traits. in "Genetic Analysis of Common Diseases: Application to Predictive Factors in Coronary Disease" (C.F. Sing and M. Skolnick, eds), pp. 307-342, Alan R. Liss, New York, 1979.

39. Morton, N.E. Diseases determined by major genes. *Soc. Biol.* 26:94-103, 1979.

40. Morton, N.E. Outline of genetic epidemiology, Karger, Basel, 252pp 1982.

41. Morton, N.E., and MacLean, C.J. Analysis of family resemblance. III. Complex segregation of quantitative traits. *Am. J. Hum. Genet,* 26:489-503, 1974.

42. Morton, N.E., Gulbrandsen, C.L., Rhoads, G.G., Kagan, A., and Lew, R. Major loci for lipoprotein concentrations. *Am. J. Hum. Genet.* 30:583-589, 1978.

43. Neel, J.V. Diabetes mellitus: A "Thrifty" genotype rendered detrimental by "progress"?. *Am. J. Hum. Genet.* 14:353-362, 1962.

44. Orr, J.D., Sing, C.F., and Moll, P.P., Analysis of genetic and environmental sources of variation in serum cholesterol in Tecumseh, Michigan. VI. A search for genotype by environment interaction. *J. Chronic Dis.* in press.

45. Ott, J. Maximum likelihood estimation by counting methods under polygenic and mixed models in human pedigrees. *Am. J. Hum. Genet.* 31:161-175, 1979.

46. Ott, J. Detection of rare major genes in lipid levels. *Hum. Genet.* 51:79-91, 1979.

47. Rao, D.C., Morton, N.E., Gottesman, I.I. and Lew, R. Path Analysis of qualitative data on pairs of relatives: Applications to Schizophrenia. *Hum. Hered.* 31:325-333, 1981.

48. Rao, D.C., Morton, N.E., Gulbrandsen, C.L., Rhoads, G.G., Kagan, A., and Yee, S. Cultural and biological determinants of lipoprotein concentrations. *Ann. Hum. Genet.* 42:467-477, 1979.

49. Reich, T., Rice, J., Cloninger, C.R., Wette, R., and James, J. The use of multiple thresholds and segregation analysis in analyzing the phenotypic heterogeneity of multifactorial traits. *Ann. Hum. Genet.* 42:371-390, 1979.

50. Scheffe, H. A 'mixed model' for the analysis of variance. Ann. Math. Stat. 27:23-36, 1956.

51. Schull, W.J., Harburg, E., Erfurt, J.C., Schork, M.A., and Richard, R. A family set method for estimating heredity and disease. *J. Chron. Dis.* 23:82-96, 1970.

52. Sing, C.F., and Orr, J. D. Analysis of genetic and environmental sources of variation in serum cholesterol in Tecumseh, Michigan. IV. Separation of polygene from common environment effects. *Am. J. Hum. Genet.* 30:491-504, 1978.

53. Smouse, P.E. Statistical analysis of HLA-Disease associations. In "Genetic Analysis of Common Diseases: Applications to predictive Factors in Coronary Disease" (C. F. Sing and M. Skolnick eds.) Alan R. Liss, Inc. New York, 1979.

54. Smouse, P.E., Weiss, K.M. and Chakraborty, R. A simple test for the aggregation of disease occurrence in genealogical data. *Hum. Hered.* 31:334-338. 1981.

55. Thompson, E.A. Optimal sampling for pedigree analysis: Relatives of affected probands. *Am. J. Hum. Genet.* 33:968-977, 1981.

57. Weinberg, W. Weitere Beitrage zur Theorie der Verebung. IV. Uber Methode und Fehlerquellen der Untersuchung auf Mendelschen Zahlen beim Menschen. *Arch. Rass. Gess. Biol.,* 9:165-174, 1912.

58. Weiss, K.M., Chakraborty, R., Majumder P.P. and Smouse, P.E. Problems in the assessement of relative risk of chronic disease among biological relatives of affected individuals. *J. Chron. Dis.* (in press).

59. Williams, W.R., and Lalouel, J.M. Complex segretation analysis of hyperlipidemia in a Seattle sample. *Hum. Hered.* 32:24-36, 1982.

60. Wright, S. The application of path analysis of etiology. In "Genetic Epidemiology" (N.E. Morton and C.S. Chung, eds), pp. 13-51. Academic Press, New York, 1978.

61. Zavala, C., Morton, N.E., Rao, D.C., Lalouel, J.M., Gamboa, I.A., Tejeda, A., and Lisker, R. Complex segregation analysis of diabetes mellitus. *Hum. Hered.* 29:325-333, 1979.

DISCUSSION[1]

Blackburn opened the discussion by agreeing that dietary experiments would best be done in families, but pointed out that such studies might still be biased by the environment in which exposure is so high as to be maximal. He then questioned the statement that genetic-nutritional relationships in the hyperlipidemias may be multiplicative rather than additive, noting that the few available studies demonstrate that lipid levels distribute normally. Ward responsed to these several points. He recommended that family units or other clusters be examined across a known and measurable set of environments. He agreed that little data either way exists to test the multiplicative nature of genotype-environmental intrications, but found some of Connor's data on the differences in response to dietary cholesterol by patients with types IIA and IIB hyperlipoproteinemias provocative. Connor agreed and amplified this to include Type I in which hyperchylomicronemia is insensitive to cholesterol, but very much so to general dietary fat and type IV hyperlipoproteinemia in which weight loss seems to be of paramount importance. Connor also noted a number of family studies of blood lipid responses to dietary changes are going on and for which results may be available in several years. Scrimshaw inquired whether synergism might be a better term than multiplicative. Rosenberg also asked Ward to define the term multiplicative. Ward responded that he wished only to state that different genotypes may respond distinctly to different kinds

[1]*Summary of the discussion prepared by S. Cederbaum.*

of environments and that family studies might be one tool to uncover this. Rosenberg then pointed out that true multiplicative effects can be seen in homozygotes for inborn errors of metabolism. Using galactosemia as an example, he noted that heterozygotes are moderately different from normal when subjected to a galactose challenge, whereas the homozygotes achieve galactose blood levels twenty to forty times normal. He then asked why the cholesterol model is any different. Motulsky urged that we think of mechanisms and avoid terms like multiplicative to characterize exaggerated responses, terms which can only be confusing. Cavalli-Sforza stated that multiplicative has a very specific meaning, which is both good and bad whereas synergistic is more vague, thus also having both advantages and disadvantages. He would restrict multiplicative to situations in which the combined increments of variables increase on a log scale and use additive to describe coordinate effects on a direct scale. Synergism would describe a situation in which the result exceeds the sum of each of the individual effects. Scrimshaw notes that an illustration of synergism was the combined negative effects on growth of infection and malnutrition. Cederbaum closed the discussion by recalling Blackburns's comments and noting that genetic influences may play a more prominent role in nutrition when some of the most extreme dietary deprivation is eliminated.

PART II

INTERACTIONS BETWEEN GENETICS AND NUTRITION: CASE STUDIES

NUTRITIONAL GENETICS: CASE STUDIES

Antonio Velázquez

Unidad de Génetica de la Nutrición
Instituto de Investigaciones Biomédicas
Universidad Nacional Autónoma de México
Mexico City, Mexico

When the organizing committee first met to start planning the Workshop on Genetic Factors in Nutrition, we immediately became aware of the exciting challenges involved in gathering scientists who, specializing in different fields, generally have little or no contact with each other. We asked ourselves how to avoid sterile confrontations and trivialities and how to promote a spirit of co-operation, vital to an interdisciplinary approach encompassing genetics and nutrition. With the idea of drawing up guidelines to use in venturing into uncharted and risky seas, we have reviewed some examples of successful interactions between these fields. How have nutritionists and geneticists in the past approached the same problems from the perspective of their fields and sometimes solved them through interdisciplinary action?

We thought that perhaps these case studies would help us develop a mood of cooperation and light a spark of optimism based on previous achievements, no matter how limited they might be. We could then switch to a discussion of methods and strategies used in each field and the kinds of problems we might tackle with them. As a matter of fact, although at first glance this middle ground between genetics and nutrition seems to be a no-man's land, there have already been several successful interactions between these fields. Through them we have gained some idea of mechanisms involved, difficulties encountered, frameworks for questions, and underlying subtleties frequently found.

Geneticists have long known that genes do not act in vacuum, that their expression does not depend solely on interactions with other genes ("genetic background") and the information coded in DNA, and that the environment exerts its own, equally decisive, influence. Gene-environment interaction can be categorized into three classes (1):

57

a) direct effects of environmental agents on genetic material (mutation and carcinogenesis);
b) natural selection of genes by altered environments (evolution); and
c) influence of existing genetic variability on response to environmental agents (which Brewer (2) referred to as "ecogenetics").

One of the main environmental agents is food. Individual needs for each foodstuff for adequate development and optimal health, surely depend on numerous factors, both environmental and genetic. Simple easily-studied genetic traits are usually rare. Although geneticists have frequently used a biometrical, "black box" approach to solve biomedical puzzles (3), the most significant contributions have come from studies of individual differences that are relatively simple, clear-cut, and amenable to Mendelian analysis, a process which rather easily yields answers to simple, clear-cut questions and provides insights of responsible mechanisms. Although this approach works very well with straightforward, black-and-white traits, it is limited in its ability to resolve complex, multifactorial problems. The only way, however, to start solving a complex problem is to analyze it in a piecemeal way, reducing the problem to its simplest elements. Once those pieces are clearly in place, one proceeds to gradually fit in the other parts of the puzzle.

We will start our discussion on the relationship between genetics and nutrition by looking at the inborn errors of metabolism, more specifically at phenylketonuria (PKU), a classic example of a one-gene, one-nutrient interaction, as well as at ornithine transcarbamylase deficiency and the methylmalonic acidemias. We will then proceed to consider other examples of the relationship, such as lactose intolerance and hyperlipidemias, which involve both more complex mechanisms and epidemiology.

Genetically-determined nutritional variations may lead, not only to intolerances such as PKU or lactase deficiency, but also to new or higher nutritional requirements. For example, Hartnup's Disease, a transport disorder, increases the need for protein and for nicotinamide (4). Likewise, inherited vitamin dependencies (5), an example of which are some of the methymalonic acidemias, create new nutritional requirements. So do biosynthetic defects such as orotic aciduria (6) in which blocked pyrimidine synthesis makes uridine an essential nutrient.

Finding examples of new or increased nutritional needs is difficult, partly because screening methods for detecting inborn errors of metabolism have been designed primarily to discover those metabolic blocks, in which substrate accumulation is the predominant effect. This type of defect occurs most frequently in catabolic pathways. Furthermore, in higher organisms, there are fewer synthetic than catabolic routes. In humans, for example, each of the twenty amino acids has at least one catabolic pathway; on the other hand, only twelve amino acids can be synthesized by adults. Of course, nutritional requirements might increase with a heightened catabolic disposal. Here, too, examples are scarce, not only because we have no general methods for their detection, but also because mutations which increase flow through metabolic pathways are quite rare.

There is another type of variation that has been successfully studied by nutritionists and geneticists. Foods sometimes contain, not only nutrients, but also substances towards which idiosyncracies may be presented. Perhaps the best-known example is that of favism: a hemolytic anemia which occurs in some glucose-6-phosphate dehydrogenase (G-6-PD) deficient people who eat fava beans (*Vicia fava*) (7). Although details have not yet been completely worked out, it is known that these beans contain a substance which oxidizes erythryocytic glutathione efficiently. The oxidized metabolite combines as a mixed disulfide with hemoglobin, which it then irreversibly denatures and precipitates in the form of Heinz bodies. But not all G-6-PD deficient subjects appear to be sensitive to fava beans; several additional factors, probably metabolic (8) and genetic (9), may be involved in this hemolytic disorder.

These case studies will hopefully show that the interaction between nutritionists and geneticists is both desirable and feasible.

REFERENCES

1. Motulsky, A.G. Ecogenetics: genetic variation in susceptibility to environmental agents. *In:* Armendares and Lisker (eds). Human Genetics. Excerpta Medica, Oxford. 1976, pp. 375-385.
2. Brewer, G.J. Annotation: human ecology, an expanding role for the human geneticist. *Am. J. Hum. Genet.* 23:92-94, 1971.
3. Vogel, F. and Motulsky, A.G. Human Genetics: problems and approaches. Springer Verlag, Berlin, 1979.
4. Jepson, J.B. Hartunp Disease. *In:* The Genetic Basis of Metabolic Disease. McGraw-Hill Book Company, New York, 1978. pp. 1563-1577.
5. Rosenberg, L.E. Vitamin-dependent disease. *Hosp. Pract.* 5:59, 1970.
6. Kelly, W.N. and Smith, L.H. Hereditary orotic aciduria. *In:* The Genetic Basis of Metabolic Disease. McGraw-Hill Book Company, New York, 1978. pp. 1045-1071.
7. Kattamis, C.A., Kyriazakou, M. and Chaida, S. Favism: clinical and biochemical data. J. *Med. Genet.* 6:34-41, 1969.
8. Cassimos, C., Malaka-Zafiriu, K. and Tsiures, J. Urinary D-glutaric acid excretion in normal and G-6-PHD deficient children with favism. *J. Ped.,* 84:871-872, 1974.
9. Bottini, E., Lucarelli, P., Agostino, R., Palmarino, R., Businco, L. and Antognoni, G. Favism: association with erythrocite acid phosphatase phenotype. *Science,* 171:409-411, 1971.

INBORN ERRORS OF NUTRIENT METABOLISM: GARROD'S LESSONS AND LEGACIES

Leon E. Rosenberg

Yale University School of Medicine
Department of Human Genetics
New Haven, Connecticut

INTRODUCTION

Garrod's Insights

"The existence of chemical individuality follows of necessity from that of chemical specificity, but we should expect the differences between individuals to be still more subtle and difficult of detection. Indications of their existence are seen, even in man, in the various tints of skin, hair, and eyes, and in the quantitative differences in those portions of the end-products of metabolism which are endogenous and are not affected by diet... Even those idiosyncrasies with regard to drugs and articles of food which are summed up in the proverbial saying that what is one man's meat is another man's poison, presumably have a chemical basis" [4].

These words, like so many of Archibald Garrod's sound more current in the context of today's science and medicine than to those of his day. Garrod wrote them in his introduction to the famous Croonian lectures on inborn errors of metabolism which were delivered before the Royal College of Physicians of London in 1908. In these foreshadowing lectures, Garrod proposed that the biochemical reactions which constitute intermediary metabolism occur stepwise, each catalyzed by a specific enzyme under genetic control. Now, nearly 75 years later, we realize that Garrod's notions of gene action, of subtle chemical differences between individuals, and of idiosyncrasies to drugs and foods laid the foundation for the entire field of human biochemical genetics with its now numerous subdisciplines concerned with normal variation, inherited metabolic disease, and untoward responses to drugs and other environmental agents.

GENETIC FACTORS IN NUTRITION

61

Gene-Environment Interface in Nutrition

Surely, those environmental agents which most often confront our species (and, therefore, confront the endogenous chemical processes controlled by our genes) are found in the air we breath, the water we drink, and the food we eat. Here, then, is the link between nutrition, which considers the sum of the processes by which a living organism takes in and utilizes food substances, and genetics, which seeks to explain individual variation and heritable transmission. Human nutritional health depends on a balance between extrinsic (environmental) and intrinsic (genetic) factors (Figure 1). On the extrinsic side of the fulcrum, good nutrition depends on nutrient intake. Nutrients cannot be consumed unless they are available; they cannot be available unless there is an adequate supply. Intake, then, requires the orderly interplay between supply, availability, and consumption. These variables, in turn, are powerfully influenced by climatic, sociologic, economic, and religious forces. On the intrinsic side of this idealized nutritional equation, an even larger series of specific variables exist. Ingested nutrients are of value only if they are digested, absorbed, distributed, transformed, sorted, and excreted. These intrinsic processes depend on chemical reactions, many of which require catalysis by proteins in the form of receptors, carriers, enzymes, and hormones. In turn these proteins are the products of structural genes. Therefore, the intrinsic limb of nutrition is under genetic control. It is integral to and almost synonymous with the concept of metabolism, which refers to all of the processes by which living matter is built up or broken down.

From this schematic depiction of nutrition, it is obvious that nutritional dysfunction (or malnutrition) can result from either environmental or genetic disturbances. Clearly, the major nutritional problems in most of the world have environmental etiologies—inadequate food supply, improper distribution, ina-

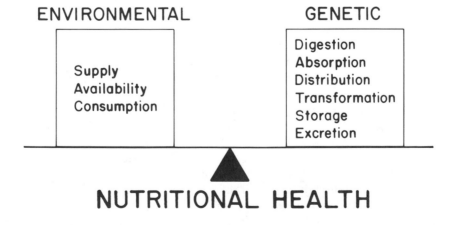

Figure 1. Scheme of nutritional health as a balance between environmental and genetic factors.

dequate consumption. However genes modify nutrient metabolism, they are of no great importance in the pathogenesis of such disorders of undernutrition as marasmus, kwashiorkor and specific vitamin deficiencies which affect millions of individuals worldwide. Obesity, the most prevalent disease of overnutrition, tilts the nutritional balance in the opposite direction but, again, the primary force is exogenous-excessive caloric intake. Faced with environmental nutritional stress, the intrinsic system concerned with nutrient metabolism compensates in many ways: absorption of a scarce nutrient may be enhanced and its excretion reduced; catabolism of a limiting nutrient may be decreased and its stores mobilized. If such compensatory mechanisms are adequate, health is maintained; if they are inadequate, nutritional dysequilibrium or malnutrition ensues.

Overview of Inborn Errors of Nutrient Metabolism

But malnutrition in its broadest sense can as well result from endogenous as exogenous disturbances. Garrod understood this brilliantly in alluding to the proverb that what is one man's meat is another man's poison. Each of the intrinsic processes required for proper nutrition (digestion, absorption, excretion) are affected selectively in the many inborn errors of nutrient metabolism, a sampling of which is shown in Table I. These disorders vary enormously with regard to the nutrient involved. These disorders, now numbering well over one hundred, vary as well in frequency, ethnic distribution, clinical severity, disease manifestation, and mode of Mendelian inheritance. Some are characterized by complete absence of a particular receptor or enzyme, others by partial deficiency. In some, the structural gene involved has been mapped to a particular autosome or sex chromosome; in others such information is lacking. Most of these disorders are inherited as autosomal recessive traits implying that clinically affected patients bear two mutant alleles at the locus in question, and, as importantly, that heterozygous carriers have no clinical problems. Only an occasional disorder is expressed dominantly in heterozygotes or shows a polymorphic population distribution, [6, 12, 15].

These disorders may interface with nutritional health in a variety of ways. They may produce deficiency of an essential macro-or micronutrient even though that substance is provided in adequate amounts in the diet. They may lead to chemical toxicity by blocking the catabolic pathway of a given nutrient ingested in usual amounts. They may interfere with formation of a needed product from an ingested nutrient. They may disrupt feedback regulatory pathways. They may lead to pathologic accumulation of macromolecules. These consequences, for which there are no general rules, depend on the site of the metabolic derangement and on its severity.

In whatever way nutritional balance is "tipped" by these disorders, one of their most important features is their potential for effective therapeutic management via modification of ingested nutrients (Table II). If intestinal absorption of a vitamin is defective, for example, effective treatment can be provided

TABLE I Selected Inborn Errors of Nutrient Metabolism

Process Affected	Disorder	Nutrients involved
Digestion	Lactose intolerance	Lactose
	Trypsinogen Deficiency	Protein
Absorption	Juvenile Pernicious Anemia	Cobalamin (Vitamin B_{12})
	Glucose-Galactose Malabsorption	Glucose; Galactose
	Chloride Diarrhea	Chloride
	Lysinuric Protein Intolerance	Dibasic Amino Acids
Distribution	Abetalipoproteinemia	Lipids
	Transcobalamin II Deficiency	Cobalamin (Vitamin B_{12})
	Familial Hypercholesterolemia	Cholesterol
Transformation	Phenylketonuria	Phenylalanine
	Homocystinuria	Methionine
	Ornithine Transcarbamylase Deficiency	Protein
	Galactosemia	Galactose
	Multiple Carboxylase Deficiency	Biotin
	Vitamin D Dependent Rickets	Vitamin D
Storage	Glycogenoses	Carbohydrates
	Refsum's Disease	Phytanic Acid
	Wolman's Disease	Cholesterol
Excretion	Hartnup Disease	Neutral Amino Acids; Nicotinamide
	Hypophosphatemic Rickets	Phosphorus
	Nephrogenic Diabetes Insipidus	Water

TABLE II Selected Inborn Errors Treated by Modification of Nutrient Intake

Therapeutic Modality	Disorder	Nutrient Modified
Avoidance	Refsum's Disease	Phytanic Acid; Phytol
Restriction	Phenylketonuria	Phenylalanine
	Citrullinemia	Protein
	Isovaleric Acidemia	Protein; Leucine
	Galactosemia	Galactose
	Hypercholesterolemia	Cholesterol
Supplementation	Cystinuria	Water
	Hypophosphatemic Rickets	Phosphate
	Methylmalonic Acidemia	Cobalamin (Vitamin B_{12})
	Multiple Carboxylase Deficiency	Biotin
	Homocystinuria	Pyridoxine; Folate
	Orotic Aciduria	Uridine

by parenteral administration of physiologic amounts (thereby circumventing the block). If toxicity results from a blocked catabolic pathway for an essential amino acid, dietary restriction of that amino acid may be beneficial. If derangement results from deficiency of an enzyme which requires a vitamin cofactor, vitamin supplementation may restore holoenzyme activity sufficiently to lessen or even overcome the disturbance. If the nutrient involved is unessential, it may be eliminated from the diet [6, 12].

Illustrative Disorders

For more than 20 years my laboratory has been engaged in the study of inborn errors of nutrient metabolism. During the 1960's we concentrated on disorders of amino acid, hexose, and ion transport. Specific conditions investigated included cystinuria, imino-glycinuria, renal glycosuria, glucose-galactose malabsorption and hypophosphatemic rickets. Subsequently, we have investigated a number of enzymatic disorders affecting cellular pathways of amino acid, organic acid, and vitamin utilization. From the latter group I have selected two disorders for special consideration: ornithine transcarbamylase deficiency; and the methylmalonic acidemias. These disorders have been chosen because they illustrate the principle that manipulation of administered nutrients may offer general scientific insights as well as specific therapeutic resources. (For a more detailed description of these conditions, the interested reader is referred to reference 13).

Ornithine Transcarbamylase Deficiency. In 1967 we were asked to see a 14-month-old girl admitted to the hospital with hemiplegia and coma. A lengthy work-up revealed that her neurologic dysfunction resulted from a dramatically elevated blood ammonia value (> 1000 μg/dl) which was, in turn, caused by partial deficiency of ornithine transcarbamylase (OTC). This mitochondrial matrix enzyme, found only in the liver and intestinal mucosa, is part of the Krebs-Henseleit cycle by which ammonia is detoxified and urea is formed (Figure 2). When nitrogen intake was eliminated transiently and intestinal ammoniagenesis was reduced by antibiotics and enemas, her sensorium and focal findings cleared entirely. She remained well until challenged transiently with a diet containing 3 gm protein per kg body wt per day, on which she promptly became ataxic, lethargic and hyperammonemic. Reduction of dietary protein to 1.5 gm/kg/day led to prompt clinical improvement which has been sustained for the past 15 years. This young woman, who now self-restricts her dietary protein, has a normal I.Q., height, and weight; her periodically obtained blood ammonia determinations are regularly within the normal range.

Detailed family history revealed that this girl had two brothers and two maternal uncles who died during the first week of life. Liver from one of her deceased brothers was devoid of OTC activity. This pedigree was strongly suggestive of an X-linked trait and led to further appraisal of family members [14]. *In vitro* oral loads of ammonium chloride, followed by serial blood ammonia determinations, revealed that her mother and maternal aunt had distincly abnormal ammonia tole-

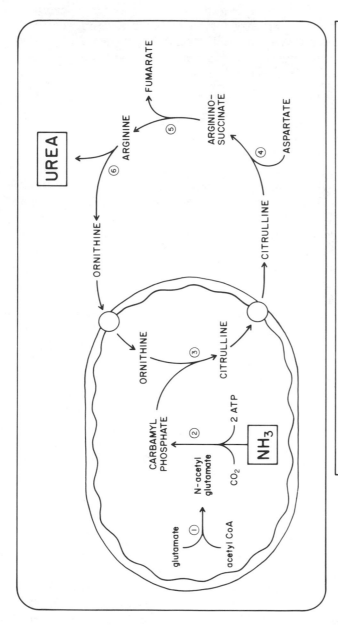

Figure 2. The hepatic urea cylce by which ammonia is detoxified. Six enzymes are required, three in the mitochondrion (NAG synthetase, CPS I, and OTC), and three in the cytosol (ASA synthetase, ASA lyase, and arginase). Inherited defects of each of these enzymes result in hyperammonemia in humans: ① N-acetyl glutamate synthetase ② Carbamyl phosphate synthetase I ③ Ornithine transcarbamylase ④ Argininosuccinate synthetase ⑤ Argininosuccinate lyase ⑥ Arginase

rance tests (Figure 3), consistent with each of them being heterozygous for an X-linked trait. Subsequently, their hepatic OTC activities were noted to be distincly reduced as well (Figure 3). Ultimately, this combination of *in vivo* oral ammonia or protein loads and *in vitro* hepatic OTC assays in other families established: that the structural gene for OTC is located on the X chromosome, that males with complete (or nearly complete) OTC deficiency are hemizygous for a mutant allele whereas females with partial deficiency are heterozygotes, and that OTC deficiency is genetically heterogeneous (*i.e.,* that many different mutant alleles exist at this locus).

This disorder, for which there is an analagous mouse model [2], is now treated by a variety of nutrionally-based regimens. Females with partial OTC deficiency may do well, as our proposita has, on a diet only moderately restricted in protein. Depending on the degree of OTC deficiency, other heterozygotes may need arginine supplements to replete urea cycle intermediates, or sodium benzoate to "siphon" waste nitrogen into hippurate. The latter adjuncts may permit less rigorous dietary protein restriction [1]. Hemizygous affected males present a much more difficult therapeutic challenge. Neither severe protein restriction nor protein restriction plus the use of arginine or keto acid analogues of essential amino acids have permitted long-term growth and viability. It remains to be seen whether a combination of protein restriction, arginine supplementation, and benzoate administration will alter the dismal prognosis in these boys [1]. If such treatment is successful, it would constitute a most dramatic pronouncement that humans can detoxify ammonia successfully without an intact urea cycle.

The Methylmalonic Acidemias. Soon after working up the young girl described in the section above, we saw an 8-month-old boy who was admitted in coma with ketosis and a blood pH below 7.0. After correcting his ketoacidosis by usual measures (parental glucose and bicarbonate administration), we challenged him with protein and reproduced his admitting complaints in milder form. Ultimately we showed that his protein intolerance reflected an inherited catabolic block in methylmalonate isomerization to succinate [10]. The specific reaction involved, through which several essential amino acids (isoleucine, methionine, threonine, valine) and odd chain fatty acids feeds, is catalyzed by the enzyme, methylmalonyl CoA mutase, which rewires a cobalamin (vitamin B_{12}) cofactor for activity (Figure 4). When this child was given 1 mg of cyanocobalamin daily parenterally (about 1000 times the estimated human daily requirement), his urinary methylmalonate content fell markedly (Figure 5) and his ability to tolerate valine improved [7, 11]. Such cobalamin responsiveness was studied in considerable detail subsequently, with the following major conclusions: his *in vivo* requirement was at least 500 times the normal; the defect in his cells was in the mitochondrial pathway of cellular cobalamin metabolism by which ingested and transported vitamin is converted to active coenzyme [8]; there are at least four biochemically and genetically distinct disorders in the cobalamin pathway, each leading to a cobalamin-responsive form of methylmalonic acidemia [3]; such

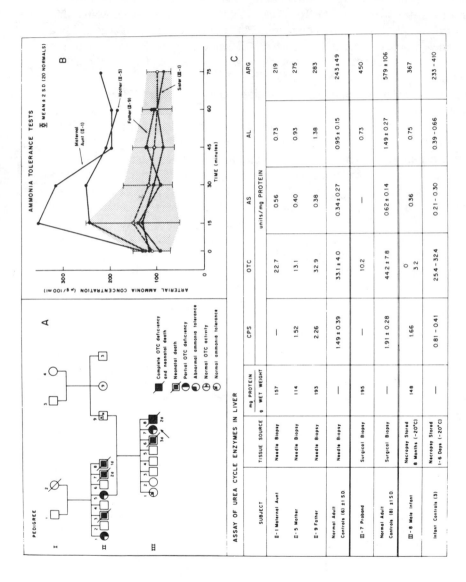

Figure 3. (A) Pedigree of proposita (shown by arrow) with OTC deficiency. (B) Results of ammonia tolerance tests in several family members (C) Assays of urea cycle enzymes in liver of subjects denoted in (a). From Short et al. [14].

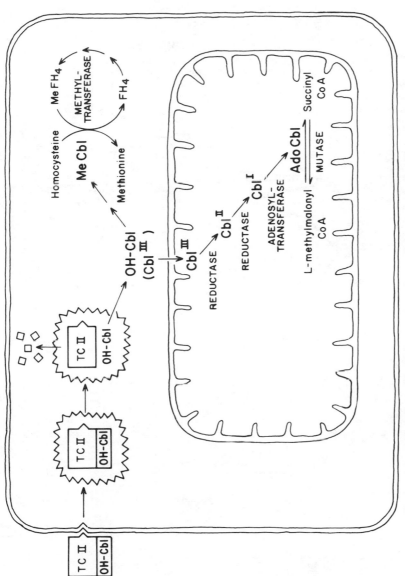

Figure 4. General pathway of cellular uptake and subcellular compartmentation of cobalamins, and of intracellular distribution and enzymatic synthesis of cobalamins; MeCbl, methylcobalamin; AdoCbl, adenosylcobalamin; Cbl^{III}, Cbl^{II}, Cbl^{I}, cobalamins with cobalt valence of 3+, 2+, and 1+, respectively. See reference 13 for details.

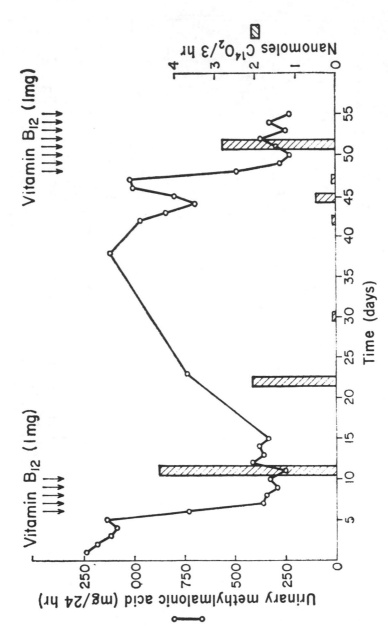

Figure 5. Effect of parenteral vitamin B_{12} (cobalamin adminstration on urinary methylmalonic acid excretion (left ordinate) and ^{14}C-propionate oxidation by peripheral blood leukocytes (right ordinate) in index patient with cobalamin-responsive methylmalonic acidemia. Each vertical arrow represents single daily injection of vitamin. From Rosenberg et al [11].

vitamin-responsive children may constitute close to half of all children with inherited methylmalonic acidemia, the remainder having primary apomutase abnormalities. Finally, this line of clinical investigation has prognostic significance as well in that children with cobalamin-responsive forms of methylmalonic acidemia tend to thrive better, live longer, and have fewer medical problems than their vitamin-unresponsive counterparts [9].

Concluding Remarks

Patients with overt inherited disorders of nutrient metabolism challenge the clinician upon whose acumen their very lives depend. Moreover, they offer biochemists cell biologists, and geneticists unique puzzles whose solutions define new reactions and delimit old ones. Most germane to this volume, however, these patients remind those interested in nutritional epidemiology of the limits of our information. They represent the exception to our rules; the outlyers in our Gaussian distributions. Take, for example, the notion of essential nutrients. Whereas most humans must ingest only nine amino acids because we cannot make them, a child with cystathionine synthase dificiency is unable to form cysteine from methionine, thereby adding cystine to his/her list of essential nutrients. Similarly, tyrosine is an essential amino acid for patients with PKU, and arginine for individuals with urea cycle defects. In this instance an inborn error results in a qualitative redefinition of the word "essential". Quantitative alterations in nutritional requirement, too, derive from patients with inherited disorders. Thus, a patient with cobalamin-responsive methylmalonic acidemia requires ~ 500 μg of parenteral cobalamin daily—not the 1-3 μg usually needed. Further, these rare "experiments of nature" remind us that nutrients harmless to most of us may cause serious toxicity in a rare "sport". Patient with polyneuropathy due to Refsum's Disease, for example, are unable to catabolize phylanic acid, a long chain fatty acid found exclusively in dairy and ruminant fats; dietary exclusion of this fatty acid leads to neurologic improvement.

It seems certain that the extreme variations in nutritional requirements demonstrated by patients with inborn errors of metabolism bear witness to variation in nutritional needs found among and between different populations. Such variation will reflect, at least in part, the unexpectedly large amount of heterozygosity now known to exist at as many as one-third of all human loci [5]. The challenge remaining is to identify these more subtle genetic determinants of individual nutritional requirements and to determine their significance on human health, disease and longevity. This will not be easy for the differences will undoubtedly be subtle enough to require sophisticated in vivo or in vitro tools. Nonetheless, the reward of more rational nutritional advice for individuals, ethnic groups, and races are likely to be worth the effort. Garrod certainly would applaud the attempt.

REFERENCES

1. Batshaw, M.L., Brusilow, S., Waber, L., Blom, W., Brubakk, A.M., Burton, B.K., Cann. H.M., Kerr, D., Mamunes, P., Matalon, R., Myerberg, D., and Schafer, I.A. Treatment of inborn errors of urea synthesis. Activation of alternative pathways of waste nitrogen sinthesis and excretion. *New Engl. J. Med.* 306: 1387, 1982.

2. DeMars, R., LeVan, S.L., Trend, B.L., and Russell, L.B. Abnormal ornithine carbamoyltransferase in mice having the sparse-fur mutation. *Proc. Natl. Acad. Sci. USA* 73: 1693, 1976.

3. Fenton, W.A., and Rosenberg, L.E. Genetic and biochemical analysis of human cobalamin mutants in cell culture. *Annu. Rev. Genet.* 12: 233, 1978.

4. Garrod, A.E.' Introduction to the Croonian lectures on inborn errors of metabolism. *Lancet* 2: 1, 1908.

5. Harris, H. Enzyme and protein diversity in human population. *In* "Principles of Human Biochemical Genetics". 3rd Edition (H. Harris, ed.), pp. 316-406. Elsevier/North-Holland, Amsterdam, 1980.

6. Holtzman, N.A., Batshaw, M.L., and Valle, D.L. Genetic aspects of human nutrition. *In* "Modern Nutrition in Health and Disease", 6th Edition (R.S. Goodhart, and M.E. Shils, eds.), pp. 1193-1219. Lea and Febiger, Philadelphia, 1980.

7. Hsia, Y.E., Lilljeqvist, A.C., and Rosenberg, L.E., Vitamin B_{12}-dependent methylmalonicaciduria: Amino acid toxicity, long-chain ketonuria and protective effect of vitamin B_{12}. *Pediatrics* 46: 497, 1970.

8. Mahoney, M.J., Hart, A.C., Steen, V.D., and Rosenberg, L.E. Methylmalonicacidemia: Biochemical heterogeneity in defects of 5'-deoxyadenosylcobalamin synthesis. *Proc. Nat. Acad. Sci.* 72: 2799, 1975.

9. Matsui, S.M., Mahoney, M.J., and Rosenberg, L.E. The natural history of the inherited methylmalonic acidemias. *New Engl. J. Med.* (in press).

10. Rosenberg, L.E., Lilljeqvist, A.C., and Hsia, Y.E. Methylmalonic aciduria: An inborn error leading to metabolic acidosis, long-chain ketonuria and intermittent hyperglycinemia. *New Engl. J. Med.* 278: 1319, 1968.

11. Rosenberg, L.E., Lilljeqvist, A.C., and Hsia, Y.E. Methylmalonic aciduria: metabolic block localization and vitamin B_{12} dependency. *Science* 162: 805, 1968.

12. Rosenberg, L.E. Inborn errors of metabolism. *In* "Metabolic Control and Disease". 8th Edition (P.K. Bondy and L.E. Rosenberg, eds.), pp. 73-103. W.B. Saunders, Philadelphia, 1980.

13. Rosenberg, L.E. and Scriver, C.R. disorders of amino acid metabolism. *In* "Metabolic Control and Disease", 8th Edition (P.K. Bondy and L.E. Rosenberg, eds.), pp. 583-776. W.B. Saunders, Philadelphia, 1980.

14. Short, E.M., Conn, H.O., Snodgrass, P.J., Campbell, A.G.M., and Rosenberg, L.E. Evidence of X-linked dominant inheritance of ornithine transcarbamylase deficiency. *New Engl. J. Med.* 288: 7, 1973.

15. Stanbury, J.B., Wyngaarden, J.B., and Fredrickson, D.S. Inherited variation and metabolic abnormality. *In* "The Metabolic Basis of Inherited Disease", 4th Edition (J.B. Stanbury, J.B. Wyngaarden, and D.S. Fredrickson, eds.), pp. 1-32. McGraw-Hill, New York, 1978.

DISCUSSION[1]

Even though the homozygous state of the "inborn metabolic errors" is too infrequent in the general population to account for the variability in nutrient requirements, Motulsky wondered if the heterozygotes for those errors —or perhaps different capacity isoalleles at a given locus related to the error— could be in higher risk and thus explain some outlying cases.

Rosenberg replied that there is lack of evidence of deleterious effects in carriers of "classical" errors. We recalled that large surveys done on obligate carriers of galactosemia (parents of sick children) and of the cystathione synthetase defect in homocystinuria have failed to show increased incidence of some of the corresponding clinical manifestations (cataract in galactosemia and premature atherosclerotic disease and thrombosis in homocystinuria); nevertheless, increased levels of urinary cysteine and occasional cysteine calculi are found in carriers of the mutant allele for cystinuria. In Rosenberg's opinion, even though higher risk is likely in heterozygote carriers for some particular loci and disorders, these individuals do not represent a group large enough to explain outlying requirements found in nutritional surveys. A potentially rich source of information could be the 20-25 Mendelian disorders associated with unusually high vitamin requirements in homozygotes, if appropiate studies are done on their obligate carriers.

Hillman pointed out that the vitamin dependence syndromes as well as transport errors and other auxotrophic defects should be more suitable models to prove the "heterozygote effect" than the catabolic errors in breakdown pathways, since in the latter, low nutrient intakes tend to obscure the clinical picture.

Coleman indicated that in his mice studies he finds many loci which have multialleles producing a great variety of syndromes, from the very severe to the very mild, and suggested this could also apply to human populations, especially when exposed to a variety of environmental conditions. Harper called attention to other factors, such as hormonal and nutritional variables which modify ify enzyme activity, and to the fact that some enzymes may be controlled by more than one gene; all these factors, apart from the simple presence or absence of a single gene, could produce variability, at least for some nutrient requirements.

Accepting the importance of the factors mentioned by Harper, Motulsky insisted in stressing that, for many enzymes, different isoalleles with varying activity within the normal range may explain much variability, as in the case of acid phosphatase previously presented by Ward. The concept of multiple genes determining low and high activity enzymes as clearly seen in Coleman's mice studies — will greatly help to understand variability. Special techniques — electrophoresis, DNA studies or careful breeding experiments — capable of clearly distinguishing the different capacities of enzymes are needed to disentangle the differences; twin or family studies are inadequate for that purpose.

[1]*Summary of the discussion prepared by H. Bourges*

Garby asked the group to specify in each case whether reference was made to enzyme activity or enzyme amount, two concepts that should not be confused. Rosenberg reacted mentioning that it is not simply the issue of amount versus native activity; some other distinctions were necessary. In biochemical genetics studies of a large number of enzymes focusing on genetic variation, several different mechanisms can be found: there are mutant alleles, at the same locus, giving essentially no enzyme production; others giving normal production of a catalytically inactive enzyme or normal production of a rapidly-degraded enzyme; there may be increased production of a catalytically poor enzyme and even synthesis of an enzyme molecule with exaggerated catalytic activity.

In Rosenberg's opinion, there are surely far more numerous alleles than those identified through intensive investigation of severely defficient individuals. Indeed, this group is viewed as the "tip of the iceberg". As an example, for the methylmalonyl mutase locus, there may be twenty different mutase alleles in patients with enzyme defficiency. Therefore, there is no reason to believe that isoalleles producing modest variations in enzyme activity do not exist in normal populations.

Cohen added several comments to illustrate the extreme complexity of the picture further. Reduction of activity —for instance by 50%— of an enzyme normally present in amounts 100-fold greater than needed, as is the case for carbonic anhydrase, makes no metabolic difference. It is necessary to recognize that each enzyme step is a self-regulated system; we need to understand these steps in terms of, for example, their coenzymes, or of reactions in which end-products never become free, but become substrates of other enzymes, which are frequently integrated into enzyme complexes. Furthermore, the end-product of one system may be a cofactor or a regulator of other systems.

For example, carbamyl-phosphate-synthetase-1 —catalyzing the first step of urea biosynthesis— is totally dependent on the availability of N-acetyl glutamate; in turn, the concentrarion of this activator depends on the capacity of the mitochondrion to make glutamate react with Acetyl Co A. Any reaction competing for coenzyme A or glutamate has consequences on carbamyl phosphate synthesis.

In each particular pathway, there are many overlapping and interdigitating steps on which to focus. Perhaps, subsequent effects are not revealed because they manifest themselves in obscure ways, and have therefore not been looked for.

There are claims in literature about changes in enzyme level which are unimpressive because the decrease in enzyme activity or amount is not enough to make the step rate-limiting. On the other hand, it must be realized that we should be dealing with cell functions more than with rates of enzyme-activity in a test tube with conditions set for optimal rates, which may or may not represent the steady state rate in the cell. We have yet to understand steady state kinetics of a number of enzyme systems *in situ*.

Also, DNA is not as stable as previously considered. It forms and reforms; components separated by introns seem to associate and rejoin to finally express themselves in transcription. There are also postranslational changes. Repressed genes can be derepressed. So, DNA may be quite vulnerable to the influx of noxious agents. We do not know the amount of daily dietary insults and whether their effects are transient or semipermanent. In chronic diabetes mellitus, for example, hemoglobin and albumin are glucosylated; there is no reason for the amino groups of the DNA bases not to be glycosylated as well.

We are in an era —Cohen concluded— with skills and technology to understand DNA, how the gene sequence finds its expression, and how it is regulated. Time has come to lend the necessary attention to dietary factors influencing genetic expression.

In relation to one of Cohen's remarks, Cederbaum recalled studies where a fairly close correlation between *in vivo* activity and residual enzyme activity *in vitro* has been found. He mentioned studies on patients with phenylketonuria or hyperalanincmia and on the obligate heterozygotes, done in Germany and published in 1975. Enzyme was measured in liver biopsies and the *in vivo* conversion of deuterated phenylalanine to tyrosine was followed. Correlation was very high except in one patient with severe accumulation of phenylalanine, but with high residual activity of an enzyme which was surely altered in its kinetic porperties.

Torún proposed to discuss the very practical issue of iodine deficiency in relation to goiter and cretinism and asked if anybody had a hint concerning a genetic answer to the problem. Iodine deficiency is widespread and even endemic in some regions. Goiter is practically its only manifestation, but in some groups, for no clear reason, it is accompanied by cretinism. Scrimshaw added that the prevalence of goiter before the iodination of salt had reached 30% in Nicaragua and 38% in Guatemala, and as high as 66% and 80% in affected communities in the respective countries. In spite of such high frequency, not a single case of cretinism was detected in communities with very low inbreeding, while cretinism appeared in populations where inbreeding was common. Inbreeding may also have a role in deaf mutism and feeblemindedness but the different factors, including the role of iodine deficiency and goitrogens in the environment, have never been adequately sorted out. Torún and Scrimshaw stressed their belief that this issue provides an outstanding opportunity for future development on the interphase between genetics and nutrition.

Neel commented that Marcel Roche and John Stanbury, working with Yanomama and Macutari Indians of the Amazon region in 1960, observed that euthyroid individuals, with no goiter, had ^{131}I uptakes as high as 85% in 24 hours. The finding was attibuted to methodological problems, but the observation was confirmed in 1967 and presented at a PAHO meeting; high uptakes were not found anymore in groups who had contacted the outside world during the 7 year period. Neel feels that goiter was probably much less common in precontact times in the continent, and that a factor —most likely a molecule— which travels with civilization, blocks the extremely effective iodine uptake mechanisms of these populations. Individuals whose genotype unables them to handle this molecule, develop goiter with contact. Certainly, in a given goiter area, many but not all individuals develop the disease.

Cavalli-Sforza asked Rosenberg two questions. First, if he could guess the proportion of cases of inherited metabolic disorders without diagnosis in the United States; and second, what number of metabolic errors did he expect to exist.

Rosenberg opined that only a very small fraction of cases in the population are detected; only phenylketonuria is systematically screened for in medically developed societies. Some disorders such as certain urea cycle defects are so severe, that they cannot be missed because affected individuals are challeged by the environmental side of the nutrition paradigm, and show illness very early in life. But for each one of these severe diseases there are probably twenty with no known effects until later in life, such as acute intermittent porphyria manifested in the "teens".

Regarding the second questions, Rosenberg stated that the number of possible inborn errors is as large as the number of structural loci in the human genome — between 10,000 and 100,000. Cohen expressed that if we live long enough and the population keeps increasing at the present rate, other pathways controlled by genetic components will eventually join up in the list.

Rosenberg added that, for the branched chain amino acid pathways, there are some 15 disorders for 15 different loci, almost one disease for every enzymatic step.

Waterlow proposed to include hemoglobinopathies in the discussion. Neel commented that there are several hundred variants but only a few have been shown to have deleterious effects, such as S, C and E; for many of the rarer variants the homozygous condition, which would probably show a significant handicap, has not been observed. Motulsky mentioned the thalassemias, which are quite severe in the homozygous state; according to recent studies, there are 12 different lesions known only for beta thalassemia, slicing lesions in terms of introns and exons. This area of research is extremely exciting. In some affected regions with high incidence of these disorders, the disease is diagnosed *in utero* and, through selective abortion, the frequency of the disease is being decreased.

Regarding the abnormal hemoglobins Lisker commented that many —probably about 50 or 60— can produce pathology; at least ten of them produce metahemoglobin, about 15 are unstable hemoglobins and others produce thalassemia or anemia through different mechanisms.

Velázquez, turning back to the question of the number of possible inborn errors, pointed out that many mutations produce abortion so that, unless they are looked for prenatally, the complete spectrum will not be covered. Neel added that it is now accepted that around 50% of all conceptions terminate prior to term, a much higher proportion that usually thought. He has been specially interested in the mutation-selection balance in man but the present understanding on how frequently genes give rise to disease is incomplete. Looking at the frequency of a dozen unselected enzymes, by two-dimensional electrophoresis, he found 3 to 4 individuals per 1000 who were heterozygous for the null genes (with no activity) at these loci; considering the number of existent enzymes, it may be estimated that 3 to 4% of all conceptuses would be homozygous for null alleles. Since the frequency of unrecognized disease is quite below that figure, Neel speculated, a high proportion of these inborn errors may be eliminated *in utero*. In relation to this, recent results show that about 7% of all conceptuses have a serious chromosomal abnormality; but only 0.5% of live-born infants carry a chromosomal abnormality; the rest are spontaneously aborted.

Motulsky then insisted that there are several enzymes with the null allele in the homozygous state, with no activity whatsoever, and the person is perfectly normal, as is the case for cholinesterase, paraoxonase and many others. Although there are at least 7 or 8 important functions known for albumin, albuminemia coexists with health in the 15 patients known to have this disease in the World. There may either be a physiologic compensation or it may have no physiological significance within our environment. Lisker doubted that absence of proteins could equal lack of disease; he opined that it simply depends on the lack or presence of environmental challenges.

Hillman commented that there are many common genetic disorders important in nutrition and growth which fall out of the realm of geneticists because of their frequency. Such is the case of cystic fibrosis, adrenal hyperplasia, a host of muscle diseases, genetic variations in growth and bone metabolism, and others. Adrenal hyperplasia, for instance, has a reported incidence of 1 in 1200 in Switzerland, but the carrier rate is 1 in 12 in that population. Geneticists seem to prefer rarer diseases leaving the more common ones to other physicians.

PHENYLKETONURIA

Stephen D. Cederbaum*

Departments of Psychiatry and Pediatrics
The Mental Retardation Research Center
Los Angeles, California

INTRODUCTION

Phenylketonuria (PKU) is a disease at the interface of genetics and nutrition. In its classical form, the inherited deficiency of phenylalanine hydroxylase results in excess accumulation of phenylalanine in the body fluids when dietary intake exceeds its incorporation into protein and the amino acid pool, its obligatory loss in urine, feces, or its conversion to breakdown products [6,41,42]. The clinical hall-mark of PKU, mental retardation, is largely prevented if early detection and nutritional therapy reduce plasma phenylalanine levels toward the normal range [6,41,42]. Yet the broad spectrum of phenylalanine levels in the untreated patient, the variable degree of mental retardation from patient to patient, the individuality of daily phenylalanine tolerance and the several inherited causes of hyperphenylalaninemia have created a degree of clinical, genetic, and molecular heterogeneity sufficient to assure preeminence for this disorder as a prototype for understanding biochemical genetics and the medical aspects of inherited metabolic disordes.

This discussion will include an outline of the phenylalanine hydroxylating system, of the different forms of hyperphenylalaninemia, of neonatal screening and finally of the therapy of this family of disorders.

Phenylalanine Hydroxylation

The normal North American diet contains two to three times as much phenylalanine as is needed to maintain positive nitrogen balance and the protein synthesis required for growth and cellular renewal. The vast majority of this

* *Supported in part by the Mental Retardation Research Program at UCLA and USPHS grants HD-11298, AM-25983, HD-06576, HD-05615, HD-04612, and RR-00865.*

excess is hydroxylated to form tyrosine and then metabolized further to substrates of energy metabolism [4,22]. Phenylalanine hydroxylation is know to occur with certainty in the liver and may also occur in the kidneys [22]. Although other pathways for phenylalanine metabolism are present in man, they lack the capacity to handle the metabolic excess occasioned by the deficiency of phenylalanine hydroxylase [22,42].

The linchpin of the penylalanine hydroxylating system (Fig. 1) is the enzyme phenylalanine hydroxylase (PH; EC 1.14.16.1) which in the presence of tetrahydrobiopterin (BH₄) and oxygen converts phenylalanine to tyrosine, H_2O and dihydrobiopterin (BH₂). BH₄ is regenerated when BH₂ is reduced by NADH in the presence of dihydropteridine reductase (DHPR; EC 1.6.99.7), an enzyme that is relatively stable as compared with PH. 7,8-BH₂ is synthesized *de novo* in man from guanosine triphosphate in a series or reactions which for the sake of simplicity in this discussion will be refered to as the synthetic reactions. Other more arcane enzyme and substrate components of this system are discussed elsewhere [22,40,42].

Clinical Hyperphenylalaninemia

Both logic and experience have taught us that defects in all steps of an inherited metabolic pathway will be found if appropriate study methods are applied to a large enough population. The truth of this contention is exemplfied by

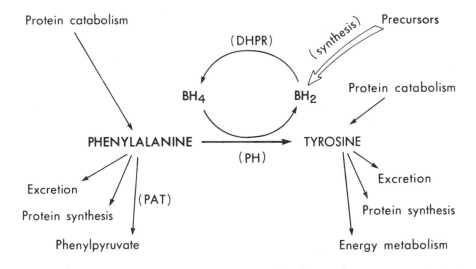

Figure 1. A simplified schematic representation of phenylalanine hydroxylation and the production and fate of phenylalanine and tyrosine in man (adapted from Seriver and Clow [42] and others. PH-phenylalanine hydroxylase; DHPR-dihydropteridine reductase; BH₄-tetrohydrobiopterin; BH₂-dihydrobiopterin; synthesis-the aggregate of biosynthetic reactions responsible for the endogenous production of dihydrobiopterin; and PAT-phenylalanine amniotransferase.

study of the hyperphenylalaninemias. Enzymatic defects of variable severity have been found in each component arm of the phenylalanine hydroxylating system (Table I).

Classical Phenylketonuria

The most frequent and clinically significant form of hyperphenylalaninemia is "classical" phenylketonuria (PKU) first described by Folling in 1934 in two retarded sisters [46]. This has been shown to be due to a profound deficiency of phenylalanine hydroxylase activity, *in vitro,* in tissue obtained at biopsy [3] and *in vivo* when deuterated phenylalanine is administered to the patients and tyrosine formation measured [45]. As a consequence of this deficiency, phenylalanine accumulates in the blood at levels of 20 mg/100 ml (1.25 mM) or more

TABLE I. Clinical and Biochemical forms of Hyperphenylalaninemia

Name	Enzymatic Defect	Clinical Aspects	Serum Phenylalanine	Urinary Findings
"Classical" Phenylketonuria	Phenylalanine Hydroxylase (severe)	Mental Retardation, Neurological Disability, pigment dilution and eczema, if untreated	Persistently greater than 20 mg/100 ml (1.25 mM)	Phenylpyruvate ("phenyl-ketone") and its its metabolites
Persistent hyper-phenylalaninemia	Phenylalanine hydroxilase partial in most instances	Often phenotypically normal without therapy	4-20 mg/100 ml (0.25-1.25 mM)	Usually normal
Dihydropteridine reductase deficiency	Dihydropteri-dine reductase	Mental Retardation, neurological disa-bility-progressive and potentialy fatal	So far always greater than 4 mg/100 ml (0.25 mM)	Those of classical PKU or persistent hyperphenylalani-nemia depending on phenylanine le-vel: reduced level of neurotrams-mitter metaboli-tes: elevated dihydrobiopterin
Neopterin (BH₂) synthetic defects	Synthetic enzyme defect inferred	Same as dihydropter-dine deficiency	So far always greater than 4 mM/100 ml (0.25 mM)	Same as dihy-dropteridine reductase defi-ciency except elevated urinary levels of neopterin

(10 times normal levels) [41,42] and to a lesser degree in the tissues. Excess phenylalanine activates or avails itself of secondary metabolic pathways and greatly increased plasma and urinary levels of phenylpyruvic acid and urinary levels, at least, of phenylacetate, phenylacetyl glutamine and other metabolites as well [41,42]. Secondary changes in other compounds not directly related to phenylalanine metabolism are also seen [42].

The untreated patient was typically perceived as normal for the first three or more months of life after which progressive mental delay, neurological deterioration, pigmentary dilution (hair and skin) and eczema developed, leaving most patients quite severely retarded and behaviorally and neurologically impaired [26]. With the advent of early diagnosis in the impaired child or more commonly presymptomatic chemical diagnosis at birth and preemptive therapy, this full clinical phenotype has become a historical oddity virtually unknown to the general pediatrician and rarely seen even by specialist in inborn errors of metabolism, especially in developed countries [41]. Previously 0.5-1.0% of patients in hospital for the mentally retarded were affected by this disorder [49].

Persistent Hyperphenylalaninemia

Our current understanding of molecular biology leads logically to the prediction that a significant proportion of gene mutations would encode proteins with normal or only partially impaired function or stability. Thus, the discovery of patients with hyperphenylalaninemia and substantially greater phenylalanine tolerance than those with true PKU comes as no surprise [41,42]. Of those few studied in depth, most have seemed to have partial defects of phenylalanine hydroxylase activity, and partial impairment of phenylalanine hydroxylation when assessed *in vivo* using heavy-labelled substrates [45]. Most of these patients, and especially those with phenylalanine levels below 15 mg/100 ml (about 1.0 mM) will show no increase in the products of the secondary phenylalanine pathways [41]. There is some debate as to whether phenylalanine levels below 20 mg/100 ml (about 1.25 mM) leads to suboptimal intellectual and neurologic function, but a consensus of conservative opinion favors treatment of all patients with levels persistently greater than 10-12 mg/100 ml (0.62-0.75 mM) bringing then below/100 ml (0.62 mM) at least during the early years in which brain development and myelination is occurring [35].

Tetrahydrobiopterin Deficiency

The clinical features of dihydopteridine reductase deficiency and biopterin synthetic defects are similar as both are due, ultimately, to a deficiency of tetrahydrobiopterin (BH_4), as shown in Figure 1 [13]. Deficiency of BH_4 causes reduced functional activity of phenylalanine hydroxylation when judged by plasma phenylalanine levels, but normal activity of phenylalanine hydroxylase is found when the customary assay is performed on fresh liver specimens, in the presence of excess reduced biopterin [2,24]. DHPR is assayed directly and its deficiency demonstrated, *in vitro*, using either liver tissue, white blood cells or cultured skin fibroblasts [2, 16, 24, 25, 38]. The synthetic defects were first ascertained in hyperphenylalanemic patient with normal levels of both PH and DHPR [13,25]. Evaluation of pterin levels in the urine as well as the response of plasma phenylalanine levels to administered BH_4 [12] permit presumptive enzymatic diagnoses in these disorders. In both DHPR and BH_2 synthesis deficiencies, phenylalanine levels fall transiently to normal in response to exogenous BH_4. In DHPR deficiency, BH_2 levels in urine are augmented, whereas they are grossly deficient in BH_2 synthesis deficiences [40]. BH_4 deficiency may make up 1-2% of all cases of hyperphenylalaninemia [13] or more in some isolated populations.

The degree of impairment of phenylalanine hydroxylation is variable, sometimes causing the biochemical picture of classical phenylketonuria and at others that of hyperphenylalaninemia [18,13]. A presentation with no detectable abnormality of phenylalanine metabolism appears possible, but would prove quite difficult to ascertain. The pathogenesis of the clinical phenotype in these deficiences is more complex. BH_4 is the reducing agent in two other aromatic hydroxylation reactions in the nervous system, that of tryptophan to 5-hydroxytrytophan and that of tyrosine to L-Dopa [31]. These hydroxylated compounds are converted ultimately to serotonin and epinephrine and norepinephrine and their metabolites are deficient in the urine and CSF of patients unable to generate adequate amounts of BH_4 [13,31]. Like patients with classical PKU, they appear normal at birth, but after some months show signs of mental retardation, and neurological symptoms such as seizures, hypo-or hypertonia and extrapyramidal signs. Death often ensues within the first year [13]. Not surprisingly, the first patients were ascertained amoungst PKU and hyperphenylalaninemic patients who failed to develop normally despite adequate control of plasma phenylalaline levels by diet or appropriate conservative therapy [13].

Newborn Screening for Hyperphenylalaninemia

The treatment of hyperphenylalaninemia proved to be preventative, sometimes palliative, but rarely partially or completely curative [6,41,42]. The efficacy of the diet was demonstrated particularly in the younger siblings of PKU patients who were ascertained at birth and in whom the increase in IQ above those with untreated PKU convinced all but the most extreme skeptics [15,18,44]. Because younger siblings of late diagnosed and treated PKU patients represented fewer than 25% of the case total, 75% of all patients were destined to some degree of retardation unless presymptomatic screening was introduced. The ferric chloride test for urinary phenylpyruvate was simple and inexpensive, but proved inadequate in PKU infants, in many of whom the appearance of positive test might be delayed until three months of age [33]. The Guthrie microbiological inhibition assay for phenylalanine in dried blood spots overcame these defects and proved to be a highly specific and inexpensive test with low false positive and false negative rates [17]. With this test, newborn screening for metabolic disorders was introduced to modern medicine and is virtually universal in the economically and medically developed countries of the world [33]. Experience suggests that when screening is properly planned and executed, 95% or more of cases are ascertained and treated preemptively [46]. At UCLA participating in the California State program, this usually is accomplished in the first ten days if life. With this approach, PKU and more recently cretinism are likely to disappear as causes of serious mental retardation in our society. Moreover, a considerable amount of our awareness and knowledge of the variants of hyperphenylalaninemia has ocurred as a direct result of the screening program [42].

The Dietary Treatment of Phenylketonuria

Although efforts to develop alternative methods of treatment for PKU have recently been explored, the phenylalanine-restricted or elimination diet, remains the only proven therapeutic approach [42]. The concept of an elimination diet, eschewing the precursor of the missing reaction for the treatment of an inborn error of metabolism was introduced for galactosemia in 1935 [37]. It was for PKU, however, that the semisynthetic diet was developed and it is from this disorder that we have learned so much about these diets and their risks [6,7,11]. The aim of the diet is to lower the elevated phenylalanine levels depending on this effect to lower the levels of the associated metabolites. It is sobering to contemplate that as we approach the 30th anniversary of this highly successful therapy, we still are uncertain as to whether it is phenylalanine and/or one of its metabolites that is the principal neurotoxin in PKU and, in fact, unclear as to how this neurotoxin might work. When one considers the nearly unanimous acceptance of the efficacy of the diet today, it is difficult to believe that as little as 10-12 years ago, this was a subject of a vigorous polemic [6, 41,42].

Phenylalanine constitute about 5% of animal protein and somewhat less of those derived from plants. From the begining it was apparent that restricted intake of protein alone could not reduce phenylalanine levels in PKU without causing malnutrition. Because large quantities of purified L-amino acids were both unavailable and expensive, it was indeed fortunate that activated charcoal treatment of protein hydrolysates removed aromatic groups and yielded material with substantially reduced levels of phenylalanine [6]. When tryptophan and tyrosine were supplemented, the final product was suitable as the source of the bulk of the amino acids of growth by these patients [6,41,42]. Natural protein was used to raise phenylalanine levels to the minimum daily requirements. When supplemented with fat carbohydrate, minerals, and vitamins, a diet complete in all major nutrients was available. Lofenelac, produced by

Mead-Johnson is a complete low-phenylalanine powdered formula and is used to treat virtually all North American infants with PKU, in combination with either breast milk, normal infant formula, or cows milk.

Dietary treatment for PKU was tested simultaneously by several groups in the early 1950's, but Boikel *et al* are generally given credit as the pioneers [7]. They found that the diet lowered plasma phenylalanine levels, eliminated the positive ferric chloride test in the urine and when used in young enough patients, albeit with well established mental retardation and neurologic disease, a clear remission of symptoms was noted [7,11]. During this period the striking developmental success of younger siblings of PKU patients treated from the age of one month or less was the impetus of the development of the neonatal screening test noted above.

Several aspects of the early treatment protocols seem related to suboptimal clinical outcome and helped to fuel the controversy surrounding the therapeutic efficacy of the diet that did not subside until recently [5,11,14,18]. Firstly, the diet was often started later than one month of age as neither the laboratory techniques for diagnosis nor the dietary expertise for treatment was so widely and readily available [11,18]; and secondly, inexperience with semisynthetic diets and the mortal growth requirements led to overtreatment and iatrogenic undernutrition [1,18]. Thus, many early patients had IQ results 10-20 points below normal and had small stature and small head circumferences [11,14,19].

When dietary therapy was initiated, normal phenylalanine requirements were known only for adults. This intake, about 25 mg/kg/day was used for newborn infants whose requirements we now know are 70-90 mg/kg/day and in some instances more [11]. The impact of this ignorance was exaggerated by the belief that appropriate therapy required phenylalanine levels in the normal range, tolerating values sometimes below the lower limits of normal. We now know that values on the low side of normal are more dangerous than those that are moderately elevated, an understanding that developed empirically as well as from the ascertainment and study of healthy normal patients with persistent hyperphenylalaninemia [11,42]. Finally, it became clear that at least some patients with PKU had received formulas with inadequate amounts of vitamins and had true deficiency syndromes [11].

The lessons of these early deficiencies have been incorporated into the modern products and treatment protocols and the improved results are best exemplified by the outcomes recorded in patients enrolled in the PKU Collaborative Study directed by Dr. Richard Koch at Childrens Hospital of Los Angeles [47]. Briefly stated, early-treated PKU patients (1 month of age or less) when studied at four years have mean height and weight at the 50th percentile, mean head circumference at that level for boys and slightly below for girls [2]. IQ scores are slightly reduced as compared with those of their parents and normal siblings at age 6, but above the population mean [48]. Episodes of lethargy and listlessness, skin rash and generalized aminoaciduria previously associated with undernutrition are unknown. All other physical and chemical studies are in the normal range as well. Plasma phenylalanine levels of therapy now fall most often in a range of 5-10 mg/dl (0.25-0.5 mM) [48]. These patients seem to do no worse than those with therapeutic levels nearer the normal upper limit of 2.0 mg/100 ml. (0.1 mM), but precise comparisons are unavailable.

The enormous progress made in the treatment of PKU should not be allowed to obscure the fact that the disease is far from benign, exacts a considerable toll on the family, and is still associated with many unsettling doubts. Despite the normalized IQ, treated PKU is associated with a significantly increased incidence of perceptual-motor problems and learning disabilities [27,28,42]. These difficulties appear in patients who have benefitted from early diagnosis and apparently optimal therapy, as well as those who have encountered therapeutic problems.

The maintenance of the diet itself is a manageable challenge for the physician and staff. It is tecnically more demanding for the family, but this problem is dwarfed by the psychological challenges imposed. Parents confront a diet whose complete failure would result in mental retardation, and they abandon a considerable degree of latitude and discipline to insure an adequate intake whithin restricted bounds. Although adequate nutrition and phenylalanine levels may be maintained with some variability of intake, this provides little relief to the anxiety of many parents. After the age of five, substantial responsibility shifts to the patients who must mature and adapt to a complex world while maintaining disciplined control of phenylalanine intake.

Despite the excellent growth and clinical outcome in the patients, uncertainties in the therapy persist and are reinforced by the recognition of our early failures. We have not solved the problem of educational failures and don't know if earlier treatment or more stringent therapy would help. If they did matter, it is unclear how appropriate changes in screening and therapy would be implemented. The composition of natural protein in the diet varies from patient to patient and would in all cases exclude animal proteins in those patients who adhere to their diet between the ages of 1-1/2 and 10. Only recently rather profound deficiency of blood selenium was found in treated PKU patients, and with it a proportional decrease in glutathione, peroxidase, a selenium dependent enzyme [36]. Zinc and copper levels are reduced as well in treated PKU [1]. Lowered bioavailability of selenium and zinc is thought, in part, to be the cause of their reduced levels in blood [1]. These examples underscore the risk of still other unknown deficiences, especially as they may have special impact on a genetically susceptible host. Finally, two important issues of dietary therapy remain unresolved: the age (if any) at which dietary therapy may be safely terminated; and the appropriate approach to the treatment of hyperphenylalaninemia in the pregnant PKU patient.

The practical application of elimination diet is straighforward. Current methods of diagnosis in California usually permit the identification of patients and establish the need for therapy by 10 days of age. Because of the technical and emotional demands made by the diagnosis of PKU, patients are generally admitted to the hospital for the initiation of therapy. During this admission, diet regulation is begun and the parents are taught record keeping and are given considerable conselling and reassurance. Lofenelac alone is used at first to bring elevated levels of plasma phenylalanine into the normal range. Subsequently, whole or evaporated milk is added back to the diet in small amounts to bring daily phenylalanine intake into the range of 270-300 mg. Because of its low protein content, breast milk may constitute the majority of the nutritional intake during the early months of treatment.

Phenylalanine levels are obtained semiweekly and then weekly for the first six months with formula and natural protein varied to meet normal nutritional needs and individualized phenylalanine requirements and tolerances. After this time, patients with stable eating habits and phenylalanine levels are seen biweekly and then monthly. Juices and solid foods are introduced at appropriate times and food variety is enhanced by recipes and food products. High protein foods are avoided. Parents must calculate the protein intake from solid foods and reduce milk consumption to maintain phenylalanine intake at the prescribed leved. As noted above, whole milk intake usually ceases in the second year.

As the patients reach the age of four, meeting hunger demands using Lofenelac becomes increasingly difficult. The substantial, albeit reduced, phenylalanine content of Lofenelac requires limitation even of low protein foods. Substitution of Mead-Johnson formula 3229 (Phenyl-free) or other similar products, in which crystalline amino acids replace casein hydrolysate and which contain no phenylalanine, increases the permissible intake of natural foods and is an important adjunct to therapy. In addition, older patients may find this more palatable, although taste does not appear to be a major problem in dietary compliance.

The treatment of hyperphenylalaninemia due to partial phenylalanine hydroxylase deficiency is similar to that in classical PKU, but greater tolerance for dietary phenylalanine is usually observed. Treatment of biopterin defects is aimed at controlling phenylalanine levels and replacing the products of tyrosine and tryptophan hydroxylases, 5-hydroxytrytophan and L-Dopa. These considerations are not germane to this discussion and are discussed extensively elsewhere [6,12,13,23].

Diet Termination

The phenylalanine restricted diet is quite limited in scope and is an onerous burden to the patient and family. It becomes particularly difficult when the patient enters school and a far less isolated environment. In this setting, the wider availability of forbidden temptations and the desire to conform often create major conflicts within the patient and family, and pressure to diminish or terminate dietary restriction. In addition, the early supplements (especially) were expensive and provided an added impetus to return to a normal diet. Because of these pressures and with the knowledge that brain growth was largely complete by age five or six, physicians frequently capitulated and allowed special therapy to be stopped. Striking deterioration in clinical status was not observed [21,29]. Recent systematic studies suggest that certain patients may experience considerable deterioration when the diet is terminated and may, in turn, benefit by its reinstitution [10,43]. Others appear to fare quite well without dietary regulation after this age. We believe that this differential susceptibility, like that to the adverse impact of the untreated cases, is due probably to a combination of genetic characteristics and environmental factors, such as the normal amount of unregulated protein intake. Whatever the mechanism, the arrival of the school years places new tension on both physician and family, each wishing to take the easier route, but fearing that the harder one might be safer.

I believe a consensus of conservative thought on dietary termination might be as follows: the ideal would be the indefinite maitenance of phenylalanine levels below 10 mg/100 ml (0.625 mM). Recognizing this as impractical, an attempt is made to maintain tight control until age 10, accepting that episodic relaxation between ages 5 and 10 may be required to insure overall compliance. Subsequently, an attempt should be made to keep levels below 20 mg/100 ml (1.25 mM) by continuing dietary supplements and a high intake of low protein foods. All patients are seen semiannually and those who discontinue dietary therapy are observed more closely for indications of diminished school performance and acceptable home behavior, without the imposition of a rigid formal testing schedule. Dietary therapy must be reinstituted in PKU women who wish to have children (see below).

Maternal Phenylketonuria

The adverse impact of hyperphenylalaninemia in the mother on the development of non-PKU children was recognized first in 1957, and since then more than 100 instances were recorded independently [6]. As many as 90% of liveborn off-spring of women with serum phenylalanine levels <20 mg/100 ml (1.25 mM) may have some abnormality including mental retardation; microcephaly; congenital heart disease; other congenital anomalies; and low birth weight [32].

The problem was quantitatively unimportant when retarded women of childbearing age became pregnant infrequently and only accidentally. Now however, as a result of newborn screening and successful therapy, a generation of PKU women with normal intelligence and aspirations is approaching childbearing age. Given the average family size, the number of individuals retarded as a result of PKU would rapidly return to pretreatment levels unless adequate therapy were developed. Unfortunately, the solution to his problem is not easy.

Lenke and Levy have demonstrated that the severity of measurable damage in maternal hyperphenylalaninemia is roughly proportional to the plasma levels of the amino acid [32]. They and others have shown that plasma phenylalanine levels may be readily brought into the therapeutic range and controlled in a stable manner during pregnancy [9,30,32,34]. The outcomes of pregnancy may be apparently normal especially if the diet is begun prior to conception and abnormalities may be reduced in treatment begun later [9,39,32,34,39]. More discouraging are reports of damaged children born to mothers with well-controlled phenylalanine levels during the first and second trimesters of pregnancy, and that women at risk seem to resist the admonitions that they avoid pregnancy prior to the reinstitution of therapy [9,30,32,34]. It seems likely that experience with dietary therapy and more intense and continuous counselling of teenage females will increase our success still further, but how much is unknown. Many questions remain to be answered. Studies in rats, in higher primates, and in man have established that the placenta is a phenylalanine (and an amino acid) pump, allowing fetal plasma concentrations about twice those of the parent [41]. Yet we know little of the fetal tolerances for deviations from the norm. Levels of 7-8 mg/100 ml (0.5 mM) are relatively harmless to the neonate and developing infant, and can be achieved in the pregnant PKU mother. Some or many featuses may be intolerant of these levels. Similarly the fetus may be less tolerant of low phenylalanine levels, rendering it particularly susceptible to overzealous therapy. We are sitting on a time bomb that threatents the lustre and success of 30 years of continuous progress.

SUMMARY

PKU and hyperphenylalaninemia represent a family of disorders with a high degree of intra-and intergenic heterogeneity. Many of the conditions lead to mental retardation and serious neurological impairment. The largest proportion of these patients can be ascentained in the presymptomatic stage and neurological impairment can be prevented by the institution of dietary therapy aimed at lowering plasma phenylalanine levels. The application of this therapy has taught us much about the nutritional requirements of infants and adults, the individual variability in dietary phenylalanine requirements and tolerance. This information has proven applicable to a variety of other inherited metabolic disorders and, we hope, to the normal population as well.

REFERENCES

1. Acosta, P.B., Fernhoff, P.M., Warshaw, H.S., Hambidge, K.M., Ernest, A., McCabe, E.R.B., and Elsas, II, L.J. Zinc and copper status of treated children with phenylketonuria. *JPEN* 5:406, 1981.
2. Bartholome, K., Byrd, D.J., Kaufman, S., and Milstien, S. Atypical phenylketonuria with normal phenylalanine hydroxylase and dihydropteridine reductase activity *in vitro*. *Pediatrics* 59:757, 1977.
3. Bartholome, K., Lutz, P., and Bickel, H. Determination of phenylalanine hydroxylase activity in patients with phenylketonuria and hyperphenylalaninemia and hyperphenylaninemia. *Pediatr. Res.* 9:899, 1975.

4. Bernheim, M.L.C. and Bernheim, F. The production of a hydroxyphenyl compound from L-phenylalanine incubated with liver slices. *J. Biol. Chem.* 152:481, 1944.

5. Bessman, S.P. Legislation and advances in medical knowledge-acceleration or inhibition. *J. Pediatr.* 69:344, 1966.

6. Bickel, H. Phenylketonuria: past, present, future. *J. Inher. Metab. Dis.* 3:123, 1980.

7. Bickel, H., Gerrard, J., and Hickman, E.M. Influence of phenylalanine intake on phenylketonuria. *Lancet* 2:812, 1953.

8. Brewster, T.G., Moskowitz, M.A., Kaufman, S. Breslow, J.L., Milstien, S., and Abroms, I. F. Dihydropteridine reductase deficiency associated with severe neurologic disease and mild hyperphenylalaninemia. *Pediatrics* 63:94, 1979.

9. Buist, N.R.M., Lis, E.W., Tuerck, J.M., and Muphey, W.H. Maternal phenylketonuria. *Lancet* 2:589, 1979.

10. Cabalska, B., Dusynska, N., Borzymowska, J., Zorska, K., Koslacz-Folga, A., and Bozkowa, K. Termination of dietary treatment in phenylketonuria. *Eur. J. Pediatr.* 126:253, 1977.

11. Clayton, B.C. The principles of treatment by dietary restriction as illustrated by phenylketonuria. *In,* "The Treatment of Inherited Metabolic Disease", (D.N. Raine, Ed.), pp. 1-32. American Elsevier, N.Y., 1974.

12. Curtius, H. Ch., Niederwieser, A., Viscontini, M., Otten, A., Schaub, J., Scheibenreiter, S. and Schmidt, H. Atypical phenylketonuria due to tetrahydrobiopterin deficiency. Diagnosis and treatment with tetrahydrobiopterin, dihydrobiopterin and sepiapterin. *Clin. Chim. Acta.* 93:251, 1979.

13. Danks, D.M., Bartholome, K., Clayton, B.E., Curtius, H. Grobe, H., Kaufman, S., Leeming, R., Pfleiderer, W., Rembold, H., and Rey, F. Malignat hyperphenylalaninemia. *J. Inher. Metab. Dis.* 1:49, 1978.

14. Dobson, J., Koch, R., Williamson, M., Spector, R., Frankenberg, W., O' Flynn, M., Warner, R., and Hudson, F. Cognitive development and dietary therapy in phenylketonuric children. *New Engl. J. Med.* 278:1142, 1968.

15. Dobson, J.C., Kushida, E., Williamson, M.L., and Friedman, E.A. Intellectual performance of 36 phenylketonuria patients and theri non-affected siblings. *Pediatrics* 58:53, 1976.

16. Figaira, F.A., Cotton, R.G.H., and Danks, D.M. Dihydropteridine reductase deficiency: diagnosis by assays on peripheral blood cells. *Lancet* 2:1260, 1979.

17. Guthrie, R. and Susi, A. A simple phenylalanine method for detecting phenylketonuria in large populations of newborn infants. *Pediatrics* 32:338, 1963.

18. Hanley, W.B., Linsao, L.S., and Netley, C. The efficacy of dietary therapy. *Canad. Med. Assoc. J.* 104:1089, 1971.

19. Holm, V.A. and Knox, W.E. Physical growth in phenylketonuria I. A retrospective study. *Pediatrics* 63:694, 1979.

20. Holm, V.A., Kronmal, R.A., Williamson, M. and Roche, A.F. Physical growth in the PKU collaborative study from birth to 4 years of age. *Pediatrics* 63:700, 1979.

21. Holtzman, N.A., Welcher, D.W., and Mellets, E.P. Termination of restricted diet in children with phenylketonuria: a randomized control study. *New Engl. J. Med.* 293:1121, 1975.

22. Kaufman, S. Phenylketonuria: biochemical mechanisms. *Adv. Neurochem.* 2:1, 1976.

23. Kaufman, S. Progress in phenylketonuria: defects in the metabolism of biopterin. *Pediatrics* 65:837, 1980.

24. Kaufman, S., Berlow, S., Summer, G.K., Milstien, S., Schulman, J., Orloff, S., Spielberg, S., and Pueschel, S. Hyperphenylalaninemia due to a deficiency of biopterin. *New Engl. J. Med.* 299:673, 1978.

25. Kaufman, S., Holtzman, N.A., Milstien, S., Butler, I.J., and Krumholz, A. Phenylketonuria due to a deficiency of dihydropteridine reductase. *New Engl. J. Med.* 293:785, 1975.

26. Knox, W.E. Phenylketonuria *In* "the Metabolic Basis of Inherited Disease" (J.B. Stanbury, J.B. Wyngaarden, and D.S. Fredrickson, eds.) 3rd ed. pp. 266-295, McGraw-Hill, New York, 1972.

27. Koch, R., Blascovics, M., Wenz, E., Fishler, K., and SChaeffler, G. Phenylalaninemia and phenylketonuria. *In* "Heritable Disorders of Amino Acid Metabolism" (W.L. Nyhan, ed), 109-140, Wiley, New York, 1974.

28. Koff, E., Boyle, P., and Peuschel, S.M. Perceptural-motor functioning in children with phenylketonuria. *Am. J. Dis. Child.* 131:1084, 1977.

29. Koff, E., Kammerer, B., Boyle, P., and Peuschel, S.M. Intelligence and phenylketonuria: effects of dietary termination. *J. Pediatr.* 94:534, 1979.

30. Komrower, G.M., Sardharwalla, I.B., Coutts, J.M.J., and Ingham, D. Management of maternal phenylketonuria: an emerging clinical problem. *Br. Med. J.* 1:1383, 1979.

31. Koslow, S.H. and Butler, I.J. Biogenic amine synthesis defect in dihydropteridine reductase deficiency. *Science* 198:522, 1977.

32. Lenke, R.R. and Levy, H.L. Maternal phenylketonuria and hyperphenylalaninemia. New *Eng. J. Med.* 303:1202, 1980.

33. Levy, H.L. Genetic screening. *Adv. Hum. Genet.* 4:1, 1973.

34. Levy, H.L., Kaplan, G.N., and Erickson, A.M. Comparison of treated and untreated pregnancies in a mother will phenylketonuria. *J. Pediatr.* 100:876, 1982.

35. Levy, H.L., Shih, V.E., Karolkewicz, V., French, W.A., Carr, J.R., Cass, V., Kennedy, Jr., J.L. and McCready, R.A. Persintent mild hyperphenylalaninemia in the untreated state. *New Engl. J. Med.* 285:424, 1971.

36. Lombeck, I., Kasperek, K., Bachmann, D., Feinendegen, L.E., and Bremer, H.J. Selenium deficiency. *Eur. J. Pediatr.* 134:65, 1980.

37. Mason, H.H. and Turner, M.E. Chronic galactemia. *Amer. J. Dis. Child.* 50:359, 1935.

38. Milstien, S., Holtzman, N.A., O' Flynn, M.E., Thomas, G.H., Butler, I.J., and Kaufman, S. Hyperphenylalaninemia due to dihydropteridine reductase deficiency: assay of enzyme in fibroblasts from affected infants heterozygotes and in normal aminotic fluid cell. *J. Pediatr.* 89:763, 1976.

39. Nielsen, K.B. Wamburg, E., and Weber, J. Successful of pregnancy in a phenylketonuric mother after a low pehylalanine diet introduce before conception. *Lancet* 1:1245, 1979.

40. Nixon, J.C., Lee, C-L, Milstien, S., Kaufman, S., Bartholome, L. Neopterin and biopterin levels in patients with atypical froms of phenylketonuria. *J. Neurochem.* 35:898, 1980.

41. Rosenberg, L.E. and Scriver, C.R. Disorders of amino acid metabolism. *In* "Metabolic Control and Disease" (P.K. Bondy and L.E. Rosenberg, eds.) pp. 583-776, Saunders, Philadelphia, 1980.

42. Scriver, C.R. and Clow, C.L. Phenylketonuria: epitome of human biochemical genetics *New Engl. J. Med.* 303:1336, 1394, 1980.

43. Smith, I., Lobascher, M.E., Stevenson, J.E., Wolff, O.H., Schmidt, H. Grubel-Kaiser, S., and Bickel, H. Effect of stopping low-phenylalanine diet on intellectual progress of children with phenylketonuria. *Br. Med. J.* 2:723, 1978.

44. Smith, I., and Wolff, O.H. Natural history of phenylketonuria and influence of early treatment. *Lancet* 2:540, 1974.

45. Trefz, F., Bartholome, K., Bickel, H., Lutz, P., and Schmidt, H. *In vivo* determination of phenylalanine hydroxylase activity using heptadeuterated phenylalanine and comparison to the *in vitro* assay values. *Monogr. Hum. Genet.* 9:108, 1978.

46. Veale, A.M.O. Screening for hereditary metabolic disorders: screening for phenylketonuria. *In:* "Neonatal Screening For Inborn Errors of Metabolism" (H. Bickel, R. Guthrie, and G. Hammersen, eds.) pp. 7-18, Springer-Verlag, New York, 1980.

47. Williamson, M., Dobson, J.C., and Koch, R. Collaborative study on children treated for phenylketonuria: study design. *Pediatrics* 60:815, 1977.

48. Williamson, M.L., Koch, R., Azen, C., and Chang, C. Correlates of intelligence test results in treated phenylketonuric children. *Pediatrics* 68:161, 1981.

49. Wright, S.W. and Tarjan, G. Phenylketonuria. *Amer. J. Dis. Child.* 93:405, 1957.

LACTASE DEFICIENCY

Ruben Lisker

Department of Genetics
Instituto Nacional de la Nutrición Salvador Zubirán
Mexico City

INTRODUCTION

The carbohydrate of milk, lactose, is a disaccharide composed of glucose and galactose. In order to be absorbed, lactose must be hydrolyzed by lactase which is present in the brush border of the epithelial cells in the small intestine. Most newborns have adequate amounts of lactase to metabolize the lactose contained in human milk. However, after the weaning period, its concentration begins to decrease in the majority of humans [1], as well as in most other mammals, and in our species it reaches its lowest concentration (around 10 percent of the initial values) between the age of 6 to 16 years. This form of lactase deficiency is known as the "primary adult type", and it must be distinguished from the secondary type which may occur following injury to the small intestinal mucosa by a variety of diseases, including malnutrition [2].

The low lactase level present after the weaning period is a matter of concern because most nutritional supplementation programs are based on the administration of milk, and it is possible that such programs may be rejected by the participants because of milk intolerance.

We have been working in this area for several years with the following objectives:

1. To determine if lactase deficiency is frequent in Mexico.
2. To find out if the deficiency is an inherited phenomenon, and
3. To evaluate the relationship between the deficiency and milk drinking habits and capacity.

Supported in part by grant PCADNAL 790128 from the Consejo Nacional de Ciencia y Tecnología of México.

At this point I would like to introduce a few definitions:

Lactose malabsorption: a decrease of lactose absorption measured by an objective method.

Intolerance to lactose: presence of gastrointestinal symptomatology (diarrhea, abdominal pain, flatulence and bloating) following the ingestion of lactose.

Intolerance to milk: presence of gastrointestinal symptomatology following the ingestion of milk. It may or may not be due to lactase deficiency.

Lactase malabsorption is *not equal* to milk intolerance.

Materials and methods

Throughout this work we have employed a uniform methodology in several aspects which will be described below. Whatever variations were included in individual studies are clarified in the text.

Measurement of lactase activity

The direct measurement of lactase activity can be done in small intestinal mucosa obtained by byopsy. It is considered an accurate and precise measurement, but impractical in field studies. There are several indirect techniques to determine lactase activity and some, like the hydrogen concentration measured in expired air after a lactose load, correlate almost perfectly with the direct method [3].

We have used throughout our work the so called lactose tolerance test (LTT) for which a standard dose of 50 g of lactose is given to each individual, and capillary blood samples for glucose measurements are obtained before, and 15 and 30 minutes after the lactose load.

All our cases have been studied after an overnight fast, and a field reflectometer has been used to measure blood glucose. If the post load blood glucose increases 25 mg/dl or more above the basal level, the subject was considered to be a lactose absorber; increases smaller than 20 mg/dl indicates lactose malabsorption and if the increase is between 20 and 25 mg/dl it is considered a doubtful result and is either restested or interpreted utilizing the clinical response to the lactose load i.e., those having gastrointestinal (GI) symptomatology were classified as malabsorbers and the asymptomatic ones as absorbers. The frequency of doubtful results is less than 10%.

To validate the methodology we performed glucose assays in two samples taken at 3 minute intervals in 20 individuals: the intrapair differences were found to be minimal. In addition, in another 20 subjects the LTT was done simultaneously measuring blood glucose by the capillary method and from venous samples using an autoanalyzer. Only one individual classified as absorber by the capillary samples, was found to be malabsorber with the autoanalyzer, suggesting a rate of 5% of false negative results. Similar findings have been reported by others [4] and a good review of the different techniques employed to measure lactase activity can be found in the paper of Newcomer *et al* [3].

Milks employed

Powdered milk was used in all of our experiments. Lactose free milk contained 7.1 g of glucose per 100 ml and had an osmolality of 421 miliosmoles/L. Ordinary milk contained 5 g of lactose per 100 ml with an osmolality of 370 miliosmoles/L. They were prepared the afternoon before administration following the instructions of the manufacturers (Nestle of Mexico) and were maintained overnight at 4°C. To minimize differences in flavor both milks contained 4 g of lactose free powdered chocolate/100 ml. The milks were codified and given in a double blind manner and a bacteriological culture performed before starting the experiment and at the end of it. In no case was the milk found to be contaminated.

Questionnaire

In children studies, the questionnaire contained in addition to questions directly related to lactose intolerance, several other questions with two main objectives: a) to have an internal control of the questionnaires validity; and b) to prevent suspicion of the children as to which questions we were more interestted in, to minimize biased answers.

Assessment of clinical response to lactose ingestion

The individuals studied were interviewed between 6 Hs and 24 Hs after the ingestion of lactose to evaluate the clinical response: the presence of diarrhea alone or a cumulative rating of 4 + or more of the other symptoms was considered as severe symptomatology, while from 1 + to 3 + it was scored as mild. A score of 0 was required to consider a response asymptomatic. The other symptoms were abdominal pain, flatulence and bloating, each receiving 1 + if mild, 2 + if moderate and 3 + if severe.

Frequency of lactase deficiency

Johnson [5] has divided the world's population, in regard to their frequencies of lactose malabsorption into two main groups: the first one is composed of populations in which 60% to 100% of the people are malabsorbers and includes the following geographical areas:
a) Near East and Mediterranean: Arabs, Jews, Greek Cypriots and Southern Italians; b) Asia: Thais, Indonesians, Chinese and Koreans; c) Africa: South Nigerian peoples, Hausa and Bantu; d) North and South America:

TABLE I. Frequency of lactose-malabsorbers in several Mexican groups

| Location | Subjects studied | | | References |
	Total (No.)	Malabsorbers (No.)	(%)	
Mexico City I	105	76	72.4	6
Mexico City II	171	114	66.7	7
Mexico City III	150	97	64.7	8
Mexico City IV	200	131	65.5	9
Huamantla I	193	148	76.7	10
Huamantla II	100	74	74.0	10
Ixtenco	108	74	68.5	10
Tenango	122	94	77.0	11
S. Francisco Oxtotilpa	48	39	81.2	12
S. Juan Atzingo	52	40	76.9	12
Tenango del Valle	90	68	75.5	12
Ixmiquilpan, El Cardonal	117	90	76.9	13
Total	1,447	1,045	72.2	

$X^2_{11} = 19.60; p > 20.05$

Eskimos, Canadian and U.S. Indians and Chami Indians. We can add the Mexican population [6-13] to this list, and as can be seen in Table I twelve Mexican studies have been performed: four in Mexico City and the rest in rural areas. The proportion of deficient individuals range from 64.7% to 81.2% with an average of 72.2%. In addition we know of two studies in South America, one in Colombia [14] and the other in Peru [15], showing that both populations belong to this group.

The second group of Johnson includes the populations with only 2% to 30% of malabsorbers. The following geographical areas are considered:

a) Europe: Danes, Finns, Germans, French, Dutch, Poles, Czechs and Northern Italians; b) Africa: Hima, Tussi and nomadic Fulani; c) India: Punjab and New Dehli areas.

The fact that all groups whose origins stem from non milking areas are predominantly malabsorbers while the reverse is true for the groups where absorbers predominate, suggested a cultural historical hypothesis to explain the phenomenon [16]. During the hunting and gathering stage humans were like all other mammals in that their lactase activity would diminish after the weaning period. With the onset of dairying, a selective advantage might have been enjoyed by people with high lactase activity, specially in situations where milk was a critical nutrient. In this way, individuals with high activity would have more children than malabsorbers, and therefore they would be selected for.

Time elapsed since the begining of dairying to present day, is enough to have produced the differences now observed in the frequency of lactase deficiency assuming a 1% to 3% selective advantage [17]. The advantage could have been a general nutritional one or specific for some nutrients as suggested by Flatz and Rotthauwe in relation to calcium [18].

Genetics of lactase deficiency

It used to be argued whether lactase deficiency is an adaptive phenomenon or a genetic one. The adaptive hypothesis, championed by Bolin, David and coworkers [19], states that lactase deficiency after the weaning period is present only in populations that do not consume milk after this period, and that the enzyme activity can be induced by drinking milk. There are a few animal experiments suggesting that lactase activity can be induced in deficient rats [20], but there is no evidence in humans that such is the case.

On the other hand, there are two lines of evidence that support the genetic hypothesis. The first is the observation that human groups of the same origin but living in societies with different milk drinking habits, such as blacks living in Africa versus those in the United States, have the same frequency of lactose malabsorbers [21] although milk consumption in the U.S. is much greater than in Africa.

The second line of evidence stems from family studies. Johnson et al in 1977 [22] summarized the family studies of inheritance of lactase malabsorption reported in the literature (Table II) including our own data [11]. They found that the observed proportion of lactose absorbers in the progeny of the three possible combinations of matings of absorbers and malabsorbers agreed very well with the expected proportions, which were calculated under the hypothesis that lactose absorption is inherited as a autosomal dominant trait and under the assumption that all absorbers in these studies were heterozygotes. The latter assumption is debatable, but perhaps acceptable in view of the low frequency of the "absorber gene" in most of the populations where these studies were done. The main discrepancy from genetic theory in the above results is that among the 220 children of the malabsorber by malabsorber matings, all were expected to be malabsorbers but only 208 were. This discrepancy might be due

TABLE II. Inheritance of lactose malabsorption (modified from reference 22)

| Matings | Families (No.) | Children (No.) | No. of children | | | | X^2 | $p >$ |
| | | | Absorbers | | Malabsorbers | | | |
			Obs	Exp	Obs	Exp		
Absorbers × absorbers	10	31	23	23.25	8	7.75	0.01	0.90
Absorbers × malabsrorbers	60	196	95	98.0	101	98.0	0.18	0.50
Malabsorbers × malabsrorbers	76	220	12	0.0	208	220.0	——	——
Total	146	447	130	121.25	317	325.75	0.86	0.30

to several reasons, including misclassification of some individuals and we have already mentioned that in our experience a 5% of false negative results are obtained with the LTT.

Milk drinking habits and capacity

Regarding milk drinking habits we have studied [7] the presence of lactase deficiency by the LTT in 94 adults who ingested daily 750 ml or more of milk versus 67 individuals who drank no milk at all because of gastrointestinal intolerance. 44% of the milk drinkers were malabsorbers as compared to 88% of the non drinkers, the difference being highly significant ($X_1^2 = 34.2$; $p < 0.0005$. In a similar study we investigated 182 girls from a foster home. They are normaly offered 500 ml of milk daily, half in the morning and half in the evening and although they are supposed to drink it all, in fact some drink less and some more than the 500 ml. We were able to divide them in three groups: a) 21 drank more than 500 ml, b) 114 drank their 500 ml; and c) 47 who ingested less than that amount. The proportion of malabsorbers in these groups was, contrary to our expectations, 80.9%, 65.8% and 55.3%, respectively. Although these differences were not significant ($X_2^2 = 4.3$; $p > 0.10$) the trend observed is contrary to the hypothesis that malabsorbers drink less milk than absorbers. The literature in this regard is conflicting: Paige, Bayless, and Graham [23] found that black children reject milk twice as frequently as whites, and that the frequency of malabsorbers is higher in those who reject milk that in those who drink it. However in white children there was no difference in the prevalence of malabsorbers amongst milk drinkers and non drinkers.

As our information regarding milk drinking habits in our initial study was obtained through a very simple questionnaire and we did not take into account its validity, we decided to use another approach in an investigation aimed specifically to evaluate experimental milk drinking capacity in relation to absorber status [9]. It was performed in 200 healthy adults who were given, in 4 consecutive days, 250 ml, 500 ml, 750 ml and 1000 ml of milk. If untoward G.I. symptoms appeared in any amount, the following day instead of increasing it, the subject was given the same amount which produced symptoms but in two doses rather than one, separated by an 8 hour interval, ending this part of the experiment at this point. Five days after the last milk dose, and LTT was performed to evaluate lactose absorption and the milk drinking habits were determined.

93% of the absorbers tolerated well 1000 ml of milk against only 25.2% of the malabsorbers. In addition, 5.3% of the latter had severe GI symptomatology and 9.2% a mild on with the ingestion of 250 ml of milk while all the absorbers tolerated this amount well. Ninety percent of the individuals who received in two doses the same amount of milk that produced symptoms the previous day, tolerated it well.

The correlation between milk drinking capacity and milk drinking habits was poor. Of the 97 individuals that were able to drink 1 liter of milk, 8 drank no milk, 11 one glass per day, 33 two glasses, 17 three and 28 four or more. Of the seven malabsorbers who manifested GI symptomatology with 250 ml of milk, one regularly drank three glasses per day. One important point of these results is that they strongly suggest that absorbers can indeed ingest more milk than malabsorbers, which is a critical fact in order to sustain the possible selective advantage of absorbers in situations where milk was of critical importance in the diet, as suggested by the cultural-historical hypothesis.

Much confusion exists in the literature regarding the clinical effect of 250 ml of milk or its equivalent of lactose in malabsorbers, the range of symptomatic individuals varying from 0% to 75% in different reports [24]. We decided to perform several double blind studies to obtain information in this regard and to simultaneously study the tolerance to lactose free milk. The first one [8] was performed in 150 adults of high socioeconomic status. Each subject received in three separate days, 250 ml of one of three different milks, one was lactose free, another was regular milk, and the third was lactose enriched milk so that 250 ml had the lactose usually present in 750 ml of regular milk. Subjects were interviewed 6 hours later to determine their clinical response with the criteria previously stated. One week later an LTT was performed. The results showed that lactose free milk produced no severe G.I. symptoms in the 53 absorbers and the 97 malabsorbers, while regular milk produced symptomatology in two of the absorbers and in 36 of the malabsorbers, the difference being highly significant ($X^2 = 19.9$; $p < 0.0001$). The better tolerance to lactose free milk agrees with other studies [25, 26] and is an alternative to consider in supplementation programs of populations where the prevalence of lactose intolerance is high. On the other hand in this double blind study 36% of the malabsorbers had symptoms with 250 ml of regular milk, while in a previous one we had found 14.5% of clinical responders to this dose. The latter figure is similar to the 12% found by Newcomer, in a double blind study [27] but in contrast, in three different double blind studies from Scrimshaw's group [28-30], the proportion of symptomatic individuals was of 0%. The reasons for these differences are difficult to understand.

Our next study was performed in rural children [31] who are most in need of nutritional supplementation. The study was conducted in escentially the same way as that of the adults, and the participants were 240 children of very low socio-economic status between 5 and 14 years old. Again lactose free milk was significantly better tolerated than regular milk ($X^2 = 14.47$; $p < 0.0001$), but surprisingly only 49.6% of the children were asymptomatic to lactose free milk, the rest manifesting mild or severe symptomatology. This led us to investigate another group of children in the same age group and ethnicity than the former, but enjoying good nutrition and sanitary conditions. In this study we added a control period after giving the milk, which consisted in solving the same questionnaire used after giving the milk, but no milk was given on the previous day. The results showed statistical differences in the clinical response to lactose free milk as compared to regular milk ($X^2 = 16.4$; $p < 0.0001$) and the proportion of asymptomatic individuals with the former was of 83.2% intermediate between adults of high socioeconomic status (100%) and poor rural children (49.6%). A very interesting finding was that during the control period, there were 78.3% asymptomatic individuals, a figure very similar to that after lactose free milk ingestion. These results suggest that: 1) lactose free milk does not increase the background of GI symptomatology present in children; and 2) that the differences observed in the response to milk ingestion in rural and other children and adults, might be due in part to the different health status of these groups.

With the above in mind, we performed another three double blind studies which included control periods, in three different schools. The results of the first school have been published [32] and what follows is the summary of the results obtained in the two latest ones, which have not been reported so far, and which are quite similar to the others.

We studied 92 children from a grammar school in Puerto Morelos, State of Quintana Roo in South East Mexico, and 102 children from a grammar school in Mexico City. Both belonged to a low socioeconomic status, and their ages ranged between 8 and 13 years. Boys and girls were included in both schools and as the results showed no statistical differences between the schools; they will be presented together.

The experiment consisted in giving each child 250 ml of lactose free milk and 250 of regular milk on two different days of the same week. 24 hours after each milk ingestion, the children were interviewed to evaluate the clinical response to the milk. In addition, each child had a control period which consisted in solving the same questionnaire but without receiving milk the previous day. Before the field work, the sequence of milk and control periods were assigned by random numbers.

Table III shows that there was a significant difference in the response to both types of milks, and that roughly half of the group manifested GI symp-

TABLE III. Clinical response to lactose free milk, regular milk and the control period in 194 school children of low socioeconomic status

	Milk					
Clinical response	Lactose Free (No.)	%	Regular		Control	
			No.	%	No.	%
Asymptomatic	120	61.9	92	47.4	96	49.5
Mild symptoms	61	31.4	72	37.1	78	40.2
Severe symptoms	13	6.7	30	15.5	20	10.3
Total	194	100.0	194	100.0	194	100.0

$X_2^2 = 11.32; p < 0.01$. It compares clinical response of lactose free vs regular milk.

toms of intolerance during the control period. Thus it would seem that lactose free milk does not increase this background symptomatology, and confirms previous findings [31, 32]. Tables IV and V show the clinical response to both types of milk, dividing the group in individuals that had an asymptomatic control period (Table IV) and those that had symptoms during the control period (Table V). It is clear types of that the proportion of asymptomatic individuals with both milk is higher when the control period was also asymptomatic than in the other situation, the differences being highly significant for both milks. We believe this means that the GI symptoms present in this groups are due in some individuals, around 14.5% (substracting the proportion of asymptomatic individuals with regular milk to that found with lactose free milk), to the ingestion of 250 ml of regular milk, and the rest are probably due to a host of other conditions unrelated to milk intolerance.

To validate the questionnaire employed, we could show that the frequency of symptoms unrelated to milk intolerance in relation to the ingestion of both types of milk and the control period were not significant in the case of cough,

TABLE IV. Clinical response in children who were asymptomatic during the control period

| Clinical response | Milk | | | |
	Lactose Free (No.)	%	Regular No.	%
Asymptomatic	71	73.9	59	61.5
Mild symptoms	21	21.9	24	25.0
Severe symptoms	4	4.2	13	13.5
Total	96	100.0	96	100.0

$X_2^2 = 6.07; p < 0.05.$

TABLE V. Clinical response in children who were symptomatic during the control period

| Clinical response | Milk | | | |
	Lactose Free (No.)	%	Regular No.	%
Asymptomatic	48	49.0	35	35.7
Mild symptoms	40	40.8	46	46.9
Severe symptoms	10	10.2	17	17.4
Total	98	100.0	98	100.0

$X_2^2 = 4.26; p > 0.1.$

palpitations, headache and vomiting, and marginally significant in the case of arthralgia. The lack of significance of most variables unrelated to milk intolerance suggests that the questionnaire is trustworthy. The finding, that there is no significant difference in the clinical response to lactose free milk, regular milk and the control period in relation to their sequence of administration, can be interpreted similarly.

Currently we believe that lactose free milk is better tolerated than regular milk in populations such as ours with a prevalence of lactase deficiency, and that around 15% of individuals drinking 250 ml of regular milk will show variable degrees of GI symptomatology. Whether this symptomatology means that lactose is not being absorbed in these individuals or that the nutritional value of regular milk in them is impaired, should not be infered from our results, and constitutes an area where more work should be done. Some preliminary data [33] suggest that low dose milk supplements are well utilized by lactose-malabsorbing children.

ACKNOWLEDGEMENTS

The field work of the last two schools investigated was done by Alicia Ríos, Magali Daltabuit, Edna Aizpuru, Jesús de Rubens and María del Carmen Rodríguez. Alicia Ríos used the material for a thesis to obtain her diploma of Physical Anthropologists. Nestle de Mexico kindly supplied us with lactose free and regular milk.

REFERENCES

1. McCracken, R.: Lactase deficiency: an example of dietary evolution. *Curr. Anthropol.* 12:479-517, 1971.
2. Lisfshitz, F.: Acquired carbohydrate intolerance in children. *In* "Lactose Digestion. Clinical and Nutritional Implications" (D. Paige and Th. Bayless, eds.), pp 182-193. J. Hopkins University Press, Baltimore, 1981.
3. Newcomer, A., McGill, D., Thomas, P. and Hofman, A.: Prospective comparison of indirect methods for detecting lactase deficiency. *New Eng. J. Med.* 293:1232-1236, 1975.
4. Gilat, T., Kuhn, R., Gelman, E. and Mizrahy, O.: Lactase deficiency in Jewish communities in Israel. *Am. J. Dig. Dis.* 15:895-904, 1970.
5. Johnson, J.: The regional and ethnic distribution of lactose malabsorption. *In* "Lactose Digestion. Clinical and Nutritional Implications" (D. Paige and Th. Bayless, eds.), pp 11-22. J. Hopkins University Press, Baltimore, 1981.
6. Lisker, R., López-Habib, G., Mora, M.A. and Pitol, A.: Correlation in the diagnosis of intestinal lactase deficiency between the radiological method and the lactose tolerance test. *Rev. Invest. Clín.* (Méx.) 27:1-5, 1975.
7. Lisker, R. and Meza-Calix, A.: Intestinal lactase deficiency and milk drinking habits. *Rev. Invest. Clín.* (Méx.) 28:109-112, 1976.
8. Lisker, R. and Aguilar, L.: Double blind study of milk lactose intolerance. *Gastroenterology* 74:1283-1285, 1978.
9. Lisker, R. Aguilar L. and Zavala, C.: Intestinal lactase deficiency and milk drinking capacity in the adult. *Am. J. Clin. Nutr.* 31:1499-1503, 1978.
10. Lisker, R., López-Habib, G., Daltabuit, M., Rostenberg, I. and Arroyo, P.: Lactase deficiency in a rural area of Mexico. *Am. J. Clin. Nutr.* 27:756-759, 1974.

11. Lisker, R., González, B. and Daltabuit, M.: Recessive inheritance of the adult type of intestinal lactase deficiency. *Am. J. Hum. Genet.* 27:662-664, 1975.
12. Serrano, C., Daltabuit, M. and González, B.: Algunos aspectos genéticos de la Población Matlatzinca del Estado de México. *In* Teotenango: El Antiguo Lugar de la Muralla (R. Piña-Chan, ed.), pp 476-483, Dirección de Turismo, Estado de México, 1975.
13. Daltabuit, M. and Sáenz, M.E.: Hábitos de consumo de leche y deficiencia de lactasa intestinal en el Valle del Mezquital. *An. Antropología* (Mex.) 15:267-292, 1978.
14. Alzate, H. Ramírez, E. and Echeverri, M.: Intolerancia a la lactosa en un grupo de estudiantes de medicina. *Antioquía Med.* 18:237-246, 1968.
15. Figueroa, R., Melgar, E., Jó, N. and García, O.: Intestinal lactase deficiency in an apparently normal Peruvian population. *Dig. Dis.* 16:881-889, 1971.
16. Simoons, F.: The geographic hypothesis and lactose malabsorption. A weighing of the evidence. *Dig. Dis.* 23:963-980, 1978.
17. Cavalli-Sforza, L.: Analytic review: Some current problems of human population genetics. *Am. J. Hum. Genet.* 25:82-104, 1973.
18. Flatz, G. and Rotthauwe, H.: Lactose nutrition and natural selection. *Lancet* 2:76-77, 1973.
19. Bolin, T. and Davis, A.: Primary lactase deficiency: Genetic or acquired? *Am. J. Dig. Dis.* 15:679-692, 1970.
20. Bolin, T., Mckern, A. and Davis, A.: The effect of diet on lactase activity in the rat. *Gastroenterology* 60:432-437, 1971.
21. Stephenson, L., Latham, M. and Jones, O.: Milk consumption by black and by white pupils in two primary schools. *J. Am. Diet. Ass.* 71:258-262, 1977.
22. Johnson, J., Simoons, F., Hurwitz, R., Grange, A., Mitchell, Ch., Sinatra, F., Sunshine, P., Robertson, W., Bennett, P. and Kretchmer, N.: Lactose malabsorption among the Pima Indians of Arizona. *Gastroenterology* 73:1299-1304, 1977.
23. Paige, D., Bayless, Th. and Graham, G.: Milk programs: Helpful or harmful to Negro children? *Am. J. Publ. Health.* 62:1486-1489, 1972.
24. Torún, B., Solomons, N. and Viteri, F.: Lactose malabsorption and lactose intolerance: Implications for general milk consumption. *Arch. Latino Nutr.* 29:445-494, 1979.
25. Paige, D., Bayless, Th., Huang, S. and Wexler, R.: Lactose hydrolyzed milk. *Am. J. Clin. Nutr.* 28:818-822, 1975.
26. Turner, S., Daily, T., Hourigan, J., Rand, A. and Thayor, W.: Utilization of low lactose milk. *Am. J. Clin. Nutr.* 29:739-744, 1976.
27. Newcomer, A., McGill, D., Thomas, P. and Hoffman, A.: Tolerance to lactose among lactase-deficient American Indians. *Gastroenterology,* 74:44-46, 1978.
28. Garza, C. and Scrimshaw, N.: Relationship of lactose intolerance to milk intolerance in young children. *Am. J. Clin. Nutr.* 29:192-196, 1976.
29. Haverberb, L., Kwon, P. and Scrimshaw, N.: Comparative tolerance of adolescents of differing ethnic bacground to lactose-containing and lactose-free milk. I. Initial experience with a double-blind procedure. *Am. J. Clin. Nutr.* 33:17-21, 1980.
30. Rorick, M. and Scrimshaw, N.: Comparative tolerance of elderly from different ethnic backgrounds to lactose-containing and lactose-free dairy drinks: a double blind study. *J. Gerontol.* 34:191-200, 1979.
31. Lisker, R., Aguilar, L., Lares, I. and Cravioto, J.: Double blind study of milk lactose intolerance in a group of rural and urban children. *Am. J. Clin. Nutr.* 33:1049-1053. 1980.
32. Lisker, R. and Moreno-Terrazas, O.: Estudio doble ciego sobre la tolerancia a la lactosa de la leche en un grupo de niños rurales. *Rev. Invest. Clin.* (Méx.) 32:363-368, 1980.
33. Brown, K., Khatun, M., Parry, L. and Ahmed, G.: Nutritional consequences of low dose milk supplements consumed by lactose-malabsorbing children. *Am. J. Clin. Nutr.* 33:1054-1063, 1980.

DISCUSSION[1]

Torún emphasized the non-physiological nature of the 2 g/kg body weight lactose load used for diagnosis of lactose malabsorption. In a recent review[1][(Torún, B., Solomons, N.W. and Viteri, F. *Arch. Latinoamer. Nutr.* 29:445-494, 1979)] he and his colleagues pointed out that the epidemiological conception of lactose malabsorption should be reassessed by using a more physiological, smaller dose of lactose, not exceding 18 g, administered as part of a meal. In any case, milk is not the ideal type in food distribution programs to adults, except for pregnant or lactating women and then mostly as a good source of calcium. As for children, care should be taken so that spurious diagnoses of lactose malabsorption are not considered as a contraindication for using milk as a food supplement. Lisker emphasized his view that 14.5% of the children in his study showed lactose intolerance as judged from the appearance of clinical signs after drinking a normal amount of milk. For him the concept of lactose malabsorption rests on the results of an objective test such as breath hydrogen excretion or the lactose tolerance, as carried out in his investigation.

[1]*Summary of the discussion prepared by S. Frenk.*

DETERMINANTS OF INDIVIDUAL AND POPULATION BLOOD LIPOPROTEIN LEVELS

Henry Blackburn

Laboratory of Physiological Hygiene
School of Public Health
University of Minnesota
Minneapolis, Minnesota

INTRODUCTION

One of the greatest needs for understanding of the blood lipoprotein levels in humans, their responses to habitual diet and their relationships to atherosclerosis, is a model which accounts at the same time for large differences in distributions between populations and for a wide range of individual variation. Here an attempt is made to describe these correlations in individuals and between populations and to reconcile the departures from prediction of diet, blood lipoprotein levels, and coronary heart disease rates (CHD). The concept is developed that environmental factors most determine the averages and the positions of the population distributions of blood lipoproteins and their associated disease rates-under the condition where susceptibility is widespread and similar. On the other hand, genetic or intrinsic factors most determine individual lipoprotein levels and the associated risk, as well as the range of individual variations in a population, under the condition where the cultural influence is powerful and ubiquitous (that is mainly the diet).

The shape of the relationship between individual CHD risk and blood lipoprotein levels as represented by total cholesterol (TC) is re-examined here with the conclusion that no model fits the data better than any other and most fit relatively well. The author comes down on the side of a continuous relationship of CHD risk to TC level and opines that "the principle of biological continuity"is a better *a priori* assumption than a discontinuous relationship or a "threshold effect".

Individual CHD risk attributable to TC level involves the bulk of the TC distribution in high incidence cultures. Thus, whatever the model adopted for the diet-lipid-CHD relationship, the population-wide approach to prevention, now occurring spontaneously and abetted by health advice, is probably necessary for the continued reduction of disease. And whatever educational or other preventive strategy is used, change in the health behavior of many if not most people of affluent cultures will be needed to reduce further the frequency of coronary events and deaths.

One of the greatest needs for understanding of the blood lipoprotein levels and their responses to habitual diet and relationships to atherosclerosis, is a model which accounts at the same time for large differences in distributions between populations and for a wide range of individual variations. Construction of such a model in detail is not yet feasible. New protein subfractions of the lipoproteins are being discovered at frequent intervals and the individual variations possible are not even estimable. Moreover, distributions of even the major lipoprotein fractions have rarely been collected systematically. This is now needed from defined populations which differ in culture. Until such data are available we may nevertheless learn much from a fresh look at the excellent older data on nutrition and blood lipoprotein levels as approximated by measures of total serum or plasma cholesterol (TC). I would like to solicit criticism of some ideas and models based on TC data in populations and on predictions of TC response to diet from the long series of metabolic ward studies carried out in the past in this and others' laboratories. I invite informed speculation on what magnitude population differences *could* be attributable to unequal distributions of the polygenic factors which most affect blood lipoprotein responses to diet and culture. I will focus on current questions about, and apparent inconsistencies in, the generally well-established triangular relationship between diet, TC and coronary heart disease (CHD). That fundamental relationship will be reviewed first, after which I will treat the instances which appear to depart from established predictions. I will also consider the detailed shapes of the diet-TC-CHD relationship and alternative causes and mechanisms for the correlations and departures from them. I will attempt to model diet-genetic interactions as they determine differences in the lipoprotein levels of individuals and of populations. Finally, I will discuss the implications of these findings for a population-wide versus an individual approach to disease prevention.

Genetic Dyslipoproteinemias and Diet

With respect to the more or less classifiable, genetic dyslipoproteinemias, diet influences their expression and their severity in ways just beginning to be elaborated.

In the very rare form, old Frederickson-Lee's Type I chylomicronemia, a lipoprotein lipase deficiency, the affluent eating pattern influences the levels of chylomicrons in the circulation and they can be substantially reduced by decreasing the total fat content of diet and the addition of small doses of heparin.

In another rare form, old Type III, associated with high levels of intermediate density lipoprotein (IDL), a low fat diet may influence the levels favorably but the picture is often complicated by glucose intolerance.

The more common disorders formerly classified as Type IIa and b and Type IV all are unfavorably affected by an eating pattern characterized by relatively high fat, high sugar, and high alcohol intake. The Type IIa familial endogenous hypercholesterolemia is variably influenced by a "one diet" strategy consisting of lower saturated fat, lower dietary cholesterol and weight reduction.

Type IIb familial combined hyperlipidemia in which LDL an VLDL are both elevated is affected by the same diet, both positively and negatively, and often requires specific attention to sugar and alcohol intake for its readjustment.

Type IV, the more common endogenous hypertriglyceridemia, responds in the same way to a diet abundant in fat and calories. Here again a one-diet strategy can be extremely effective in changing the levels, but special attention is required to sugar, alcohol and body weight.

Old Type V is a rare form in which I and IV are combined with elevated chylomicrons and VLDL, associated with low HDL and with atherosclerosis. The diet which most favorably affects this rare type is a low fat, weight loss diet to which heparin is added in treatment.

Genetics is clearly the more crucial issue in these entities compared to the nutritional components. However, this is a rapidly developing field and the genetic mechanisms and the genetic-nutrition interactions are increasingly understood. The frequency of cell receptors to apoprotein B and E seems to be a primary determinant of the ability of plasma to clear LDL and they regulate both cell permeability and synthesis of LDL. Genetic defects in the frequency of these receptors results in elevation of LDL, or combined dyslipoproteinemias, which, in turn, are exaggerated by the common affluent diet, high in dietary cholesterol and saturated fat and calories.

Now let us turn to the larger issue of genetic-diet interactions in the general population.

Epidemiological Evidence

The epidemiological evidence about diet, blood lipid levels and atherosclerosis involves population comparisons as well as information on individual risk within populations. It includes their changes over time. The Seven Countries Study provides contrasts of dietary composition and energy expenditure among men of stable rural, farming, logging and fishing populations having similar socioeconomic status [10]. Data were collected with careful attention to adequate sample size, standardized measurements, training and quality control, central standard chemical analyses of blood lipids and of foods eaten, and central data analysis. Chemical analysis of the diet was performed on lyophilized specimens shipped from the field, prepared from locally

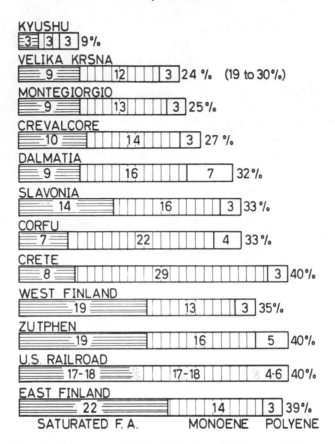

Figure 1 Average percent daily calories from fats in men 40-59 years old.

purchased food, in precise quantities as recorded by trained dieticians living in randomly selected households of each geographic area. Diets were measured seasonally in families during one week. Figure 1 shows the large contrast between populations in the fatty acid composition of diet. The variation is great for the proportion of daily calories as saturated and monounsaturated fat. Dietary cholesterol was not measured. These "natural experiments" include extremely low total fat in Japan, and relatively high fat in Greece but of a very different composition than in Northern Europe. In Figure 2a and b are the population (ecologic) correlations of diet with levels of total serum cholesterol (TC), and with CHD, as studied across a wide range of saturated fat calories (3 to 22%).

Figure 3 shows the correlation between median TC values for the population and the 10-year coronary disease rates. Eastern Finland deviates on the high side of the prediction with the highest average TC level of all the Seven Countries areas. In contrast, West Finland and the Greek Island of Crete are on the low side of expectation for 16 areas [11].

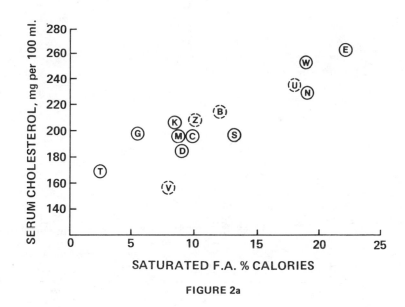

FIGURE 2a

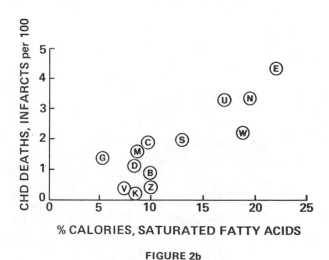

FIGURE 2b

Figure 2a and 2b B = Belgrade Faculty, C = Crevalcore,
D = Dalmatia, E = East Finland,
G = Corfu, K = Crete, N = Zutphen,
M = Montegiorgio, S = Slavonia,
U = U.S. Railroad, V = Velika Krsna,
W = West Finland, Z = Zrenjanin.

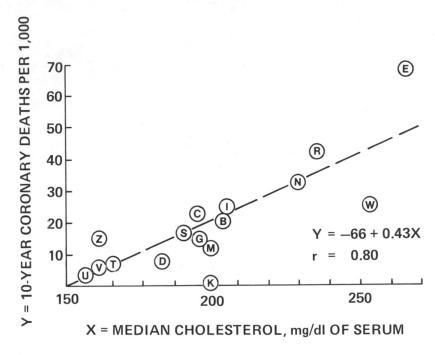

Figure 3 Median total cholesterol level is related to CHD incidence in men aged 40 to 59 followed 10 years.

TABLE I: *Seven countries study: total serum cholesterol and 10-year CHD incidence and deaths in men 40-59*

Population	% Sat. fat	5	50	95	CHD deaths	Any CHD	All deaths
E. Finland	22	182	265	356	681	2868	1511
W. Finland	19	184	253	338	251	1582	1270
U.S. Railway	18	173	236	318	146	—	861
Netherlands	19	169	230	317	317	1066	1134
Crete	8	151	206	279	0	210	627
S. Italy	9	150	198	274	125	966	1007
Corfu	7	141	198	283	149	686	847
W. Yugoslavia	9	128	186	259	74	629	775
Japan (T)	3	106	171	304	71	354	1052
Serbia	9	115	156	217	71	452	1136
Japan (U)	3	96	141	194	50	458	1349

Table I provides the detailed distribution of TC, ranked by descending order of median TC value, along with 10-year coronary disease and total death rates for Seven Countries populations [11]. Here a generally unfavorable experience of northern European countries and the United States is contrasted to the better experience in the Mediterranean Basin and Japan. Again, there is the remarkable absence of clinical atherosclerotic manifestations on the island Crete where the 10-year rate of dying from any cause, among men initially ages 40-59 is only half that of other areas. All except one of the very low CHD incidence areas, Crete (having CHD deaths from 0.5 to 1.5 per thousand per year) have median TC values under 200 mg/dl. All high incidence areas (having 3-7 cases per 1000 men per year) have TC medians greater than 235 mg/dl. Areas in the intermediate range of the mean population TC levels show wide variation in CHD rates. All diet analysis are chemical measurements of the major nutrients. However, there are differences between Northern Europe, the United States and the other populations in the actual foodstuffs consumed, including simple sugars, complex carbohydrates, dietary fiber, vegetable protein and alcohol.

Population (Ecologic) Correlations

Relevant diet-lipid-CHD correlations in the Seven Countries data between 14-16 geographic areas are as follows: Population TC level is strongly related to population CHD deaths and nonfatal infarction, with an r value of 0.76 while percent calories from total fats is less strong, r = 0.40; percent calories as saturated fats has the strongest correlation with disease rates, r = 0.84; for percent calories as protein, not illustrated, r = 0.14. Total calories consumed per kg body weight is not correlated with serum cholesterol, r = -0.07, and physical activity calories/kg burned daily is highly negatively correlated with skinfold obesity, r = -0.75. Thus, with a few individual population departures from prediction, to be discussed in detail later, the Seven Countries evidence is clear and consistent. The strength of these relationships between populations (ecological correlations) and the "dose-effect" of diet and TC on CHD, support the inference of causality.

The U.S.P.H.S. International Study of the relationship of diet, serum lipid levels, and coronary disease rates has made comparisons similar to Seven Countries [8]. The Framingham Heart Study, the Honolulu Heart Program and the Puerto Rico Heart Health program were compared using standardized laboratory and clinical assessments. These populations differ widely in socioeconomic status and otherwise. Framingham rates of CHD are somewhat higher than expectation based on blood lipids or combined baseline risk characteristics for all areas. The comparative data are compatible with a contribution of habitual diet to average population blood lipid levels and to CHD rates; they suggest the absence of a direct effect of serum triglycerides on CHD incidence.

The Ni-Hon-San Study provides comparisons based on acculturation of Japanese migrants from the mainland to Hawaii and California [14]. This study is the major source of epidemiological evidence in which there is a semblance of control for genetic factors; standard genetic markers are similar among the 3 groups. Table II summarizes these findings. The acculturation in diet was reported least in elderly mainland Japanese and most in the California Japanese. The migrant populations are seen to take in fewer calories per Kg, presumably because they are less active, but to consume substantially more protein, animal protein, fat, saturated fat, dietary cholesterol and simple carbohydrates while they drink less alcohol than the mainland Japanese. Mean values for TC go up according to the degree of eastward migration and Western acculturation, as does the frequency of elevated TC and mean levels of triglycerides. There are surely many other aspects of acculturation than diet and physical activity in these populations. Nevertheless, the data on diet, lipids and CHD incidence are compatible with a strong dietary and acculturation effect on populations having similar genetic composition.

We interpret these findings to indicate a wide susceptibility to hyperlipidemia in human populations, presumably as a mass response to habitual differences in diet. Apparently the exhibition of a maximal number of "supermarket" phenotypes among susceptible genotypes is encouraged, as well as a shift upward in population distributions, by mass exposure to high saturated fat diets and calorie abundance.

Hunter-Gatherers and Vegetarians

Other types of human populations are of interest in testing the diet-TC-heart disease relationship. Truswell has divided humans into four nutritional groups: the hunter-gatherer, the peasant-farmer-pastoralist, the urban ghetto

TABLE II: Japanese migrant studies: risk factor differences

Variable	Japan	Hawaii	California
Relative weight (%)	109	122	126
Calorie intake/kg.	40	37	35
Sat. fat % cal.	7	23	26
CHO % cal.	63	46	44
Alcohol % cal.	9	4	3
T.S. cholesterol (mg/dl)	181	218	228
TSC 260 (%)	3	12	16
S. triglycerdies (mg/dl)	134	240	234
CHD deaths/1000	1.3	2.2	3.7

dweller, an affluent man. In the Seven Countries, The Minnesota Laboratory of Physiological Hygiene has studied the rural farmer and affluent man "Primitive" populations may provide other important evidence of the relationship between diet and serum lipid levels, but observations about their atherosclerosis and disease rates are mainly anecdotal. For example, the general experience among pathological observations in primitive populations is that they appear to have the same distribution of fatty steaks in younger years, along with moderate amounts of aortic atherosclerosis as adults, but very little coronary atherosclerosis at any age. There is extensive evidence that diets of hunter-gatherers in Africa, South America and Australia are extremely low in animal fat (because of the composition of wild game), very high in plant protein, complex carbohydrates and fiber, and low in simple sugars and salt. Such diets are consistently associated with very low values of TC, from means of less than 100 to 140 mg/dl and with seasonal differences related to the abundance of calories and weight change (Table 3). Data on urban construction workers in Ethiopia indicate how TC levels may be very low in otherwise healthy, active people (average TC levels of 104 mg%).

The relevance of anthropological and rural epidemiological studies to the predicament of modern, urban affluent humans may, of course, be questioned. However, modern man is very likely a "hunter-gatherer" still, at least in respect to his evolutionary metabolic adaptations [2]. The 100,000 or more generations prior to agriculture and civilization were certainly more influential in physical evolution than the mere 500 generations since. The food available and the physical activity patterns required to obtain it during major phases of evolution were probably central to the physiological adaptations for survival. Thus, while it may be infeasible to return to subsistence economies, insights may be gained into the "modern maladaptations" of hyperlipidemia, hypertension, hyperinsulinemia, obesity, diabetes, hypercoagulability, and hyperuricemia by study of extant hunter-gatherers. The evidence suggests that, compared to affluent man, they are lean and active, with a more varied diet than early agricultural groups, have low blood pressure and blood lipids and little apparent atherosclerosis. They may have the same capacity for longevity as modern affluent humans.

How about vegetarianism in "high incident" cultures? Studies among Seventh Day Adventists in the United States and New Zealand provide evidence that blood lipid levels and CHD incidence vary according to diet habits of non-vegetarians, lacto-ovo-vegetarians, and pure vegetarians. Compared to age-matched Californians, non-vegetarian SDA men, aged 35 and over, have CHD mortality rates 44% lower than the general population, the lacto-ovo group 57% lower, and the pure vegetarian group 77% lower. Though these people have many differences in lifestyle other than eating habits, the other factors appear to account for little of the variation in mortality [22].

In addition to the importance of TC levels, do the lipoprotein fractions contribute to population differences? Epidemiological data suggest strongly that average population TC values generally reflect LDL or beta-lipoprotein and correlate more strongly with diet and CHD findings than does HDL or alphalipoprotein level [2]. Table III attempts to summarize interesting discrepancies between total and HDL cholesterol levels in populations. Generally, HDL values are higher in affluent Western cultures where LDL and TC are also higher. Usually, also, the HDL/TC ratio is lower. One fascinating "natural experiment" departs substantially from this rule as Connor reports here [4]. Tarahumara Indians, who have among the lowest TC and LDL values yet measured in adults and youth, also have among the lowest HDL values reported and low HDL/TC ratios. The Tarahumara are almost entirely vegetarian and are among the more active ethnic groups on earth. Also, they are lean and consume considerable amounts of alcohol as fermented corn beer. They do not smoke heavily, All these characteristics would be associated, in western affluent societies, with *higher* values of HDL and lower HDL/TC ratios than those found in these Indians. So, the issue of "protective" levels of lipoproteins and their ratios is not yet clear from ecologic correlations. The data suggest that, generally, LDL and TC follow the population diet an CHD rates much more closely than HDL. They may also be more responsive to change than is HDL and new data about the effect on HDL cholesterol of experimental change in dietary composition are confirmatory. VLDL is assumed to have

TABLE III: *Population comparisons of serum cholesterol fractions (mg/dl)*

	TC	LDL	VLDL	HDL
Norway	250	—	—	51
Minnesota	239	—	—	41
Tromso	229	—	—	39
USSR - LRC	219	—	—	53
Belgium	213	—	—	42
US - LRC	206	—	—	45
Maoris	188	122	15	51
New Zealand	176	115	12	49
South Korea	168	—	—	46
Iowa youth	163	103	8	50
Japan	—	120	—	40
South Africa	154	—	—	70
Bogalusa youth	139	—	—	50
U.S. vegetarians	126	73	12	43
Tarahumara adults	134	87	22	25
Tarahumara youth	118	75	20	23
Ethiopian workers	104	48	16	32
Honolulu Japanese	—	183	—	40
Los Angeles Japanese	—	213	—	35

mainly an intermediate role. These cross-cultural differences contribute to a public health view which focuses on population TC levels (LDL) as the main pathogen and predictor of mass hyperlipidemia and atherosclerosis. This view does not mitigate the important individual correlations and clinical predictive value of HDL, but this is primarily for older *individuals* living in high CHD incident cultures.

The baseline TC distributions in the Seven Countries cohorts of Table I also contribute to models for "existing, feasible and ideal" population TC distributions (Figure 4a and b). These curves are thought to be reasonable because the population data are congruent with clinical and laboratory evidence and other independent estimates. "Ideal" TC distributions center around 160 mg/dl as for Velika Krsna, Ushibuka and Tanushimaru and are associated

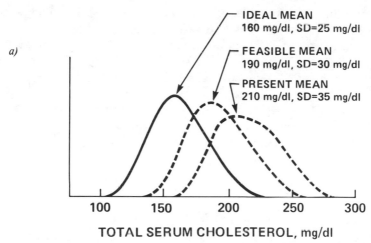

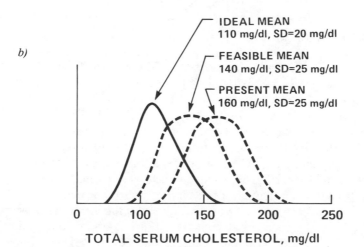

Figure 4

with the lowest CHD rates. "Desirable-feasible" TC curves center around 190 mg/dl as in the Greek Island and Adriatic coast of Italy and Yugoslavia. These levels are associated with wide variation in CHD rates which are generally less than half of U.S. and Northern European rates. "Existing" TC curves of adults in the U.S. now center around 215 mg/dl and represent recently measured population samples. It will be recalled that U.S. samples in the 50's and 60's gave TC means around 235 mg/dl and in Finland and other Northern European countries means were, and still are, around 265 mg/dl for middle-aged adults [2].

Experimental Evidence (Individual Correlations)

Experimental diets provide other major evidence concerning the relationship between diet and blood cholesterol and lipid fractions. They show mathematically predictable relationships between *dietary change* and *group change* in TC levels. They provide classic examples of defining a relationship by a predictive equation, tested for validity in populations different from those in which developed. The derivations are nearly identical among independent investigators in four separate laboratories, resulting in equations widely known in "lipid circles" as the Keys, Hegsted, Mattson, and Connor equations relating dietary lipids to blood lipids, illustrated here by the Keys equation:

$$\text{CHOL.} = 1.35\ (2\ S - P) + 1.52\ Z$$

Where CHOL. = estimated change in serum cholesterol in mg/dl; S = change in percent daily calories from saturated fat; P = change in percent daily calories from polyunsaturated fat; P = change in percent daily calories from polyunsaturated fat; z = change in the square root of daily dietary cholesterol in mg/1000 kcal.

Work is needed to establish prediction equations involving not only other components of diet than fatty acids and cholesterol, but diet effects on lipoprotein fractions. Whether the older equations will be greatly improved thereupon depends on the incompletely known HDL response to diet, the proportion of LDL and TC changes obtainable by dietary manipulation, and the likelihood of significant effects of other diet factors occurring in the range of usual affluent diets. It is likely that the contribution to TC change of vegetable protein, fiber and complex carbohydrates would give relatively small coefficients of partial correlation *in the presence of* the major contributions of dietary fatty acids and cholesterol. The individual and population importance of other dietary components may however be quite substantial, as suggested by Barry Lewis [12]. Dietary fat composition fails to explain all the variation in population levels of TC or CHD. It is not clear whether unexplained population TC-CHD discrepancies might have to do with the early age of onset of a given diet pattern and the duration of that pattern, or might relate to the usually encountered high association of low saturated fat diets with high vegetable protein, high complex carbohydrate and fiber diets and the absence of excess calories. Alternatively, the relatively greater energy expenditure of most rural populations may be involved. These are important areas for detailed search not now being adequately pursued (or approved, or funded!).

Epidemiological Evidence in Populations (Individual Correlations)

Why are zero correlations found between individually measured diet intake and serum lipid levels in U.S. studies? Does this negate the importance of the dietlipid-atherosclerosis relationship? Correlations between a personal characteristic and subsequent disease, and between personal behavior and level of the risk charactcristic, are powerful links in the chain of epidemiological evidence. In most reported North American studies, the relationship between measured individual diet and TC levels is near zero. This has been interpreted by a few to negate the "diet-heart theory." Such an interpretation is probably in error and surely misleading because a) dietary intake varies, along with its measurment and that of blood lipid levels: intra-individual variation in diet es about equal to the variation *between* individuals in the U.S. Under these circumstances, even several measurements of diet and blood lipids would be unlikely to demonstrate a true relationship if it existed. The solution to his problem includes the development of diet methods which reduce technical sources of variability to a minimum and which more accurately characterize current individual eating patterns, This might be obtained by experimentally controlling that pattern, by chemical diet analysis, and by other morc reliable, precise and representative measures of individual diet. The usual 24-hour dietary recall meets none of these criteria, nor do 3-day of 7-day diaries. It is likely that a dozen such measurements is required to improve individual diet characterization [13], b) there is an insufficient range of the variables correlated.

The range of dietary fat intake or fatty acid composition of the diet in U.S. population studies of the 1950's and 60s, in which these zero correlations with TC were derived, is small. Diets among these affluent, volunteer participants were characterized by homogeneity and an excess of calories and fat. The solution for this problem might be 1) to seek cultures and populations in which there is a much wider range, or 2) to specifically select subgroups in the U.S. population to represent a physiologic range in intake from, say, total vegetarianism and fat intake of less than 10% of total calories, up to 40 and 50% levels. Under the first condition, significant correlations of individual diet intake and serum cholesterol levels have been demonstrated in Italy, among the Tarahumara Indians and among Seventh Day Adventists in New Zealand and the United States where differences in TC levels are related to pure vegetarian, lacto-ovo-vegetarian, and nonvegetarian eating practices. The following factors, then, "guarantee" the near zero correlation found between individual blood lipid levels and diet in the diet in the U.S.: high individual variability due to technical and biological sources; poor reliability and validity of the instrument to characterize a person's diet; the homogeneity of the U.S. diet in respect to lipid-raising characteristics. These ideas were recently confirmed by the important work of Shekelle and colleagues from diet-TC-CHD data in an industrial population [19]. With careful attention to minimize measurement variability by standard methods and to reduce individual variance by repeat measures, significant individual correlations have now been demonstrated within an affluent, relatively high fat diet, relatively hypercholesterolemic U.S. industrial population. TC levels and CHD risk for *individuals* were significantly correlated, with prediction of 17 year CHD risk from averages of diet and TC values for individuals measured in the early years of observation.

In contrast, TC levels are strongly correlated with individual CHD risk in all reported studies [2]. Pooling Project data are among the more relevant and representative sources of epidimiological evidence in the United States, or from any high CHD incidence population, about personal levels of TC and subsequent risk of a coronary event [15]. In all eight U.S. studies shown in Table 4 there is greater CHD risk for higher levels of TC. Risk ratios between the top quintile and lower two quintiles vary from 1.5 to 4.9, averaging 2.4. When quintiles 1 and 2 are combined, the risk increases uniformily and smoothly with TC level, and the findings are consistent with a continuous relationship between TC level and CHD risk. But it is also noted that there is no statistically significant difference in the rates of CHD events between the first there quintiles of TC values. A slight but insignificantly greater number of events occurs in the lowest quintile in 4 of 8 studies. This finding will be discussed later in detail.

TABLE IV: AHA Pooling Project Serum Cholesterol Standardized Incidence Ratio First CHD Event

Q	TC	POOL 5	ALE	CH-GAS	CH-WE	FRAM	TECUM	LA	MN CVD	MN RR
I	≤194	72	72	100	62	74	10	37	64	47
II	194-218	61	67	61	57	50	83	46	78	50
III	218-240	78	72	89	70	88	56	116	117	77
IV	240-268	129	129	124	99	160	145	73	117	96
V	> 268	158	177	118	159	167	242	143	189	194
RR		2.4	2.5	1.5	2.7	2.7	4.9	—	—	4.0
#		647	156	123	142	177	49	72	28	112

Pooling Project Research Group, 1978

In Figure 5, across all areas and TC levels in the Seven Countries Study, the individual risk of CHD death rises from TC levels of 160 mg/dl upward, over a wide range of age-adjusted values and different populations. These data too are consistent with a continuous increase in risk with TC level.

HDL cholesterol is also strongly associated with *individual* CHD risk, based on evidence from clinical, experimental and population studies. Epidemiological studies show that the future individual risk of coronary disease in middle-aged and older men and women in high risk societies is significantly lower the greater the level of HDL cholesterol (HDL-C) [7]. All studies find little correlation between individual HDL-C values and LDL-C or TC. Individual CHD risk prediction is improved by use of the radio of HDL-C to either TC or LDL-C. [7].

Change in CHD Incidence, Diet and Blood Lipid Levels

Data on *change* is an important epidemiological source of evidence bearing on optimal lipid levels for populations, on the diet-lipid-atherosclerosis relationship and on the nutritional factors in hyperlipidemia. Cultural differences and changes in these measures provide part of the rationale for diet and lipid recommendations in preventive action and public policy but only when they are confirmatory of other findings from clinical and experimental disciplines. When all is congruent the whole provides powerful inference of cause and a basis for policy in the absent feasibility of obtaining "experimental proof."

Epidemiological data on change come from government data on diet and on Vital Statistics on Causes of Death, from sample surveys showing "spontaneous" time trends in diet, lipid levels and disease rates, from "natural experiments" such as wars and migration, and from man-made experiments such as large preventive trials.

The following countries appear to have experienced an *increase* in CHD deaths reported in their Vital Statistics between 1968 and 1976:

Sweden	Poland	Bulgaria	Republic of Ireland
Denmark	Yugoslavia	Hungary	Northern Ireland
France	Romania		

These have experienced *no* apparent *change:*

Czechoslovakia	Netherlands	Switzerland
New Zealand	F.R. Germany	Austria
Italy		

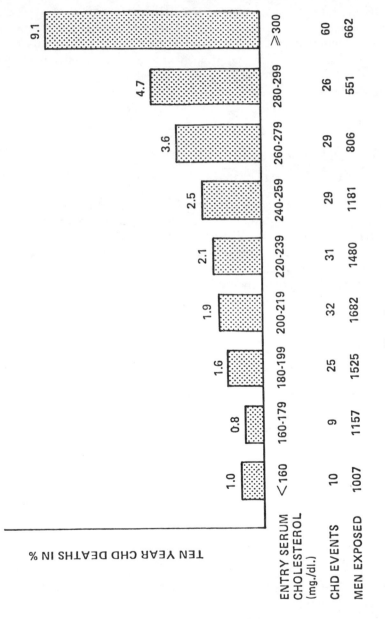

ENTRY SERUM CHOLESTEROL (mg./dl.)	<160	160-179	180-199	200-219	220-239	240-259	260-279	280-299	≥300
TEN YEAR CHD DEATHS IN %	1.0	0.8	1.6	1.9	2.1	2.5	3.6	4.7	9.1
CHD EVENTS	10	9	25	32	31	29	29	26	60
MEN EXPOSED	1007	1157	1525	1682	1480	1181	806	551	662

Figure 5

These countries have apparently experienced a significant *decrease* in annual reported CHD mortality rates for the period:

United States	Finland	Israel (males)
Canada	United Kingdom	Japan
Australia	Belgium	Norway

Some of these trends are uncertain, and in no case are representative data available on national CHD *incidence,* on case-fatality rate, or on risk factor and risk behavior changes which may precede or accompany these changes in CHD mortality.

The epidemiological evidence about change in population TC distributions derives from several sources: different populations examined at intervals, from true national samples taken at intervals, and from population cohorts followed over time. HES and HANES studies in the U.S. are national probability samples while Lipid Research Center data are from representative local samples [2]. Age adjustment of their data results in the suggestion that a 2 to 6 mg/dl or 1 to 3 percent change may exist in representative U.S. groups measured at two different times. But methodologic questions render it uncertain whether the difference is real. TC trends in cohorts followed in the Tecumseh Community Study, in Framingham and Minnesota, and in Framingham children, suggest a 10 to 20 mg/dl [5-10%] lowering over the last 10-15 years which preceded the inflection in national CHD mortality data. In contrast, a significant 10 year increase from roughly 1960 to 1970 occurred in average TC in several populations of the Seven Countries Study. The mean increase for 1,939 Northern European men was 6.9 mg/dl and among 3,928 Southern European was 28.4 mg/dl [11]. The Northern European findings are compatible with the known TC age trend between 50 and 60 years in the West and with *No* major environmental change. In contrast, the highly significant *change* in Southern Europeans is compatible with a documented rapid change in their lifestyle and economy. Thus, population surveys, making little or no intervention on health practice, indicate that mean values and distributions of TC can, and do, change among entire populations and that the change has generally been in the same direction as CHD death rates. But in the absence of a truly "dynamic" epidemiology, with regional and simultaneous measures of deaths, incidence, medical care change, risk factor levels and community behavior, causal inference is uncertain.

Change in TC as a result of experimental changes in diet is "mathematically" established for small groups under metabolic ward conditions and also for large numbers in the mass preventive trials of Diet-Heart, LRC and MR-FIT. It is possible to apply the Keys-Minnesota equation to reported national food consumption data as well as using a multivariate model of changes predicted in CHD mortality from observed risk factor trends. In Stamler's view, a substantial part of the predicted CHD mortality change is "accounted for" by the decrease in mean TC and risk factors [21].

TABLE V: A model of individual diet-serum cholesterol relationships with individual examples

Intrinsic value (mg/dl)	Mean diet-cholesterol effect (mg/dl)				
	0	+25	+50	+75	+100
75	75	100	125	150	175
150	150	175	200	225	250
300	300	325	350	375	400

Note: It is assumed that a minimal genetic or instrinsic regulatory value exists for each individual and is developed usually in the first year of life. On this intrinsic value is superposed the effect of habitual diet, which is neither neutral nor cholesterol-raising, acccording to properties determined in controlled Minneota diet experiments.

TABLE VI: A model of population diet-serum cholesterol relationships with population examples

	Mean diet-cholesterol effect (mg/dl)				
	Japan 0	Greece +25	Italy +50	USA +75	Finland +100
Population mean	150	175	200	225	250
Lower limit (2.5%)	75	100	125	150	175
Upper limit (97.5%)	225	250	275	300	325

Note: It is assumed that the polygenic determinants of blood-cholesterol levels are randomly and equally distributed among large heterogeneous populations, such that a mean population serum-cholesterol value of 150 mg/dl would prevail (S.D. ± 37.5 mg/dl) in the presence of anhabitual average diet having neutral properties in respect of cholesterol. On this mean and population distribution of intrinsic responsiveness if superposed the average habitual diet effect for a population, which is either neutral or cholesterol-raising according to the country's measured diet composition and properties determined in controlled Minnesota diet experiments.

Nutritional-Genetic Interaction

The interaction of genetic and environmental factors in lipid regulation is among the more difficult and controversial issues in the diet-heart matter [3]. A simplified model is given here in Table V, for pedagogical purposes and for readers to critique, of the relatively predominant importance to the *individual* of genetic factors, and in Table VI, for the relative importance to *population* differences of environmental factors (diet). These models can help clarify the matter and reduce controversy even if they are imprecise. In Table 5 it is suggested that an hypothetical genotype, an individual having "ideal" heredity in respect to TC level in childhood, who is exposed to *maximally* cholesterol-elevating diets during life and who responds in experimentally predicted way, might end up with and adult average TC of 175 mg%, thus below average for the U.S. population. Similarly, individuals who inherit the major gene defect of familial type IIa hypercholesteremia may eat the world's *best* (non-cholesterol-raising) diet for a lifetime and yet have an adult blood cholesterol level in the upper 1% of the population. This model demonstrates why individuals on the same diet may have different blood cholesterol levels and why individuals with the same cholesterol level may have different diets, due to their intrinsic metabolic regulation and dietary response. It emphasizes the important effect of inherent lipid regulatory factors in determining the *individual* mean TC level. It assumes, correctly or incorrectly, a simple additive model. In contrast, Table VI makes the assumption that there are no "magnitude" differences between large heterogeneous populations (such as North America, Europe and Asia) in the distributions of the multiple genes which affect intrinsic regulation of the blood lipoproteins. This assumption may well be challenged, and we invite response. However, under these assumed conditions, the habitual diet of the whole population influences the frequency of hyperlipidemias exhibited, and in addition largely determines the population TC mean and distribution. This model emphasizes the overriding importance to population differences, in the presence of widespread susceptibility, of environmental, cultura, behavioral, and dietary factors. These latter are the factors which are the major concern of the public health, i.e., the determinants of mass phenomena, mass disease, and the potential for mass primary prevention.

The Keys, Hegsted, Mattson, and Connor equations describe most elegantly the average TC responses to change in diet composition of small groups of metabolically normal individuals. Yet there is almost no detailed consideration anywhere of the range of intrinsic variation in individual dietary responsiveness, despite the many precisely controlled feeding experiments and therapeutic interventions on hyperlipoproteinemic patients studied down the years. The simplistic model of Table V illustrates the widely different achieved TC levels observable for individuals on a diet of similar composition. But what experimental evidence do we have of the range of intrinsic response to nutritional factors? With Drs. Jacobs and Anderson in our laboratory we have compiled the only sizable body of data available having many measurement points, that is, multiple TC measurements during six controlled experimental changes in diet composition, in the same individual and on a substantial number of individuals [9].

Table VII summarizes the responsiveness in 57 men defined by less than 0.5 and more than 1.5 of the response predicted by the Keys-Minnesota equation. Practically, only 7% were "hypo-" and 7% "hyper responders." No individuals failed to show a response to diet change under controlled conditions. The intrinsic (genetic) diet response is normally distributed.

TABLE VII: *Serum cholesterol response to dietary change frequency distribution of b, the estimate of responsiveness of serum cholesterol to dietary change in 57 men*

b	Number	Percent	Cumulative percent
≤ .5	4	7	7
.5 — .59	1	2	9
.6 — .69	4	7	16
.7 — .79	7	12	28
.8 — .89	5	9	37
.9 — .99	9	16	53
1.0 — 1.99	8	14	67
1.10 — 1.19	6	11	78
1.20 — 1.29	3	5	83
1.30 — 1.39	4	7	90
1.40 — 1.49	2	3	93
≥ 1.50	4	7	100
TOTAL	57	100	

Note: *By arbitrary definition of clinically important responses to diet, 7 percent of these men were "hypo-responders" (less than half of prediction), and 7 percent "hyper-responders" (more than 1.5 times prediction).*

Departures and Discrepancies in Diet-TC-CHD Relationships

The shape of the relationship

Let us consider first the shape of the TC-CHD relationship in some of the Seven Countries Study populations as shown in Figure 6. In U.S. railworkers and in Finland, CHD rates tend to meander below the 7th decile. They appear to increase regularly and rapidly from the 7th to the 10th decile. There is even a suggestion of lower rates in the middle deciles of the distribution, though statistical tests comparing them never reach significance. In fact, no monotonic model, either linear or exponential, fits these data better than any other. Each fits relatively well. A model with a zero slope for deciles one to six would be just as accurate as the other models. However, the *priori* assumption of a threshold value for TC denies what might be called "the principle of biological continuity," that is, the underlying mathematical behavior for the lower deciles is a less obvious version of the sharply increasing rates in the upper deciles. We believe that we have demonstrated it is not possible in these, or in most other data, to distinguish between zero relationships and small positive slopes in this part of the distribution [3]. Therefore, though these findings do not

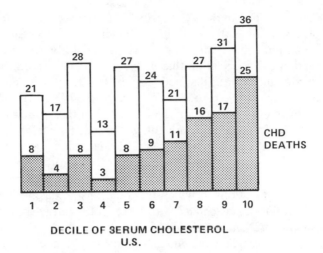

DECILE OF SERUM CHOLESTEROL
U.S.

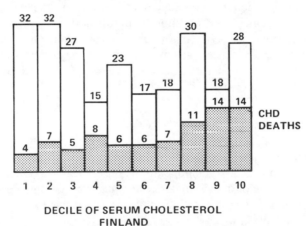

DECILE OF SERUM CHOLESTEROL
FINLAND

Figure 6

support a strong effect of TC in the lower part of the distribution, neither do they support no effect at all. It is a philosophical matter whether to put faith in a model which averages out the variation and adheres to "biological continuity" or to trust only the observed data, subject as they are to random variation.

The risk of the "low side"

Is there an excess risk at the lower end of the TC distribution, and, if so, what might be its explanations and implications? An increasing number of studies show a small excess of CHD and non-CHD mortality associated with the

lowest *relative* position in the TC distribution, irrespective of the actual TC values. This suggests to us the possibility of a general phenomenon of excess risk
of hypocholesterolemic individuals. We particularly welcome your experienced reaction to a speculation that individuals found toward the lower end of
any distribution might be as distinctive as those at the upper end. Each extreme
represents a departure from heterogeneity, from that genetic admixture
thought to have evolutionary survival value. In other words, monogenic, or
"mutant low TC" may have disadvantages of a different sort than monogenic
high TC (or LDL), i.e., familial hypercholesterolemia.

In Framingham data, much of the slight excess mortality in men in the lower part of the TC distribution is accounted for by excess cancer deaths. In
about half the populations in which this relationship has been examined, low
individual TC values are associated with excess colon cancer risk, thus the finding
is not consistent. In addition, it is found only for men and in several studies the effect disappears on excluding individuals who died within the first year or two after
the low cholesterol finding. This suggests that in this negative individual correlation the cancer "caused" the low cholesterol rather than the reverse. Additionally,
population correlations between low cholesterol values and population cancer
rates, including colon cancer, are insignificant or negative; in other words, the
lower the mean population TC value, the lower the population cancer rates [5, 18,
20]. What might the disparities mean?

Individual and Population Correlations

The finding of significant individual correlations *within* populations and absent
or inverse correlations *between* populations raises the more general and interesting
issue of the meaning of individual and ecological correlations. Let us start by considering alternative phenomena that may exist when these major correlations are
concordant or otherwise:

Case No. 1

Consonance of population and individual risk correlations, both positive:

When individuals within a culture, and when whole populations having
higher risk factor values experience, in fact, a higher disease incidence, it
would seem likely that an ubiquitous and powerful environmental influence is
in operation. The influence would have to be strong and broad enough to affect mass rates and provide the positive ecological correlation. But there would
also have to be such a wide prevalence of susceptibility in the population that
the genetic environmental interaction is sufficient to produce the significant
ecological correlation. Of course, individual, intrinsic differences, such as those
which regulate lipoprotein metabolism, would contribute importantly to the

range of values in the population distribution, whether the range were set high or low. However, susceptibility to the lipid-raising influence in the culture would have to be widely distributed to produce the positive ecological correlation.

Case No. 2

Population and individual risk correlations are not consonant:

A. In the special case where the risk factor is significantly related to disease *within* but not *between* populations, would this not suggest that an intrinsic factor were more powerfully operative than a mass, ecological one? Might such be the case for the TC-colon cancer relationship? Suppose that population TC means and distributions differ, as do the habitual population diets which are primarily responsible for the different TC distributions. Suppose that dietary patterns which result in low population TC levels are associated with a lower population risk colon cancer. Suppose also that *within* populations, individual colon cancer risk is found correlated with low TC levels. This could be either a predominantly genetic cause or an interactive effect of genes and habitual diet, for example. (Plausible mechanisms exist for either case: on the cultural side, a low TC level might depend on an individual's eating pattern being low in a co-factor such as a vitamin; on the intrinsic side, an adaptation responsible for a low individual TC level might also result in greater bile acid concentration acting as a co-carcinogen in the colon.) In fact, these suppositions appear to be the actual case for TC and colon cancer.

B. A sub-case of this condition is when internal or individual correlations are strong but population correlations are weak, or at least, there is a discrepant population having TC or disease rates which depart from the ecological regression (e.g., Masai, Tokelauans, French). Here there might be an unknown *protective* factor operating at the population level to reduce population rates of disease at a given level of the risk characteristic.

Case No. 3

Weak individual correlations and strong ecological correlations:

In the case when individual and population findings are not consonant, a powerful environmental force may exist but be difficult to demonstrate by the individual correlations which are attenuated under circumstances in which a) the whole population distribution of the risk variable is set high or exceeds some threshold effect; b) when the environment or social behavior related to the variable is homogeneous in the population; c) when intra-individual variation is virtually equal to inter-individual variation; d) and when the measurement is unreliable for individual characterization though valid for population characterization. The best known example of this phenomenon, mentioned earlier, is the habitual dietary fatty acid intake which is generally and strongly related to population TC values (and CHD rates) but significantly related to individual TC levels or CHD risk only when greatest care is taken to minimize individual variability and reduce technical error [19].

These individual and ecological correlations are expressed mathematically by the formula footnoted below[1] in which, measured over a whole population, individual differences are "averaged out." When the determinants of each factor (for example, TC and colon cancer) are little related, the ecological relationship is close to zero. In contrast, observations of individual correlations within countries tends to hold constant the factors that vary between populations.

Such apparent paradoxes between the correlations computed between populations (ecological correlations) and those computed between individuals (individual correlations) are not contradictory. The two correlations may in fact be completely different; one reflects the ecologic factors which affect all individuals in the population more or less equally and are different between populations; the other reflects individual factors which specify the usual state for each person. The "ecological fallacy" is to interpret one set of associations as the other. Stated otherwise, individual differences most determine individual risk when the ecologic influence is similarly distributed. Ecologic differences most determine population risk when individual susceptibility is similarly distributed.

Failure to look at population findings *along with* individual findings is, we believe, responsible for much of the unnecessary professional controversy in many fields, including the diet-heart matter. Those concerned only with indivi-

---

[1]*The distinction between ecologic and individual correlations is expressed mathematically in the model*

$$CA_{ij} = M_{CA} + E_{i,CA} + I_{ij,CA} + \text{error}$$

$$TC_{ij} = M_{TC} + E_{i,TC} + I_{ij,TC} + \text{error}$$

where CA refers to colon cancer (presence or absence) and TC to total serum cholesterol. The index i refers to the population, j to the individual. M is the term for the grand mean; E is the term for the ecologic factor and it sums to zero across populations. I is the term for the individual factor, and sums to zero within each population. The ecologic correlation is computed between CA and TC using population wide data from which individual variations have been removed. The individual correlation is computed between CA and TC using individual data within each population; it may be averaged across populations, if this is justified, to get a composite estimate. The computation of the individual correlation therefore does not involve the terms in E, and the ecologic correlation does not involve the terms in I. Presumably both CA and TC have multiple determinants, some of which may coincide. The factors which determine the usual levels for populations —the E terms— may be different from those which determine the usual levels for individuals— the I terms. Thus, the ecologic and individual correlations are distinct mathematical entities and may bear no resemblance to one another.

dual variations find it difficult to see the population issue or to recognize its implications to the public health, in contrast to individual health and tailored therapy. In contrast, those who look mainly at the population picture need reminding that any useful model for risk has to account for individual uniqueness and wide individual variation. We simply attempt here to show that insights can be gained by looking at population data, along with individual data within populations, and by attempting to explain or reconcile their discrepancies. Clearly, each of these views, population (ecological) and individual, is valid within its own context. It is important to put the two views together and attempt to resolve a balanced one.

An example of "the ecological fallacy" is making general recommendations for "desirable TC levels" based on individual correlations, without regard to the population correlations. Specifically, distinguished experts have suggested that it would be desirable to reduce plasma TC concentrations to a level around 220 mg/dl, but they state further that there is little evidence; it would be desirable to reduce the TC much lower than 220. Such advice, based on reasonable interpretations of the individual correlations, tends to ignore the ecological correlations and the actual population distributions required to achieve most individual values around 220 mg/dl, such as depicted in the implausible distribution of Figure 7. Thus, a well-intentioned personal recommendation

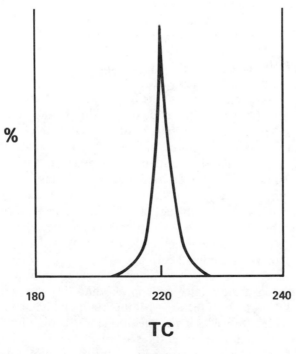

Figure 7

actually takes little account of wide individual variations in a population or of the population distribution required to achieve such an "ideal value" for most individuals. Such advice of a specified TC level would be difficult for individuals to achieve and clearly impossible for a population. We believe the population TC distribution more appropriate to optimal health would likely resemble the left-hand curve for adults seen in Figure 4. This curve is found in adult populations almost totally free of atherosclerosis and CHD, having no excess of other diseases, along with normal growth, development and longevity. It would also be compatible with the very reasonable advice for individuals to seek values below 220 mg/dl.

Other Discrepancies

Other departures from prediction occur both in individual and population (ecological) correlations. Examples are seen in the Seven Countries data in Figure 3 correlating population mean TC values and CHD rates. CHD is greater than expected in East (E) over West (W) Finland, and less than expected in Crete (K) with its high fat, predominantly olive oil intake; a fascinating "natural experiment." Only a part of these discrepancies is explained by the distribution of other known CHD risk factors. In such relatively small and insular populations genetic differences might very well exist. In fact, the greatest discrepancies claimed between diet, TC and CHD rates are from investigations among isolated "primitive" cultures. Important as they may be, the Eskimo, Samburu, and Masai experiences provide, in our view, insufficient evidence of discrepant relationships, chiefly because their field epidemiological methods and sample sizes are inadequate. However, a much better documented discrepancy between observed diet and expected blood lipid values (predicted by the Keys-Minnesota equation) is found in the South Pacific Islanders on Tokelau and Pukapuka [16]. Based on fatty acid composition of their diets, mean TC values are some 60-80 mg/dl lower than predicted, yet *differences* between the islands conform to predictions. Little or nothing is known about CHD incidence in these small populations. But the findings suggest that physiologic, metabolic, and cultural adaptations may indeed occur more rapidly in such isolates than in larger, more heterogeneous populations and that these in turn may affect the relationship between diet, blood lipid response and disease. However, it may also be that other factors operate in the diet of these islanders, including the normally different metabolic routes by which the short-chain fatty acids of coconut oil are handled.

Interesting speculation arises on considering Figure 8 in which the ecologic relationship between dietary fatty acid intake and TC levels in the Seven Countries Study departs from the Keys-Minnesota individual correlation [11]. In individuals studied for weeks under metabolic ward conditions, TC increases 1 mg/dl for every unit increase in the score 1.35 [2S-P] where S and P are the percent of daily calories consumed from saturated and polyunsaturated

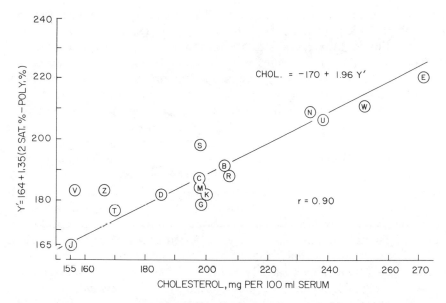

Figure 8 Relation of mean serum cholesterol concentration of the cohorts at entry to fat composition of the diet expressed in the multiple regression equation derived from controlled dietary experiments in Minnesota. B = Belgrade, C = Crevalcore, D = Dalmatia, E = East Finland, G = Corfu, J = Ushibuka, K = Crete, M = Montegiorgio, N = Zutphen, R = Rome railroad, S = Slavonia, T = Tanushimaru, U = American railroad, V = Velika krsna, W = West Finland, Z = Zrenjanin.

fatty acids respectively. Ecologic regression of TC on this score indicates a slope of 1.96 where the metabolic ward experiments in small groups would have predicted a slope of only 1. Countries as units are apparently twice as "responsive" to habitual diet as are individuals. The mean TC of populations increases 2 mg/dl for every unit increase in the dietary fat score. This suggests an ecologic factor affecting TC approximately equally in most individuals and causing TC to be higher than expected based on short-term experiments of fatty acid change. The response to a lifetime of different fat intake may result in metabolic adaptations which affect TC, or, alternatively, the dietary fat score for countries carries "information" on other dietary constituents which affect TC, i.e., fiber, complex carbohydrates and vegetable protein.

Duration of Exposure

Of the several alternative explanations for discrepant population data, one of the least known factors is the duration of exposure to risk. One can hardly know from a single measure, or even a short-term series, the true individual or population exposure to a risk factor. Similarly, slopes of the time trends in po-

pulation exposures, whether stable, ascending or descending, can usually only
be surmised. Risk predictions from the long-term observations on which we
base our estimates of risk, and infer the preventability of CHD, might well depend on whether those measures were constant or on an ascending or descending limb at the moment they were taken. Exposure may also be more crucial
in youth. On the other hand, age-specific national changes in reported CHD
mortality are, in historical terms, remarkably rapid, both upward and downward. Similarly, time trends in population TC levels are documented to change
quickly and in different directions [11]. More standardized data from
population-based samples are needed for men, women and children, with
detailed lipoprotein fractions, collected over extensive periods. A "new epidemiology" is needed for the simultaneous monitoring of trends in death, disease, risk factors and risk related behaviors [6]. Moreover, our understanding of
the interactions of risk characteristics is about as limited as that on duration of
exposure. Though we and others have suggested that a particular luxurious
diet leading to mass hyperlipidemia is a necessary factor for mass atherosclerosis and high CHD incidence rates [1], in fact, the evidence is equally compatible with *no* high CHD incidence population occurring where *any* of the three
major risk characteristics is missing or relatively low. Thus, it may be that diet,
mass elevated blood lipids, and frequent high blood pressure and cigarette
smoking may *all* be necessary to mass atherosclerosis. Obviously, there are
conceptual and factual deficiencies in all these observations and synthesis. Presumably the only solution to them is more and better data.

Attributable Risk

Consider the display in Figure 9 of relative and attributable risk based on Rose's
calculations of Framingham distributions of TC distributions is displayed
the familiar curvilinear relationship between TC level and individual CHD
risk, based on the Framingham logistic solution. The numbers imposed on the
columns are the excess CHD cases attributable to TC level, obtained by mul-
tiplying the relative risk at that level by the population exposed. The table next
to the figure shows the proportion of excess cases deriving from the several
parts of the TC distribution. It shows that relatively few excess CHD cases occur in the upper or lower extremes of the distribution, either because of low
population exposure or low relative risk. Rather it demonstrates dramatically
that 75% of the excess cases attributable to TC level come from that large
central part of the distribution having only moderately elevated TC values
(from 220 to 310 mg/dl). Would not such a mass phenomenon require
population-wide causal inferences and preventive strategies?

A Population Strategy to Shift Risk Factor Distributions

In a quantitative model of prevention in Table VIII, a first assumption is that
risk can be lowered by 25% with intensive counselling in a high risk individual

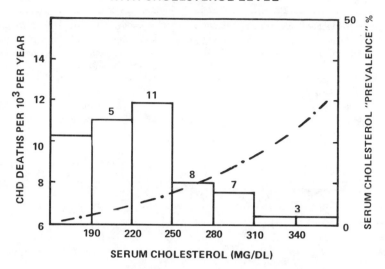

RELATIVE AND ATTRIBUTABLE RISK
WITH CHOLESTEROL LEVEL

ATTRIBUTABLE OR EXCESS CHD
DEATHS/1000/10 YEARS*
(EXCESS RISK X EXPOSURE)

TC	% POPULATION	%XS DEATHS
< 220	45	10
> 310	5	15
220-310	50	75

*ROSE: FRAMINGHAM, 26: 1970;
WHO EXPERT COMMITTEE REPORT, 1982

Figure 9

(effectively 0% of the population) but that the effectiveness of direct strategies decreases linearly thereafter. This yields estimates of 23% risk reduction in the top decile, 15% in the top half of the population risk and perhaps only 5% risk lowering applied to the entire community. People not in the prevention program are assumed to achieve no risk reduction. The decrease in risk in the whole population is the product of the columns and is smallest for intervention column (c) in which half the community is labelled as "high risk," but is limited to the higher risk group. A refinement is shown in which the considerable costs and inefficiencies of screening and placing 50% of the population on a special program is modelled to achieve the risk reduction shown. The product

TABLE VIII: A model for population risk reduction

Percentage of the population declared "at risk" and educated in risk factor lowering	Modelled linear percentage risk reduction achievable in individuals	Estimated percentage reduction in population risk	Modelled percentage risk reduction achievable in individuals (without social supports	Modelled percentage reduction in population risk	Estimated percentage risk reduction achievable in individuals (with social supports)	Estimated percentage reduction in population risk
(a)	(b)	(a) × (b)	(c)	(a) × (c)	(d)	(a) × (d)
< 1	25	< 0.1	25	0.1	N/A	N/A
10	23	2.3	23	2.3	N/A	N/A
25	20	5.0	15	3.8	N/A	N/A
50	15	7.5	10	5.0	N/A	N/A
100	5	5.0	N/A	N/A	10	10

of columns (a) and (c) show the estimated population effect. Finally, column (d) embodies the idea that a community-wide, multiple strategy program diffuses the ideas and social support for change and achieves a wider and greater effect than the medical approach to the linear model of column (b). The product of columns (a) and (d) suggests that the population-wide strategy might change community norms and values significantly and be an efficient strategy for reducing population risk.

Other Questions

What may be wrong with these data and these interpretations? I and many others suggest that taken together the evidence provides a firm base for a successful population approach to primary prevention. It is conceivable, however, that both the data and my interpretation of them are off the mark. For example, the continuous model of relative risk may be questioned. I have indicated that we find it difficult to believe that nature acts with absolute thresholds and rather incline to "the principle of biological continuity." I am not now prepared to reject the idea that risk is multifactorial and continuous. However, if exponential or other monotonic models are not the best solutions for the true relationships, and the risk is *not* smoothly and continually rising, then that basic idea of a continuum of risk is challenged. In turn, an important preventive concept also might not hold: that various *combinations* of moderate elevations of risk produce similar absolute individual risk. Again, nature does not usually present us with dichotomies and it is awfully difficult to arrive at logical mechanisms for discontinuous risk. As I have discussed extensively here, the data are actually compatible with *any* of these models, though we must consider whether the discontinuous model, if widely confirmed, would affect our proposed population strategy to shift entire risk factor distributions downward. For the nonce, it seems to us that a population strategy holds, in the face of the combined evidence of cause, safety and feasibility. The case is admittedly less arguable if we were to be concerned only with the upper tertile of TC levels in affluent populations.

It appears then that substantial numbers of people in high risk societies need to be involved in behavioral change to prevent individual incident cases and to reduce the population disease burden, whatever the risk model used or educational strategy adopted. The models suggested here for the estimated effects of downward shifts in population risk factor distributions are untested, as are the educational strategies which might lead communities of free people to make more informed and healthier choices. They are not untestable, however. The three NIH-sponsored research and demonstration projects, experiments in CHD prevention, are perhaps the closest to an experimental test of the population strategy likely to be carried out in this century [17].

Finally, it seems to me that the population observations, interpreted in the light of evolution, provide a general concept of the cause of modern mass diseases (such as atherosclerosis, diabetes, and hypertension), and their precursors (such as hyperlipoproteinemia and obesity):

If *all* diseases are the result of interaction between host and environment; then *mass* diseases are probably the result of interaction between *powerful* and ubiquitous environmental factors and *widespread* population susceptibility.

The powerful environmental factors are largely recent and manmade: socio-economic, cultural, behavioral. The widespread susceptibility is probably the legacy of evolution, i.e. survival traits to a vastly different economy and life patterns.

The corollary of this idea provides the rationale for preventive practice and public health policy:

An unfavorable environment assures maximal exhibition of susceptible phenotypes. A favorable environment encourages their minimal exibition and a reduced burden of disease in the population.

REFERENCES

1. Beaty, T.H. Discriminating among single locus models using small pedigrees. *Am. J. Med. Genet.* 6:229-240, 1980.
2. Keys, A. Seven Countries: Death and Coronary Heart Disease in Ten Years. Harvard University Press, Cambridge, 1980.
3. Gordon, T., García-Palmieri, M.R., Kagan, A., Kannel, W.B., and Schiffman, J. Differences in coronary heart disease mortality in Framingham, Honolulu, and Puerto Rico, *J. Chronic Dis.* 27:329, 1974.

 4. Marmot, M.G., Syme, S.L., Kagan, A., Kato, H., Cohen, J.B., and Belsky, J. Epidemiologic studies of coronary heart disease and stroke in Japanese men living in Japan, Hawaii and California: prevalence of coronary and hypertensive heart disease and associated risk factors. *Am. J. Epidemiol.* 102:514-525, 1975.
 5. Blackburn, H., Berenson, G.S., Christakis, G., et al. Workshop Report: epidemiological section. Conference on the health effects of blood lipids: optimal distributions for populations. *Prev. Med.* 8:612-678, 1979.
 6. West, R.O., and Hayes, O.B. Diet and serum cholesterol levels. A comparison between vegetarians and non-vegetarians in a Seventh Day Adventist group. *Am. J. Clin. Nutr.* 21:853-862, 1968.
 7. Connor, W.E., Cerqueira, M.T., Connor, R.W., Wallace, R.B., Malinow, M.R., and Casdorph, H.R. The plasma lipids, lipoproteins and diet of the Tarahumara Indians of Mexico. *Am. J. Clin. Nutr.* 32:1131-1142, 1978.
 8. Lewis, B., et al. Workshop report: clinical investigative section. The health effects of blood lipids: optimal distributions for populations. *Prev. Med.* 8, No. 6, 1979.
 9. Liu, K., Stamler, J., Dyer, A., McKeever, J., and McKeever, P. Statistical methods to assess and minimize the role of intra-individual variability in obscuring the relationship between dietary lipids and serum cholesterol. *J. Chronic Dis.* 31:399-418, 1978.
10. Shekelle, R.B., MacMillan Shryock, A., Paul, O., Lepper, M., Stamler, J., Liu, S., and Raynor, W. Diet, serum cholesterol and death from coronary heart disease. *N. Engl. J. Med.* 304:65-70, 1981.
11. The Pooling Project Research Group. Relationship of blood pressure, serum cholesterol, smoking habits, relative weight and ECG abnormalities to incidence of major coronary events: Final report of the pooling project. *J. Chronic Dis.* 31:201, 1978.
12. Gordon, T., Castelli, W.P., Hjortland, A.D., Kannel, W.B., and Dawber, T.E. High density lipoprotein as a protective factor against coronary heart disease. *Am. J. Med.* 63:707-714, 1979.
13. Stamler, J. Public health aspects of optimal lipid-lipoprotein levels. The health effects of blood lipids: optimal distributions for populations. *Prev. Med.* 8, No. 6, 1979.
14. Blackburn, H., and Jacobs Jr, D.R. Coronary heart disease risk factors: a population view. Proceedings of the Sixth International Symposium on Atherosclerosis, Springer-Verlag, Berlin, 1982.
15. Epstein, F. Cholesterol, coronary heart disease, cancer and diet. *Atherosclerosis Rev.,* 1982, (in press).
16. Jacobs Jr., D.R., Hannan, P., Keys, A., and Blackburn, H. Individual variability in serum cholesterol response to change in diet. Submitted to *Arteriosclerosis,* 1982.
17. Rose, G., Blackburn, H., et al. Colon cancer and blood cholesterol. Lancet i:181-183, 1974.
18. Sidney, S., and Farquhar, J. Cholesterol, cancer and publicy. *N. Engl. J. Med.,* 1982, (in press).
19. Prior, I.A., Davidson, F., Salmord, C.E., and Czochanska, Z. Cholesterol, coconuts, and diet on Polynesian Atolls: a natural experiment. *Am. J. Clin. Nutr.* 34:1552-1561, 1981.
20. Gillum, R.F., Prineas, R.J., Luepker, R.V., Taylor, H.L., Jacobs Jr, D.R., Kottke, T.E., and Blackburn, H. Decline in coronary death. A search for explanations. *Minn. Med.* 65:235-238, 1982.
21. Blackburn, H. Diet and mass hyperlipidemia: a public health view. In Nutrition, Lipids and Coronary Heart Disease (R. Levy, B. Rifkind, B. Dennis, N. Ernst, eds.), Raven Press, New York, 1979.
22. Report of the NIH-sponsored community research and demostration programs in primary prevention of coronary heart disease. Submitted to *Circulation,* 1982.

THE INTERACTION OF GENETIC AND NUTRITIONAL FACTORS IN HYPERLIPIDEMIA[+]

Sonja L. Connor
William E. Connor

*Section of Clinical Nutrition and Lipid Metabolism,
Department of Medicine, The Oregon Health Sciences
University, Portland, Oregon, U.S.A.*

INTRODUCTION

Mass hyperlipidemia is a significant characteristic of the affluent Western world, and particulary in the United States. Within this population, two kinds of hyperlipidemia are manifested. Purely genetic hyperlipidcmia displays itself at the time of birth or shortly after or during the first year of life. The autosomal dominant familial hypercholesterolemia (type II-a) and hyperchylo-micronemia (type I) from an inherited enzyme deficiency (lipoprotcin lipase) are two examples of genetic hyperlipidemia. These forms of hyperlipidemia affect less than 0.1 percent of the population and presumably have a worldwide distribution in less affluent countries as well.

The second kind of hyperlipidemia develops in genetically susceptible individuals exposed to nutritional excesses of total calories, cholesterol, and saturated fat over their lifetimes. This diet-induced hyperlipidemia affects well over 50 percent of the population of the United States dependent upon the arbitrary cutpoints. It is clearly manifested in school children and increases with age into the mid-thirties and early forties. The influence of genetic factors has been roughly estimated at about 50 percent [1]; dietary factors presumably account for most of the remaining variance. Let us look at two populations which illustrate dietary induced hyperlipidemia in genetically susceptible individuals.

[+]*Supported by research grant HL-20910, National Heart, Lung and Blood Institute, The Clinical Research Center (RR-34), and the National Institutes of Health.*

137

Plasma lipids and liproteins in the United States

The distribution of the plasma cholesterol concentrations of   men and women in 233 randomly selected families of Portland, Oregon, in the U.S.A. [2] is given in Fig. 1. We consider that those individuals with values over 180 mg/dl have mild to severe hyperlipidemia and that most of these people have diet-induced hyperlipidemia. A very few individuals to the far right of the distribution curves have purely genetic hyperlipidemia, i.e. familial hypercholesterolemia (above the 99th percentile). Since dietary histories have indicated a great similarity of the diets in all the individuals studied, those persons with low plasma cholesterol and LDL levels undoubtedly have "genetic" reasons for such levels.

Similar distribution curves in these same American men and women are found for an even stronger risk factor, low density lipoprotein (LDL) (Fig. 2). There is a broad range of values, from below 20 to 250 mg/dl. The LDL concentration must be considered elevated when it exceeds the 110-120 mg/dl range.

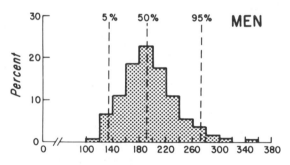

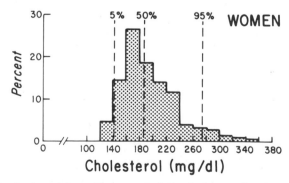

Figure 1 The distribution of the total plasma cholesterol concentrations in men and women ages 16-65 years, expressed as the percent of the total number of subjects. The fifth, fiftieth and ninety-fifth percentiles are indicated.

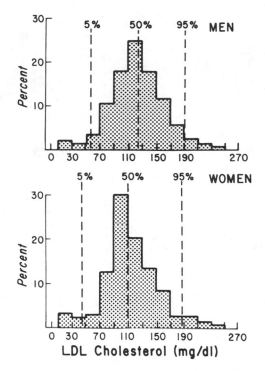

Figure 2 The distribution of the plasma low-density lipoprotein (LDL) cholesterol concentrations in men and women ages 16-65 years, expressed as the percent of the total number of subjects. The fifth, fiftieth and ninety-fifth percentiles are indicated.

HDL cholesterol ranged from 20 to more than 100 mg/dl (Fig. 3). The lower 5th percentile was 31 mg/dl for men and 36 mg/dl for women. The ninetyfifth percentile was 68 mg/dl for men and 79 mg/dl for women. In general, women were about 10 mg/dl higher than men, a factor which undoubtedly accounts for some of their relative immunity to coronary heart disease before menopause.

The plasma triglyceride levels of these families displayed a distribution curve that is skewed to the right (Fig. 4). This skewness is not seen in children. The mean triglyceride values were about 78 mg/dl for women and a little higher for men, and about 40 mg/dl for children.

A prominent characteristic of the U.S.A. population and of healthy individuals from Portland, Oregon is that the plasma lipids rise with age (Figs. 5 and 6). The mean plasma cholesterol concentrations rose steadily with age in females, from 162 mg/dl in early childhood to 35 mg/dl age 55-60 years. The mean cholesterol concentration in males was higher in childhood (169 mg/dl) and lower at post-puberty (143 mg/dl). Thereafter, it generally increased with age, attaining a maximum mean concentration of 222 mg/dl at age 55-60 years.

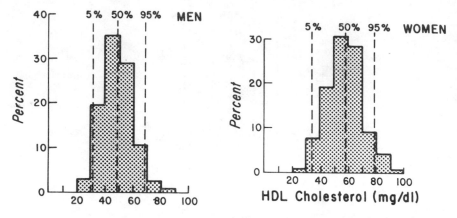

Figure 3 *The distribution of the plasma high-density lipoprotein (HDL) cholesterol levels in men and women from age 16-65 years, expressed as the percent of the total number of subjects. The fifth, fiftieth and ninety-fifth percentiles are indicated.*

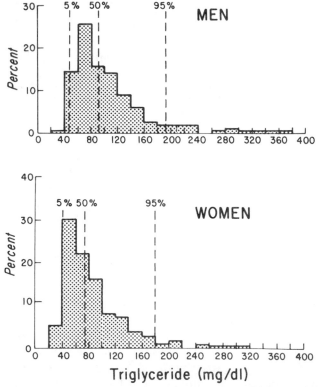

Figure 4 *The distribution in the plasma triglyceride in men and women ages 16-65 years, expressed as the percent of the total number of subjects. The fifth, fiftieth and ninety-fifth percentiles are indicated.*

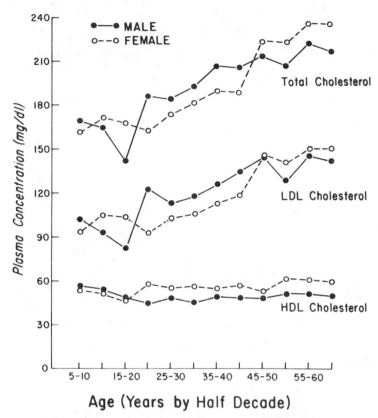

Figure 5 The age-related changes in the plasma concentrations of total cholesterol and the high- and low-density lipoprotein (HDL and LDL) in males and females ages 6-65 years.

Over the age range of 21-45 years, males had a significantly higher ($p < 0.01$) mean plasma cholesterol concentration than the females. The mean plasma LDL cholesterol concentrations paralleled the age-related increase in the total plasma cholesterol and were also significantly higher in men ($p < 0.01$).

In contrast to cholesterol and LDL, the age-related patterns for HDL cholesterol differed for males and females. Boys and girls had similar HDL values. A general drop in the HDL cholesterol level ocurred at puberty and through early adulthood, followed by an increased HDL in females and no increase in males with age. Except during childhood and late teens, the levels of HDL cholesterol in females were 9-10 mg/dl higher than those for males ($p < 0.01$).

Older subjects of both sexes had more than twice the triglyceride concentration of younger subjects. The mean concentration in males ranged from 51 mg/dl in early childhood to 132 mg/dl at ages 30-35 years, with a decreasing trend from 35-40 years through age 65 years. The plasma triglyceride levels in

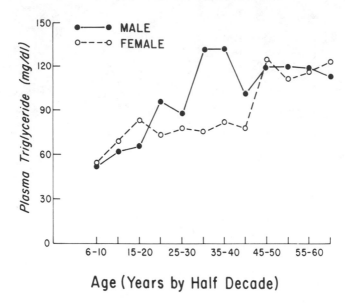

Figure 6 *The age-related changes in the plasma triglyceride concentrations in males and females ages 6-65 years.*

females increased from a mean concentration of 54 mg/dl in childhood to 125 mg/dl by ages 45-59 years, and thereafter remained at about 120 mg/dl. Between the ages of 21-45 years, the males had significantly higher triglyceride levels than females ($p < 0.01$).

Blackett *et al* [3] suggested that the rise in plasma lipids with age is related to the increasing body weight as adipose tissue so characteristic of Western populations. In the present study, the independent influence of weight and adiposity was considered in an evaluation of the circumstances that might be associated with age-lipid rise (Table I). The rise of the plasma cholesterol and LDL levels with time was generally shown to not be related to increases in body weight but to the aging process itself. Because the aging process *per se* does not seem to cause a significant rise in plasma cholesterol in other cultures (e.g. the Tarahumara Indians), the chronic exposure to quantities of dietary cholesterol and saturated fat that exceed the body's ability to maintain cholesterol might be responsible for the age-related plasma lipid rise; i.e. a progressive deterioration of metabolic homeostasis.

The relationships of the plasma HDL, plasma triglyceride and adiposity are particulary intriguing. HDL correlated negatively with all measures of adiposity in men and women and was independently related to body weight. HDL also correlated negatively with the plasma triglyceride concentrations in men, women and children.

The plasma triglyceride correlated positively with adiposity. While both age and body weight were correlated with plasma triglyceride concentrations, body

TABLE I Partial Correlation Coefficients of Age and Weight with Lipids, Lipoprotein and Anthropometric Measurements

	Choles-terol	LDL choles-terol	HDL choles-terol	Tri-Triglyce-ride	Body Mass index
Age [a]					
Men	0.382 [c]	0.325 [c]	0.120	0.151 [b]	0.265 [c]
Women	0.467 [c]	0.392 [c]	0.145 [b]	0.236 [c]	0.224 [c]
Children	0.181 [b]	0.173 [b]	0.023	−0.003	0.142
Weight [d]					
Men	0.066	0.009	−0.368 [c]	0.425 [c]	0.872 [c]
Women	0.167 [c]	0.177 [c]	−0.204 [c]	0.342 [c]	0.925 [c]
Children	−0.206 [c]	−0.214 [c]	−0.083	0.185 [b]	0.267 [c]

[a] Adjusted for weight
[b] Significantly different from zero (p < 0.05)
[c] Significantly different from zero (p < 0.01)
[d] Adjusted for age.

weight had a stronger independent association. The plasma triglyceride levels in our study correlated directly with body weight; adiposity might well be the environmental factor that affects triglyceride levels. The close relationship of hypertriglyceridemia with overweight is also a well-known clinical phenomenon [4]. This epidemiologic information fits well with the results of metabolic ward studies in which weight loss produces a lowering of plasma triglyceride levels and, frequently, a rise in HDL [5]. Weight gain or an increase in adiposity probably results in just the opposite: an increase in plasma triglyceride concentration and a decrease in HDL. Presumably, the apoproteins of HDL have been shunted into the transport of triglyceride in VLDL, and thus, HDL levels are lower when triglyceride levels rise with adiposity.

Plasma lipids and lipoproteins in the Tarahumara Indians of Mexico

Cross-cultural comparisons will further delineate the interaction of genetic and dietary influences. The Tarahumara are Indians of the high plateau and canyon country of the Sierra Madre Occidental Mountains of Mexico. Their plasma lipids and lipoproteins differed greatly from those already described for the U.S.A. [6]. Table II provides the mean values for these two populations of completely different nutritional lifestyles. Tarahumara men had mean values of 136 mg/dl vs. U.S.A. values for men of 195 mg/dl. However, the Tarahumaras were not homogeneous with regard to their admittedly lower mean plasma cholesterol levels. The Tarahumara men had cholesterol values which ranged from less than 100 to over 250 mg/dl (Fig. 7). Again, since the

TABLE II *Comparisons of the Plasma Lipids, Lipoproteins and Anthropometrics of two cultures: Tarahumara vs. U.S.A.* [a]

| | Plasma Cholesterol (mg/dl) | | | Plasma trigly- ceride mg/dl | Triceps Skinfold (mm) |
	Total	LDL	HDL		
Children					
Tarahumara	116 ± 22	83 ± 16	27 ± 10	116 ± 50	7.6 ± 3
U.S.A. [b]	167 ± 29	90 ± 31	55 ± 11	59 ± 24	13.5 ± 5
Men					
Tarahumara	136 ± 27	87 ± 22	26 ± 7	123 ± 53	6.3 ± 3
U.S.A. [b]	195 ± 40	122 ± 40	48 ± 11	111 ± 68	14.4 ± 5.6
Women					
Tarahumara	139 ± 30	89 ± 14	28 ± 14	134 ± 67	10.8 ± 4
U.S.A. [b]	192 ± 39	114 ± 40	57 ± 12	86 ± 50	23.8 ± 7.6

[a] mean ± S.D.

[b] Portland, Oregon

diets of these Tarahumaras were remarkably similar, this range indicates genetic variability. The major difference between Tarahumaras and people in the U.S.A. is that the plasma cholesterol levels of the Tarahumaras varied about a much lower mean value.

Other major differences in the plasma lipids between the Tarahumaras and the people of the U.S.A. related to higher Tarahumara plasma triglyceride

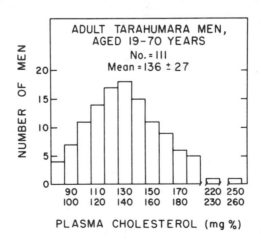

Figure 7 *Distribution of plasma cholesterol levels in adult Tarahumara men, ages 19 to 70 years old.*

levels for all three groups (children, men and women). The Tarahumara children had values of 116 vs. 50 mg/dl for U.S.A. children and higher values, too, than for U.S.A. adults (men 111 and women 86 mg/dl). This is despite the fact that the Tarahumaras had much less adipose tissue, as measured by triceps skinfold thickness, a factor which directly correlates very well with triglyceride levels in the U.S.A. We believe that the explanation for these differences lies in the very high content of dietary carbohydrate, some 75 percent of the total calories in the Tarahumara diet (Table III). High carbohydrate diets cause increased VLDL secretion by the liver because of abundant substrate for triglyceride synthesis. However, postprandial triglyceride levels are usually lower than fasting levels. In people habitually consuming a high fat diet, as in the U.S.A. where 40 per cent of total calories come from fat, the postprandial plasma triglyceride levels become grossly elevated in response to the absorbed dietary fat. Thus, the Tarahumara triglyceride response is physiologic and not pathogenic of disease.

As has been stressed, diet-induced hyperlipidemia is rare in less affluent cultures (i.e. the Tarahumara Indians or in other cultures such as the Japanese). In both of these groups the lifestyles are quite different from that of the U.S.A. Both the Japanese and the Tarahumaras have a low incidence of coronary heart disease. This is in contrast to the high incidence of coronary heart disease in the United States and other countries where diet-related hy-

TABLE III Mean Daily Nutrient Intake of American (U.S.A.) and Tarahumara Indian Men Aged 16 to 70 years

	U.S.A.(22)	Tarahumara Indians(6)
Energy (kcal)	2,674	2,818
Protein (g)	100	92
(% total calories)	15	13
Fat (g)	119	38
(% total calories)	40	12
Saturated fat (g)	42	8
(% total calories)	14	3
Monounsaturated fat (g)	45	13
(% total calories)	15	4
Polyunsaturated fat (g)	24	16
(% total calories)	8	5
Iodine Number	71	102
P/S value	0.6	2.1
Cholesterol (mg)	451	71
Carbohydrate (g)	274	528
(% total calories)	41	75
Crude Fiber (g)	2	19
Salt (NaCl) (g)	12	8

perlipidemia is very common. It should be emphasized that heart disease in even the generally affluent cultures is uncommon in at least two genetically resistant conditions: hypobetalipoproteinemia and hyperalphalipoproteinemia, which have been termed the so-called longevity syndromes [7,8].

The paramount influence of genetic factors over lipid metabolism determines what we would term the basal concentrations of the plasma lipids and lipoproteins. The environment, i.e. the diet, may shift this basal concentration upwards over the lifetime such that recognizable hyperlipidemia results and subsequent coronary heart disease develops.

A third difference in the plasma lipids of the U.S.A. and Tarahumaras relates to high density lipoprotein (HDL). The HDL levels in the Tarahumaras are close to 50 per cent lower than the values found in the U.S.A. (Table II). Children reflect this difference particulary well; HDL levels were 27 mg/dl in the Tarahumaras and 55 mg/dl in the U.S.A. This occurred despite the fact that the Tarahumaras were a slender people with much less adipose tissue and obesity than in the U.S.A. where HDL correlates inversely with adiposity [2]. HDL levels have been believed to be higher in individuals who habitually engage in more physical activity. Paradoxically, the Tarahumara culture demands much physical exertion. The word Tarahumara means "fleet of foot" and the characteristic tribal sport is the game of "kickball" over rough terrain in races up to 200 miles. Many other societies whose diet differs from the Western diet have similar low HDL levels [9].

We do not have a good explanation for these low HDL levels. Since total cholesterol and LDL cholesterol are likewise lower, perhaps the lower HDL levels share in this overall tendency, which may reflect the lifelong low intakes of dietary cholesterol and saturated fat. The low HDL cholesterol values may be, in part, related to the increased triglyceride levels and metabolic needs derived from the high carbohydrate diet. The apoproteins of HDL (AI, AII and CI, CII, CIII) are, of course, vital components of the VLDL molecule and may be shunted into VLDL instead of HDL. Because the LDL cholesterol was also low, the ratio of LDL to HDL cholesterol was still favorable from the aspect of atherosclerotic risk.

The diet of the Tarahumara Indians compared to the U.S.A. diet

The Tarahumaras are primitive agriculturalists growing most of their own foods, with the chief crops and the principal sources of calories being corn and beans. These foods contribute about 90% of the total calories. The remainder of the diet is almost completely derived from other vegetable sources. Meat is seldom eaten. The chief animal food product, consumed with some regularity, is eggs, averaging 2 per week.

The Tarahumara diet was found to be completely adequate from a nutritional point of view (Table III). A typical Tarahumara man consumed 2,818 calories with 92 g of protein (13% of total calories) which was similar to the caloric and protein intake of men in the U.S.A.; 2674 calories and protein 100 g (15% of total calories). The essential amino acid requirements for human nutrition were more than adequately met by the quantities and mixture of bean and corn protein [11,12]. The diet of the Tarahumara was very low in fat, 38 g (12% of total calories) and saturated fat, 8 g (3% of total calories). This is in contrast to that in the U.S.A. where fat intake was 119 g (40% of total calories) and saturated fat was 42 g (14% of total calories). The cholesterol intake was 71 mg/day in the Tarahumaras and 451 mg/day in men from the U.S.A. The Tarahumaras had a much higher carbohydrate intake than the men in the U.S.A., 75% of total calories versus 41% of total calories. Likewise, the crude fiber intake was much greater in the Tarahumaras, 19 g versus 2 g. The salt intake was 4 g per day, lower than the salt intake of most North Americans.

Both the diets of the Tarahumara and in the U.S.A. were nutritionally adequate in that they were not deficient in any essential nutrient. Yet these diets were very different in composition as well as in the type and quantity of foods consumed. Furthermore, the diet of the U.S.A. would contribute greatly to the risk of developing coronary heart disease because of its high saturated fat and cholesterol content. On the other hand the diet of the Tarahumaras would provide minimal risk for the development for coronary heart disease. The lesson to be learned from the Tarahumaras is not that all populations should eat largely corn and beans but rather, that the consumption patterns of food should change to reflect greater intakes of carbohydrate and fiber from vegetables and lesser intakes of saturated fat and cholesterol from animal sources.

In Western cultures the correlations between intakes of the dietary factors which elevate the plasma cholesterol levels and the actual plasma levels have tended not to be positive for reasons discussed elsewhere [6]. However, in the Tarahumaras these correlations were much more clearcut. Correlations between selected nutrients and the plasma cholesterol levels were measured for 103 adults of both sexes (Table IV). Pregnant and lactating women were excluded. Of great interest was the significantly high correlation between the dietary intakes of cholesterol and plasma cholesterol levels ($r = 0.898$, Fig. 8). Also positively correlated to the plasma cholesterol concentration were animal fat, total fat, eggs and animal protein. Sugar intakes were only marginally related to plasma cholesterol levels. No correlation was found for starch, total calories, or plant sterols. Negative correlations to vegetable protein, vegetable fat, and, to a lesser degree, fiber were seen.

Age-related differences among risk factors in the Tarahumaras surveyed were minimal. Plasma cholesterol levels and the ages of the subjects were only slightly related ($r = 0.383$). Plasma triglyceride levels were not related to age ($r = 0.121$). Body weight, plasma triglyceride, and age were also not correlated with one another. There was no correlation between body weights and plasma cholesterol levels ($r = 0.073$).

TABLE IV Correlations Between the Plasma Cholesterol Concentrations of the
Tarahumara Indians and the Intakes, of Certain Foods
and Dietary Substances *

Positive correlations (p < 0.01)	
Cholesterol	0.898
Animal fat	0.593
Total fat	0.552
Eggs	0.548
Animal Protein	0.464
Sugar	0.323
No correlations (p > 0.01)	
Starch	0.145
Total calories	0.064
Plant sterols	0.030
Negative correlations (p < 0.01)	
Vegetable protein	−0.723
Vegetable fat	−0.403
Fiber	−0.384

* *Correlation coefficients were measured for a subsample of 103 adults
(excluding pregnant and lactating women).*

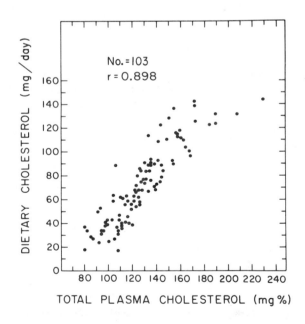

Figure 8 The correlation between the total plasma cholesterol and dietary cholesterol intake per
day (r = 0.898, p < 0.01) in a subsample of the Tarahumara study.

The addition of cholesterol to the diet of the Tarahumara Indians

A metabolic study was designed to answer the following questions: would Tarahumara Indians have a hypercholesterolemic response when given a large load of dietary cholesterol in the face of their habitual low cholesterol intake, i.e. an average of 71 mg/day? Or, conversely, would the low plasma cholesterol concentrations of the Tarahumaras have resulted from metabolic adaptations making them insensitive to a high cholesterol diet [13]?

Eight healthy adult Tarahumara men, between 20 and 45 years of age, volunteered to participate in the study in response to a general invitation to the community. On admission, baseline measurements and medical examinations were carried out. The men were found to be healthy and were short and lean (mean ± S.D. 161.0 ± 6.0 cm height, 53.8 ± 7.1 kg weight and 6 ± 1 mm triceps skinfold). Their mean blood pressures were 95 ± 13 and 60 ± 13 mm Hg and the resting pulse rate, 56 ± 11 neats per minute.

The subjects participated in the study for 6 weeks: they first consumed the baseline cholesterol-free diet for 3 weeks followed by 3 weeks of the experimental high cholesterol diet. The typical Tarahumara food pattern consisting mainly of beans, tortillas and pinole was used as the basic diet for the entire study. Local products, including dried beans and corn, vegetables, cereals and fruits were used. Three meals and one snack were served daily.

The cholesterol-free and the high cholesterol diets were identical in calories (estimated individually for each subject based on weight, height and age), in protein (15% of cal.), in fat [20% of cal. with 10% monounsaturared, 4% polyunsaturated (P) and 6% saturated (S) fat calories, P/S ratio 0.7], in carbohydrate (65% of cal. with 62% from complex and 3% from simple carbohydrate) and in fiber (78 g of dietary fiber). They differed only in cholesterol content: zero vs. 1000 mg per day.

The mean total plasma cholesterol concentration was typically low on admission, 120 ± 7 (S.E.M.) mg/dl, remained low after 3 weeks of the cholesterol free diet, 113 ± 8 mg/dl, and increased 30% after the high cholesterol feeding to 147 ± 11 mg/dl ($p < 0.01$) (Table V). This increase began during the first week of the high cholesterol diet and continued to rise until it stabilized during week 3 (Fig. 9). Such stabilization of the plasma cholesterol levels after 10 to 14 days of dietary cholesterol feeding in normocholesterolemic Caucasians has been demonstrated in previous studies [14,15] and continues indefinitely (at least for 11 weeks). All subjects had increased plasma cholesterol levels after the feeding of dietary cholesterol. The mean increase was + 34 mg/dl and the entire range of values was + 42, + 28, + 19, + 57, + 29, + 46, + 18 and + 26 mg/dl.

Most of the increase in plasma cholesterol occurred in the low-density lipoprotein (LDL) cholesterol fraction which changed from 72 ± 6 (SE) mg/dl after the cholesterol-free diet to 94 ± 9 after the high cholesterol diet ($p < 0.01$), a 31% elevation. The very low-density and high-density (HDL) lipoprotein

TABLE V The Effects of Dietary Cholesterol on the Total Plasma
Cholesterol, Triglyceride, and Lipoproteins

	Admission	Cholesterol free diet	High Cholesterol diet
Cholesterol (mg/dl)			
Total	120 ± 7 [a]	113 ± 8	147 ± 11 [b]
HDL	31 ± 3	27 ± 1	31 ± 2
LDL	72 ± 4	72 ± 6	94 ± 9 b
VLDL [c]	15 ± 12	8 ± 6	19 ± 3
LDL/HDL	2.48	2.70	3.22
Triglyceride (mg/dl)			
Total	96 ± 12	100 ± 7	111 ± 12
HDL	17 ± 2	15 ± 1	15 ± 2
LDL	27 ± 2	24 ± 2	30 ± 4
VLDL	51 ± 10	59 ± 7	68 ± 11

[a] Mean values $\pm$ S.E.M.

[b] Significantly different than admission and cholesterol-free period, $p < 0.01$

[c] Very low-density lipoprotein

cholesterol concentrations were unchanged by the dietary manipulations (Table V). Baseline mean total plasma triglyceride and the lipoprotein triglyceride fractions remained similar during the study. The ratio of cholesterol to triglyceride in LDL and VLDL did not increase statistically during the high cholesterol diet.

Mean body weight increased only slightly throughout the study, a similar minor change in both periods: +0.8 kg during cholesterol-free diet and +0.9 kg during the high cholesterol diet.

Of importance is the fact that the significant increase in plasma cholesterol and LDL concentrations to dietary cholesterol was neither exaggerated as might have been expected from the virtual absence of cholesterol in their usual diet nor attentuated as would have been predicted from the hypothesis that the dietary cholesterol in breast milk protect against cholesterol overload later in life [16]. Tarahumara infants are routinely breast-fed. Indeed, the mean plasma cholesterol increase of 34 mg/dl and the LDL cholesterol increase of 22 mg/dl were similar to increases obtained in normal American volunteers consuming a similar amount of dietary cholesterol after a cholesterol-free dietary period [15,17,18,19]. The Americans would have had a dietary background after infancy high in cholesterol content. Thus, the results of this study emphasize the universality of the increased plasma total cholesterol and LDL choles-

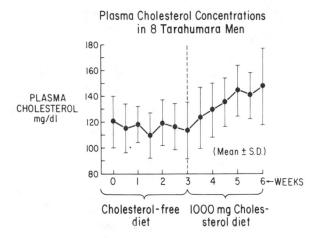

Figure 9 The plasma cholesterol concentrations in eight Tarahumara men receiving cholesterol-free and 1000 mg cholesterol diets for 3 weeks each.

terol concentrations after the ingestion of a high cholesterol diet after a cholesterol-free period. This point has been previously reviewed in depth [20,21].

The addition of cholesterol to the diet of Americans in the U.S.A.

A study was carried out in Americans (U.S.A.) fed a high cholesterol diet analogous to the diet fed to the Tarahumara Indians [21]. Twenty-five subjects previously consuming the usual American diet were given cholesterol-free diets for 3-4 weeks and then 1000 mg of dietary cholesterol per day for another 3-4 weeks. The diets were otherwise identical and contained 40 per cent of the calories as fat. All subjects exhibited a pronounced decline in plasma cholesterol concentrations following consumption of the cholesterol-free diet (Table VI). The previous typically American diet had been high in cholesterol content and saturated fat. The mildly and severely hypercholesterolemic, the hypertriglyceridemic, and the normal subjects responded similarly.

After 3-4 weeks of a cholesterol-free diet the normal subjects had plasma cholesterol levels approaching those of the Tarahumara Indians. They had decreased from 171 to 141 mg/dl. The patients with hyperlipidemia phenotype II-A, both mild and severe, decreased from 258 to 109 mg/dl and 376 to 209 mg/dl respectively, thus showing the effects of dietary manipulations in genetic hyperlipidemia as well. The patients with hypertriglyceridemia also have a considerable reduction in plasma cholesterol concentrations.

With the baseline cholesterol-free diet, the mean level of plasma cholesterol for the 25 subjects was 211 mg/dl. Egg yolk cholesterol (1000 mg/day) was then incorporated into the diet without changing the other constituents (calo-

TABLE VI Plasma Cholesterol Levels (mg/dl) after the Usual American Diet and Cholesterol-free and High Cholesterol Diets in Normal and Hyperlipoproteinemic Subjects

	Period I			Period II		
	Usual American Diet	Cholesterol-free Diet	Change	Cholesterol-free Diet	High Cholesterol Diet	Change
Normal subjects	171 ± 8 (SD)	141 ± 14	−30	141 ± 14	174 ± 20	+33
Mild hypercholesterolemia	258 ± 18	209 ± 27	−49	209 ± 27	245 ± 29	+36
Severe hypercholesterolemia	375 ± 22	338 ± 43	−38	338 ± 43	405 ± 17	+67
Hypertriglyceridemia	251 ± 36	208 ± 23	−43	208 ± 23	231 ± 23	+23
Means of all subjects				211 ± 68	247 ± 79	+36

ries, carbohydrates, fat, protein, minerals and vitamins). This dietary cholesterol caused an increase in the plasma cholesterol level to 247 mg/dl, or a net change of +36 mg/dl. All subjects changed in the upward direction. The normal subjects increased to just about where they were at baseline, from 141 to 170 mg/dl. The mild hypercholesterolemic (II-A's) increased from 209 to 245 mg/dl. The severe hypercholesterolemics (II-A's) never reached a steady state. They went up from 338 to 405 mg/dl. They were higher after four weeks of the high-cholesterol diet than they had been at baseline. These severe type II-A's were clearly much more sensitive to dietary cholesterol than were the normal individuals.

The increased plasma cholesterol was transported chiefly in LDL for the normal and hypercholesterolemic subject (Fig. 10). Slight increases occurred in HDL. In the hypertriglyceridemic subjects, however, both VLDL and LDL cholesterol increased, each accounting for about 50 per cent of the total increase.

CONCLUSIONS

Dietary factors, especially dietary cholesterol and fat, along with excessive calories, have a strong influence in affecting the plasma lipid and lipoprotein concentrations of a given individual, with or without hyperlipidemia. This is true for all populations. Dietary factors may shift the plasma cholesterol distribution curve either to the left or to the right. In other words, if the important environmental effect of diet were controlled, then a much more favorable plasma cholesterol distribution would result. The current trend in the United

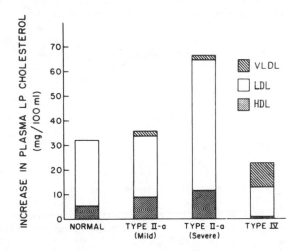

Figure 10 The effect of a 1000 mg cholesterol diet upon the plasma lipoproteins in 25 subjects.

States is that the mean plasma cholesterol level is lower and the curve is shifted a bit to the left. In societies which are currently becoming westernized, the shift is going in the opposite direction concomitantly with changes in the diet. The plasma cholesterol levels are higher and the curve is moving to the right.

Dietary factors are probably the most important in the age-rise of plasma cholesterol, LDL and triglyceride. The adult body weight also increases (and adiposity). Therefore, it would seem reasonable to consider control or prevention of a Western disease like coronary heart disease by attention to alterning the dietary factors which shift this paramount risk factor, hypercholesterolemia, to a lower range. In this manner the setpoint of genetic determination of plasma cholesterol and lipoprotein levels may be altered in a more favorable direction.

REFERENCES

1. Sing, C.F., Orr, J.D. and Moll, PP. Review of factors that predict serum cholesterol in the general population. *In* "Childhood Prevention of Atherosclerosis and Hypertension" (R.M. Lauer and R.B. Shekelle, eds.), pp. 87-97. Raven Press, New York, 1980.
2. Connor, S.L., Connor, W.E., Sexton, G., Calvin, L. and Bacon, S. The effects of age, body weight and family relationships on plasma lipoproteins and lipids in men, women and children of randomly selected families. *Circulation* 65:1290, 1982.
3. Blackett, R.B., Woodhill, J.M., Leelarthaepin, B., Palmer, A.J. Type-IV hyperlipidemia and weight gain after maturity. *Lancet* 2:517, 1975.
4. Mishkel, M.A., Stein, E. Primary type-IV hyperlipoproteinemia. *In* "Hyperlipidemia: Diagnosis and Therapy" (B.M. Rifkind and R.I. Levy, eds.), pp. 177-202. Grune and Stratton, New York, 1977.
5. Swartz, R.S., Brunzell, J.D. Increase of adipose tissue lipoprotein lipase activity with weight loss. *J. Clin. Invest.* 67:1425, 1981.

6. Connor, W.E., Cerqueira, M.T., Connor, R.W., Wallace, R.B., Malinow, M.R., Casdorph, H.R. The plasma lipids, lipoproteins and diet of the Tarahumara Indians of Mexico. *Amer. J. Clin. Nutr.* 31:1131, 1978.

7. Glueck, C.J., Fallat, R.W., Millet, R., Gartside, P., Etston, R.C., Go, R.C.P. Familial hyperalphalipoproteinemia: studies in eighteen kindreds. *Metabolism* 24:1243, 1975.

8. Glueck, C.J., Gastside, P., Fallat, R.W., Sielski, J., Steiner, P.M. Longevity syndromes: familial hypobeata and familial hyperalphalipoproteinemia. *J. Lab. Clin. Med.* 88:941, 1976.

9. Knuiman, J.T., Hermus, R.J.J., Hautvast, J.G.A.J. Serum total and HDL cholesterol concentrations in rural and urban boys from 16 countries. *Atherosclerosis* 36:529, 1980.

10. Cerqueira, M.T., Fry, M.M., Connor, W.E. The food and nutrient intale of the Tarahumara Indians of Mexico. *Amer. J. Clin. Nutr.* 32:905, 1979.

11. Urban, M.C. The food and nutrient intake of the Tarahumara Indians of Mexico. M.S. Thesis, The University of Iowa, Iowa City, Iowa, 1975.

12. FAO/WHO Expert Committee. Energy and protein requirements. FAO/Nutrition Meetings, Rep. Ser. No. 52, WHO/Techn. Rep. Ser. No. 522, 1973.

13. McMurry, M.P., Connor, W.E., Cerqueira, M.T. Dietary cholesterol and the plasma lipids and lipoproteins in the Tarahumara Indians: A people habituated to a low cholesterol diet after weaning. *Amer. J. Clin. Nutr.* 35:741, 1982.

14. Connor, W.E., Hodges, R.E., Bleiler, R.E. The serum lipids in men receiving high cholesterol and cholesterol-free diets. *J. Clin. Invest.* 43:1691, 1964.

15. Lin, D.S., Connor, W.E. The long-term effects of dietary cholesterol upon the plasma lipids. Lipoproteins,a cholesterol absorption, and the sterol balance in man: the demonstration of feedback inhibition of cholesterol biosynthesis and increased bile acid excretion. *J. Lipid Res.* 21:1042, 1981.

16. Ziegler, E.E., Fomon, S.J. Infant feeding and blood lipid levels during childhood. *In* "Childhood Prevention of Atherosclerosis and Hypertension" (R.M. Lauer and R.B. Shekelle, eds.), pp. 121-125. Raven Press, New York, 1980.

17. Beveridge, J.M.R., Connell, W.B., Mayer, G.A., Haust, H.L. The response of man to dietary cholesterol. *J. Nutr.* 71:61, 1960.

18. Mattson, F.H., Erickson, B.A., Klingman, A.M. Effect of dietary cholesterol on serum cholesterol in man. *Am. J. Clin. Nutr.* 25:589, 1972.

19. Roberts, S.L., McMurry, M.P., Connor, W.E. Does egg feeding (i.e. dietary cholesterol) affect plasma cholesterol in man? The results of a double-blind study. *Am. J. Clin. Nutr.* 34:2092, 1981.

20. Connor, W.E. Dietary sterols: their relationship to atherosclerosis. *J. Am. Dietet. Assoc.* 52:202, 1968.

21. Connor, W.E., Connor, S.L. The dietary treatment of hyperlipidemia. *In* "Lipid Disorders" (R.J. Havel, ed.), Vol. 66, No. 2, pp. 485-518. Medical Clinics of North America, 1982.

22. Connor, S.L., Vaughan, S., Gustafson, J., Artaud-Wild, S. (unpublished data).

DISCUSSION[1]

Harper saw a paradox in that while hyperlipidemia was being considered as an index of bad health with a high correlation between coronary heart disease and blood cholesterol concentration in subjects below age 65, this situation

[1]*Summary of the discussion prepared by S. Frenk.*

prevailed just in the countries enjoying the highest life expectancy and consuming diets linked with a good health. On the other hand, identical life expectancies and adequate diets coexist with vastly different incidences of coronary disease. A deeper knowledge is needed on the interaction of diet and genetic constitution, as excellently manifested in the very early age group.

DISCUSSION[1]
THE MENDELIAN HYPERLIPIDEMIAS

A.G. Motulsky

University of Washington
Division of Medical Genetics
Seattle, Washington

The human geneticist is impressed by the tremendous variability of the human species. In fact, it can be stated that every human being on this planet is genetically unique. This can be demostrated with conditions such as HLA. Mankind is a very outbred species with many different kinds of variants.

What is the nature of this variability and how can we approach it from a genetic angle?

There are problems in a very simple approach. Normally we find a bell-shaped Gaussian distribution if we look at a given characteristic of the human population. For example, let us take lipids. Appropiate genetic studies show that such variability may have an underlying multifactorial polygenic kind of variability.

A different case is when a single gene is present in a high frequency in a population, and a large percentage of the population appears on a different mode. Familial hypercholesterolemia for instance, shows a bimodal curve when similar numbers of affected and normal individuals are registered. This type of curve, however, is rarely seen in a population unless the frequency of the single gene trait is very high.

To complicate matters further, it has been shown over the last ten years, that in many situations where the bell-shaped curve arises, it may be due to the addition of various curves of similar shape which overlap. This has been shown for a variety of serum and red cell enzymes, particularly where genetic variants are inherited as single genes. One variant represents a lower part of the curve, the low-capacity allele, another a mid-capacity allele and the third a high-capacity allele; a genetic variance at the same site in the genome.

[1]*Summary prepared by Isabel Pérez-Montfort*

Red cell acid phosphatase shows this kind of curve. If the enzyme is broken down into Form-A, Form-B and Form-C, the three overlapping curves can be clearly seen.

When talking about hyperlipidemia it must be kept in mind that one may not get at this hidden simple genic kind of variability unless better methods of determination are employed.

Simple genetic approaches such as breeding for high and low responders have been used. Mice have been bred for atherosclerosis succesfully, but the mechanism requires further analysis. In some cases one gene can be identified which contributes a fairly large amount to the total variance of a specific character. This makes genetic studies easier, but much needs to be learned about this yet.

What about some of the approaches in humans? Correlation of serum cholesterol levels within families is high in siblings, and non-existent in spouses. This points to genetic predetermination. If it were entirely genetically determined, however, correlation would be higher. As it is, it can only be suggested that genetic factors are present.

The best understood single-gene hyperlipidemia is hypercholesterolemia, an autosomal dominant trait. The lipoprotein is either II-A or II-B in heterozygotes, but diagnosis is difficult, because many other conditions with high cholesterol show the same lipoprotein types.

Heredity is clearly autosomal dominant. It shows up in infancy. Goldstein and Brown have shown that it affects a cell membrane receptor for low density lipoprotein. Clinically, the condition is important because about half the affected males have some aspect of coronary heart disease by age fifty. Women, however, even though affected by the gene in the same frequency, show heart disease symptoms ten to fifteen years later. So, there seems to be some protective effect in women who carry this particular gene. The condition is also related to other factors leading to coronary heart disease such as heavy smoking, high blood pressure and others. A person combining the gene and one or more of these factors is at a much earlier risk than others.

The trait occurs in many different populations. If the trait is studied in japanese populations, one finds that the level of cholesterol of the heterozygote japanese is very similar to that of the caucasian with the disease, in spite of the low background level of cholesterol in the japanese population. Diet does not seem to have much to do in this particular condition. It is interesting to know for researchers in this area, that a rabbit strain with what looks like an identical receptor mutation has been identified in Japan. Many experiments are being done on it, which could be done on man.

There is probably significant underdiagnosis of the condition, because diagnosis is not easy. The demostration of the defect requires a research technique. In a study done on patients with myocardial infarct, about 5% appear to carry the gene.

Now, there are at least two kinds of mutations causing this condition, one that leads to complete defect in binding and another one that leads to partial defect in binding. This may serve as a model as follows: for a given enzyme or receptor specified by a gene, there are a series of isoalleles, that is, alleles of different functional capacity for receptor activity. Recent studies have identidified the severe deficiency and heritability to normal receptor activity. Also, there may be low, medium and high receptor activity, all within the normal range. This could mean that the low receptor activity could resemble familial hypercholesterolemia, and the gene frequency of this low-capacity allele may be significant.

The point is that, as Dr. Connor mentioned, the way people respond to a diet may have something to do with a monogenic variation, an isoallelic variation at a locus first demonstrated by a severe genetic deficiency. With the advent of DNA techniques, it may become easier to isolate the gene and then be able to test for it by these techniques rather than by biochemical techniques that look at the phenotype.

Another model may be set up with a condition called *familial combined hyperlipidemia*. It is also called *familial hyperlipoprotein with multiple lipoprotein types* because within the same family different lipoproteins show increased levels. It is probably more common than familial hypercholesterolemia. It seems to mendelize as an autosomal dominant character, but since it does not show up until the late twenties or thirties, family studies are difficult. Large families are necessary, and since the condition clearly leads to accelerated atherosclerosis, there are frequent young deaths. Recently it has been found, that families presumably affected by this condition show a bimodal curve of apolipoprotein-B. This could be a better marker than other lipoprotein types. One possibility is that the lesion is an abnormality in very low-density lipoprotein synthesis with different distributions of apolipoprotein-B. Studied in depth, this condition might serve as a model to help us understand some of the more frequent kinds of hyperlipidemia.

A different kind of genetic approach might be called pharmacogenetic approach. The principle behind it is that treatement of a given hyperlipidemia may vary with its biochemical nature. That is, a standard diet may have different effects on different types of hyperlipidemia. Much work needs to be done on this.

Another genetic approach is based on human genetic variability. This can be shown in many cases to be biochemical of a different nature. Apolipoprotein variants have been related to hyperlipoproteinemia. By looking for polymorphisms, such as the A-B-O blood groups, which seem to be pathophysiologically related to hyperlipidemia one might be able to construct the genetic background against which major genes may be acting. Cholesterol level varies depending on various factors. For instance, homozygotes for apolipoprotein-E have a much lower cholesterol level than heterozygotes for this particular variant, and they, in turn, have a lower level than the main population. As to the A-B-O blood groups, nonsecretors have a somewhat higher cholesterol level, the same as people with half the alpha-2 globin gene and those with GMA, another serum group system.

Of particular interest is a serologic polymorphism called LPA poly morphism. People with LPA-plus have a higher cholesterol level. In fact, Burkes has shown that people who are LPA-plus, contrasted with those who are not LPA-plus, have two to three times the rate of coronary heart disease.

Practically, this means that preventive measures might be extremely useful to treat high-risk individuals. From a clinical-medical point of view one could take relatives of premature coronary heart disease patients, test them for these conditions, and start them on an appropiate diet very early in life to defer the onset of the disease.

There are three conditions that are clearly genetic: hyperlipidemia, diabetes and hypertension. Family studies have shown that familial aggregation of coronary heart disease is not entirely accounted for by these main genetic risk factors. Other genetic factors influencing the familial aggregation are not clear. Also, there are probably environmental factors which have some influence on familial aggregation as well.

DISCUSSION[1]

Neel considered that his position had been misrepresented, since in his presentation he did not suggest that appropriate measures for management of individuals suffering from rare diseases with a simple monogenic basis should be neglected. Rather he emphasized that since multigenic inherited diseases are so common, the implementation of vigorous measures for the general population would exert a maximum impact on predisposed individuals and at the same time be more cost-effective than trying to screen out those subjects and to submit every one of them to an appropriate regime. Motulsky agreed on this, but pointed out that if those regimens are complex, then it did make sense to involve special detection methods for such a small proportion of the population. However, the problem of defining the cut-off points for the individuals who for genetic reasons have different nutritional requirements and are therefore in need of a special management still awaits solution. Harper manifested his skepticism about the approach of focusing the control of a certain disease on the basis of a mass population approach. Rather, the identification of genetically susceptible subgroups merits the highest priority; secondarily, one could deal with the distinction between the direct consequences of disease occurring in a small fraction of the population starting at an early age, and those of the aging process *per se*.

[1]*Summary of the discussion prepared by S. Frenk.*

VICTUALS AND VERSABILITY: A DISCUSSION

William J. Schull

Center for Demographic and Population Genetics
Graduate School of Biomedical Sciences
University of Texas Health Science Center
Houston, Texas

Rhubarb: (a) a broad leafed, Asiatic plant of the genus Rheum whose thick, fleshy leaf-stalks are cooked and eaten as a fruit; (b) a heated dispute or controversy (colloquial).

There seems to me something wryly appropriate to this Workshop about these two disparate meanings of a term most commonly associated with a perennial garden herb (Rheum rhaponticum) brought to Europe from Russia and the East, more specifically Tibet many centuries ago. First, it is not commonly recognized now that when originally introduced rhubarb was valued primarily for its medicinal uses. A dried extract of the rhizomes of this plant served as a purgative and paradoxically, or so it might seem as a treatment for diarrhea in England in the Renaissance. It was, of course, also eaten, indeed some 12 different species were or have been, but not apparently without some risks. Two centuries ago, for example, William Coxe [5] wrote:

The stalks of the leaves are eaten raw by the Tartars: they produce upon most persons, who are unaccustomed to them, a kind of spasmodic contraction of the throat, which goes off in a few hours; it returns however at every meal, until they become habituated to this kind of diet. The Russians make use of the leaves in their hodge-podge: accordingly, soups of this sort affect strangers in the manner above mentioned. (p. 337).

The symptoms he described may have been induced by the dangerously high amount of oxalic acid known to be present is some species of rhubarb, and which putatively at least, has been incriminated in the deaths of a number of children. Ostensibly harm arises through an interference with calcium metabolism and death, when it ensues, may be the result of renal failure [21]. But rhubarb also contains a variety of derivatives of 1,8-dihydroxyanthracene such as chrysophanic (dimethylanthraquinone) and erythrosic acid as well as a number of tannins, and illustrates well the metabolic complexities associated with the digestion of many plant substances. Its seeming paradoxic medicinal uses are a case in point. As a purgative, rhubarb's potency is directly proportional to its content of the conjugated form of rhein (1,8-dihydroxyanthroquinone-3-carboxylic acid), for normally the glucosides and quinone derivatives occur in lesser amounts in the plant than the tannins. Thus, the cathartic effect, ascribable to the anthraquinones, occurs only at larger doses whereas at smaller ones the tannins with their anti-diarrheal action prevail.

Second, disputatious though it may seem, there is a need to distinguish here between the study of those diseases, such as phenylketonuria, which as we have heard [4], may provide useful and important insights into metabolism and those disorders, e.g., lactose intolerance, favism and celiac disease, which impose or may impose much more formidable public health burdens because of their frequencies. While the former diseases are admittedly catastrophic insofar as the affected individual and his or her family is concerned, they are not singly nor collectively an important, global health problem. Our intellectual and material resource investments, however, tend not to reflect this public health imperative. As support for this assertion consider Table 1 which stems from a perusal of the Cumulated Index Medicus. Table I make two points. First, it will be noted that there has been a two-fold increase in biomedical citations overall in the last 20 years but an abolute or at least a relative decline with time in research on the nutritional disorders of which we speak. Second, there has clearly been a paucity of interest in the role genetic factors have played in

Table I. Articles indexed in the Cumulated Index Medicus under the indicated rubrics. The numbers in parentheses refer to manuscripts which are clearly genetic in orientation.

Year	Favism	Celiac Disease Gluten-Sensitive Enteropathy	Lactose Intolerance	Phenyl-ketonuria	Total Articles Indexed[a]
1960	23[b](1.5)	92 (3.5)	- -[c]	49 (4.0)	125,000
1965	18 (0.5)	94 (1.0)	- -	104 (10.0)	171,000
1970	15 (2.0)	96 (1.0)	53 (1.3)	124 (11.7)	210,000
1975	6 (0.3)	99 (2.0)	46 (4.7)	99 (11.7)	225,000
1980	3 (1.0)	77 (3.0)	48 (2.5)	85 (5.0)	254,000

[a]Articles indexed in the stated year, rounded to the nearest thousand.
[b]Articles under this rubric averaged over two (1960, 1980) or three years (1965, 1970, 1975), rounded to the nearest integer.
[c]This rubric did not exist in the years 1960, 1965.

their etiology. It can, of course, be argued that the modes of inheritance for phenylketonuria and sensitivity to the fava bean were already known in 1960, despite the disproportionate number of genetic publications seen in Table I, but this argument certainly does not apply to celiac disease or lactose malabsorption.

Many caveats to a simple interpretation of these data come to mind. Citations are equated to research work and this may not be strictly so. Moreover, the Index Medicus doesn't cite *all* of the world's biomedical research. How this may influence the results you see is uncertain, but then I'm interested only in relative effort not an absolute measure and this would seem less sensitive to some of the perturbing forces which can be identified. Finally, what is here called genetic represents either those citations under genetic or hereditary influences as a sub-heading within the individual rubrics or have been so classified by my scrutiny of the title of the individual paper. Again, these numbers may be in error somewhat but there is no reason to believe I have overlooked genetic papers preferentially by disease. These demurrers notwithstanding, it is obvious that surprisingly little research has been and is being done on these disorders, and of the research which has been undertaken little is of a genetic nature.

Rosenberg stated, "It seems certain that the extreme variations in nutritional requirements demonstrated by patients with inborn errors of metabolism bear witness to less extreme, but far more common, variation in nutritional needs found among and between different populations". I call your attention to this remark now, not solely because I believe it to be true and as a statement it has been felicitously put, but because it is a theme on which I propose to enlarge. My remarks will necessarily be speculative; virtually nothing is known about the nature-nurture interactions to which I will call your attention. The specific examples cited may-or-may not prove to be of importance ultimately. No brief is held for anyone; they are offered only to titillate.

There is an extensive and growing list of toxic factors known to occur in plants. These may be stimulants or depressants, induce hypoglycemia, inhibit absorption of vitamins or enzyme activity and influence metal-binding to cite but a few of their effects on man and his domestic animals. Neither time nor my competence allows a measured view of their collective impact on nutrition and ultimately health. We shall consider, therefore, a single class of these factors, the cholinesterase inhibitors. They are found in such diverse foodstuffs as broccoli, sugar beets, asparagus, eggplants, potatoes, celery, radishes, turnips, carrots, oranges, apples and raspberries [23]. Little is actually known about the chemistry of these natural inhibitors of cholinesterase with the single exception of the glycoalkaloid, solanine. The latter is found in greater or lesser extent in most potatoes, commercial varieties as well as wild species. It is apparently not destroyed by cooking but seemingly is by the primitive freeze-drying techniques used by the Aymara and Quechua of the Andes in the preparation of chuño negro and tunta, their traditional preserved foods. We've recognized for 20 years that this "potato inhibitor" is as effective as dibucaine in the inhibition of cholinesterase activity and hence in the recognition of different alleles at the pseudocholinesterase locus [12]. It is one of these alleles, of course, the so-called "atypical" one which is involved in suxamethonium sensitivity (a once commonly used muscle relaxant in surgical procedures; see [11] for a fuller explanation). Surprisingly little is known about the frequency of the "atypical" allele in Amerindian populations or many others too for that matter. Nor do we know whether individuals homozygous for this allele are sensitive to the cholinesterase inhibitors present in other plants. Given the natural pervasiveness of these substances and our possible increased exposure to those present in such insecticides as aldicarb, it is reasonable to be alarmed about exposures which may be cumulatively substantial, albeit small from any one source. Unfortunately, organizations such as our Environmental Protection Agency focus their concern upon single source exposures rather than cumulative ones, a more difficult task admittedly.

This brings me to a plea, an oft repeated one. Nevin Scrimshaw spoke of an individual who found eggs indigestible (at least relatively). Interestingly, Brunton [3] in his century-old treatise on Disorders of Digestion also called attention to the indigestibility of eggs for some individuals and speculated that it might be due to lecithin. He also noted, ". . . it is more difficult to say why milk should in some persons, prove poisonous. Milk also contains lecithin, but in small quantity; and all we can say about it at present is that, in some individuals, a poison is probably formed from it, which causes it to disagree." It is noteworthy that this comment precedes Jacobi's recognition of the bases for lactose intolerance in children by almost two decades [18, 20], and stems from an observation on a population where lactose intolerance is rare, presumably. The plea I wish to make to our nutritionally oriented colleagues is not to discard their atypical responders once they have satisfied themselves such responses are not artifacts of technique and the like, but to cherish them and more importantly to initiate family studies which may reveal whether a given response is inherited.

We are, even now aware of genetic differences which could affect the absorption of food or the receptivity of the gut to parasites but whose effects are, in fact, often unknown. Hillman [14] describes a number of inherited defects in the transport processes for small molecules in the intestine. Specifically, he cites the malabsorption of glucose and galactose, tryptophane, cystine, lysine, arginine and the water soluble vitamins, notably those of the B-complex. He pointedly notes that, "Since both the affinity for a particular substance and its maximal rate of transport may be genetically determined, it should, be expected that the impact of mal-nutrition in specific individuals and in specific populations may well be determined by inherited differences in the intestinal transport systems." Wostmann [38] has reminded us that man's gut is also the home of other organisms whose nutrient and energy needs interact with his own. Our bacterial flora produce smaller molecules from larger ones and may thereby facilitate transport across the intestine; however, when nutritional stress occurs, the microflora may worsen matters because of their own energy needs.

There are, of course, many enzymic systems whose roles in these processes remain speculative. Thus, an inherited sucrose and isomaltose intolerance has been reported, ostensibly an outgrowth of a deficiency of isomaltase and sucrase [36]. On a normal diet, these individuals have a persistent chronic diarrhea with frothy and liquid acid stools. How does a defect such as this impinge on the natural microflora of the intestine and what effect might it have on their normal role in the transport systems of the intestine? As another illustration, consider alkaline phosphatase. This enzyme occurs in at least three forms, one of which is intestinal. It is measurable in serum or plasma where its concentration is dependent upon the age of the individual and is functionally related fo fat absorption. The hormones secretin and cholecystokinin-pancreomyzin have been shown to release alkaline-phosphatase from the brush border into the lumen of the small intestine. Bayer and Polntner [1] have recently suggested that one of the mechanisms whereby somatostatin inhibits intestinal fat absorption is through the inhibition of intestinal alkaline phosphatase. What role, if any does this enzyme have in celiac disease? Or the occurrence of malignancies of the bowel? There is mounting albeit still equivocal evidence that malignancies generally, but lymphomas in particular are more common among the first degree relatives of individuals with celiac disease than would be expected on the basis of the age, sex and ethnic origins of the probands [10, 13, 15, 16].

As the final encouragement for a greater interest in nature-nurture interactions let me describe a situation where the geneticist and nutritionist might profitably interact to examine the nutritional implications of an unusual set of ecological circumstances. Irrigation and the rivers which arise in the mountains to the east make green many of the coastal valleys of northern Chile which lie within the Andean rain shadow. Trade winds and the stationary Pacific high to the west contribute a salubrious climate. Seasonal differences as well as the diurnal temperature cycle are small. Rain rarely falls. Eastward is the sierra. Villages here are at elevations of 3-3,500 meters. Partial oxygen pressure is approximately 100 mm. Rain, though markedly seasonal, occurs with increasing intensity from 2,500 meters upwards. Temperatures are substantially lower than on the coast, and often vary by more than 30°C between one sunrise and the next. The soil is poor and crops less diverse than in the coastal valleys. Still further eastward is the altiplano, a rolling high plain framed on the east and west by mountains which occasionally exceed 6,000 meters. Daily temperatures commonly oscillate as much as 30°C and still greater changes have been recorded. Snowfall is slight, except in the high mountains, and is confined almost exclusively to the rainy season. There are virtually no trees, save the tortuous quenua and the coarse grass and shrubby growth rarely attains a meter's height. It is a somber, yet majestic land, a land uneasy with itself, agitated by earthquakes and thrusting tectonic plates, and presided over by Guallatiri, the loftiest of the world's active volcanos. Out of this turmoil flow untold minerals-arsenic, boron, copper, lithium, potassium, sodium and sulfur to mention but a few. Their salts color the soil, taint the waters, and burden the flora and fauna.

We know the Aymara, the indigenous people of the Andean altiplano of Bolivia, Chile and Peru, to be well adapted to the hypoxia and hypocapnia which prevail at these altitudes [9, 33]. While numerous physiological and clinical measures attest to this adaptation, the underlying biochemical changes are poorly understood. We presume, however that ultimately changes in oxygen transport, or tissue utilization, or both must be involved. This adaptation did not, indeed could not have proceeded without regard to other aspects of this environment which impinge on health and reproductivity. It is these latter to which we direct your attention.

The principal foodstuffs of the Aymara are potatoes, oca and similar tubers, and quinoa supplemented to some extent with the meat of alpaca and llama. As we have already noted, their potatoes contain solanine, and many of the varieties and species they cultivate have amounts which exceed American and European standards for toxicity. The chuño negro and tunta they eat may be largely free of this glycoalkaloid, but fresh potatoes or those merely boiled are not. To the extent the latter are consumed there is a risk. Quinoa also occurs in a number of different varieties, commonly distinguished by color and taste [35]. The seeds of this plant are ground to provide a flour or eaten porridge-like. The husks contain saponin, a triserpenoid, once commonly used as an intestinal vermifuge. Important here, however, is the fact that saponins are extremely powerful hemolytic agents, and very dilute concentrations can produce conspicuous hemolysis. While saponins are apparently poorly, or virtually never absorbed at the intestinal level, presumably absorption may occur occasionally, and if so its consequences may be profound. It seems reasonable to presume that absorption may be more probable in a gut already compromised by malnutrition, parasites and recurrent episodes of diarrhea. Recently, their children have been exposed to powdered milk and dairy products, largely through food supplementation programs in schools. Although the data are limited, the Aymara are undoubtedly intolerant of lactose, since most Amerindians are [20]. Ruben Lisker [24] has described the role of genetic factors in this disorder and called attention to some of the health consequences of lactose malabsorption.

Woven through these individual challenges to health is lithium. The latter is widely albeit not abundantly distributed throughout the earth's crust. It is easily removed from rocks and sediments in weathering and tends to remain in solution because of the high solubility of most of its common compounds. Lithium can affect plant growth and development, sometimes adversely and somes beneficially. Some plants, among these are members of the families *Chenopodiaceae* and *Solanaceae,* tolerate large amounts of lithium. Potatoes and quinoa, both Andean staples as we have indicated, belong to these families. Of course, not all lithium of food is absorbed by the intestine; indeed, it is generally believed that water may constitute the major source of lithium for man and animals since medicinal lithium salts in drinking water are completely absorbed.

Toxic and adverse responses to therapeutic doses of lithium are frequent. These are of a variety of kinds; we are here concerned only with a few, namely, its effects on thyroid function and carbohydrate metabolism, and impingement on those enzymatic processes requiring magnesium or calcium. Any enzyme involved in the utilization or generation of ATP, the energy currency of metabolism, is potentially liable to lithium action because the active form of ATP is the ATP-Mg complex, and lithium is able to compete with magnesium in the formation of this complex. We do not know whether the effects on thyroid function and carbohydrate metabolism are manifest at an exposure of one milligram or so of elemental lithium per liter of water (the levels seen in numerous rivers inthe north of Chile), but an impingement on ATP production can be clearly demonstrated at these exposures.

Four lines of evidence can be mustered to show that the membrane transport of lithium is under genetic control. First, *in vivo* and *in vitro* intrapair differences in red blood cell uptake of lithium are smaller, on the average, in identical than in non-identical twins [7]. Second, there has recently been described a manic patient and some members of his family whose red blood cells revealed little or no evidence of the phloretin-sensitive Li/Na+ counterflow system which characterizes erythrocytes [28]. Third, although lithium therapy produces dramatic improvement in those individuals whom it helps, failures to respond do occur in the treatment of bipolar patients, that is, those with periods of both mania and depression. It has been found that response to lithium is significantly correlated with the presence of bipolar illness in the first degree relatives of an affected individual which argues that responsiveness is inherited [26]. Finally, we ourselves have observations that indicate the within family variability in plasma concentrations of lithium is significantly less than the between family variability. While this observation is a necessary condition for a trait to be inherited, it is not a sufficient one. Environmental factors of potential importance, diet for one, are also doubtlessly correlated. However, it appears that the intrafamily similarity persists even when family members live apart, although our evidence on this point is quite limited at present. Thus we have an interacting, multidimensional system which involves the foods these individuals eat, the water they drink, and the genes with which they are endowed. How does one separate the various signals - genetic and non-genetic -under the circumstances I have so briefly described?

Suppose, now, some of these speculations prove insightful, what is to be done to mitigate the public health burden so revealed? Health care costs escalate; containment grows progressively more imperative but difficult. Prevention of ill-health must be emphasized even more than it has been. The challenge resides, or so it seems to me in the development of new strategies of intervention which achieve these ends more cost effectively. One of the more novel approaches to the mitigation or prevention of the effects of inherited food idiosyncrasies is through plant and to a lesser extent, animal husbandry. To be successful this entails the identification and elimination through selective breeding of the substance or substances which prompt the toxic responses. Two illustrations will serve to demonstrate the feasibility of this approach. First, rapeseed, more properly the oil derived from these seeds is an important cooking ingredient in numerous areas of the world.

Occasionally, toxic, indeed fatal responses to the use of this oil have occurred. Where this has obtained, and the source of the toxicity was clearly not some inadvertent contamination of the oil with pesticides or the like, the biochemical culprit has been shown to be a natural constituent, erucic acid (cis-13-docosenoic acid), which normally makes up some 40-50%, of the total fatty acids found in rape, mustard and wallflower seeds. Through selective breeding, it has been possible to develop rape varieties which have either no erucic acid, or amounts lower than those presently, readily measurable.

Another similar illustration involves cottonseed oil. It has been suggested that the protein derived from cottonseed meal could contribute importantly to the world's needs. However, cottonseed meal contains a toxic yellow pigment, gossypol, as well as other closely allied pigments such as gossycaerulin, gossypurpurin and gossyfulion. While some of the adverse physiological effects, particulary of gossypol itself, may be offset by the use of certain minerals, especially iron salts, it is not clear whether differences exist among individuals either in the nature of the toxic response to gossypol or in the amount of gossypol which must be ingested before adverse physiological responses are apparent. Common among these responses are depressed appetite and intestinal irritation.

Gossypol and its related pigments are elaborated in glands contained in the tissue of the seed and may have a role in insect resistance. It has been possible to breed glandless seed, but such plants also lack glands in the flowers and elsewhere and seem prone to insect infestations. Efforts are now afoot to develop a plant which retains the glands which produce gossypol in the flower (which is not eaten) but lacks glands in the seed. Presumably, thereby, the toxicity would be removed but the insect resistance retained (see [2] for a much fuller discussion of these developments).

Second, and more important from a nutritional standpoint is the matter of potatoes (Solanum tuberosum) and solanine to which we have already referred briefly. Shortly after the introduction into Europe of the potato as a foodstuff instances of fatal, potato poisoning began to appear and still occur periodically [31, 37]. It was shown, in time, that the probable toxic agent was solanine, a glycoalkaloid, but chaconine, a closely related compound, one which like solanine is derivable from the alkaloidal aglycone, solanidine may also be involved. While these glycoalkaloids can be found in most tissues of the normal potato plant, it is generally conceded that the highest content is associated with potato sprouts. Presumably, the common culinary practices of discarding the sprouts and excising the eyes of the potato are empirically derived responses to this distribution of solanine and chaconine.

Potato breeders have shown that species and even varieties within a species of potatoes differ in their solanine and chaconine contents, and while temperature and other growing conditions can influence the amounts of solanine in a given potato, there remains a more-or-less characterizable species or varietal level. Somewhat differently put, the glycoalkaloid content of a potato appears highly heritable. At present, none of the commercial varieties are completely devoid of these compounds and those potatoes found to contain over 0.2% solanine are considered to be toxic. Today, in most countries such as England, Germany, Russia and the United States where potatoes are extensively cultivated, the certification of a variety for commercial purposes rests on a demonstration that its solanine content is within the nontoxic limits. Thus the content itself is one of the myriad attributes which must be borne in mind by the breeder and grower; nonetheless, occasionally important commercial varieties, such as Lenape (B5141-6), have had their certifications withdrawn because their solanine content consistently exceeded 200 mg/100 g of potato. A fuller account of glycoalkaloid content of potatoes and the factors which affect this content will be found in Maga [25].

Traditional plant breeding techniques, dependent as they have often been upon generations of breeding and selection of diploids, and thus segregating organisms have been time-consuming, but recent developments hold promise of a more rapid achievement of the breeder's aims. Thus, anther culture, more precisely pollen culture when coupled with other equally new advances in plant breeding techniques could make possible a relatively quick development of wheat strains, for example, which are either non-toxic or substantially less toxic than those presently available to the gluten sensitive individual. Indeed, more than a decade ago Chinese investigators obtained regenerated haploid plants from *Triticum aestivum* [27] and *Triticum triticale* [34] as well as such other important plants as sweet peppers *(Capsicum annum)*, maize *(Zea mays)*, eggplant *(Solanum melanogena)* and rapeseed. Hu [17] has asserted that new cereal varieties can now be developed in four or five years. Clearly, then, haploid breeding proves in practice to be a quickly effective technique for improvement of crops. While the plant breeder has generally marched to an economic drum, and sought improvements in yield more frequently than an alteration in plant composition, there certainly have been exceptions and these could be more common in the future.

We have emphasized thus far advances which might be achieved through the genetic manipulation of the plants we eat, presumably similar, albeit less dramatic strides could be achieved through animal husbandry - less dramatic for at least two reasons. First, we have as yet no animal counterpart to anther culture and the rapid establishment of homozygous lines it forfends. Presumably, however, even if similar methods obtained for animals we would still have to contend, second, with the inbreeding depression which has always loomed so large in past efforts to establish homozygous lines of cattle or pigs, for example. This depression has not been so important generally in plant breeding but this may be merely happenstance or reflect the fact that so many commercially important crops, particularly the grasses are predominantly self-pollinators. Finally, animal protein, at least that derived from domesticated animals constitutes so small a fraction of mankind's foods globally that the public health impact of manipulating the quality of animal foods seems unlikely to be large.

A rhubarb is a heated dispute you will recall, but we have seen little of this thus far. Differences of perspective have emerged, but have been bridged amicably. If a deep-seated difference exists, it must lie in the nature of nutritional recommendations. Until recently, nutritionists and nutritional epidemiologists have been so egalitarian in their approach to our collective and individual nutritional requirements that traditionally confidence limits are not even placed on their estimates of the latter. While the philosophic bases for confidence limits and those on which a presumption of inter-individual differences rest are admittedly not the same, the advocacy of a single set of nutritional needs is about as defensible in the Twentieth Century as a single valued norm for our anatomies, or oxygen requirements, or blood pressure. How are we to reconcile, then a need for nutritional guidelines, on the one hand, with an acknowledgment of important inter-individual differences, on the other? Payne [29] has addressed this issue, but possibly not to the full satisfaction of all of the geneticists present. Minimum requirements are undoubtedly a first step, but only if those minima take into account the personal differences of which we speak. But even minima fail to provide for the hyper-responders, that is, those individuals who are, in a sense, intoxicated in the presence of plenty. Is not an inelastic approach to nutritional needs responsible, at least in part for the somewhat belated concern about the dangers inherent in dairy supplements in populations where lactose intolerant children are common, or the use of Similac and its subsequent imitators where maternally-mediated immunity is important in infant survival? What justification ever existed for those extravagant statements of my childhood which made eggs, milk and tomatoes the paragons of food? And no superlative could adequately describe cream of tomato soup!

We are social animals and surely our choices of food rest not solely on need. We taste things differently, and these differences have intrigued geneticists for a half century or more; certainly at least since Fox [8] first demonstrated inherited differences in the capacity to taste phenylthiocarbamide (PTC). His studies spawned a search for other seemingly simply inherited differences. But this search was soon dampened by evidence that (a) the inheritance of these differences was not so simple as first conjectured and (b) a failure to establish a clear selective basis for their existence. Evidence has been advanced, of course, which purports to establish a relationship between PTC tasting and the occurrence of non-toxic goiter, but these data are often conflicting and unpersuasive. Purely as a paradigm, however, this uncertain relationship warrants further scrutiny. Our food preferences are unquestionably shaped by societal values as well as individual perceptions of tastiness. How soon in life the latter are established is unclear but surely deserves study for the contribution such differences could make to the understanding of nutritional needs.

Let me close this discussion on a note of levity. Recently, in a moment's idle reading, I came across the following dietary admonition. "The best general rule for diet that I can write, is to eat and drink only of such foods -at such times-and in such quantities -as experience has convinced you, agree with your constitution- and absolutely avoid all others." These are words of William Kitchener written over a century and a half ago in a book he graciously dedicated to the "nervous and bilious."

REFERENCES

1. Bayer, P.M. and Pointner, H. Action of somatostatin on intestinal alkaline phosphatase stimulated by secretin and cholecystokininpancreozymin. *Clin. Chim. Acta* 108:129, 1980.
2. Berardi, L.C. and Goldblatt, L.A. Gossypol. *In* "Toxic Constituents of Plant Foodstuffs" (I.E. Liener, ed.), pp. 184-237. Academic Press, New York, 1980.
3. Brunton, T.L. "Disorders of Digestion: Their Consequences and Treatment," MacMillan and Co., London, 1886.
4. Cederbaum. S. Phenylketonuria. In this volume, 1982.
5. Coxe, W. "Account of the Russian Discoveries between Asia and America," T. Cadell, in the Strand, London, 1780.
6. Dorus, E., Pandey, G.N., and Davis, J.M. Genetic determinant of lithium ion distribution. II. An in vitro and in vivo monozygotic-dizygotic twin study. *Arch. Gen. Psychiat.* 32:1097, 1975.
7. Dorus, E., Pandey, G.N., Frazer, A., and Mendels, J. Genetic determinant of lithiun ion distribution. I. An in vitro monozygotic-dizygotic twin study. *Arch. Gen. Psychiat.* 31:463, 1974.
8. Fox, A. L. The relationship between chemical constitution and taste. *Proc. Natl. Acad. Sci.* 18:115, 1932.
9. Frisancho, R. Functional adaptation to high altitude hypoxia. *Science* 187:313, 1975.
10. Gough, K. R., Read, A. E., and Naish, J. M. Intestinal reticulosis as a complication in idiopathic steatorrhea. *Gut* 3:232, 1962.
11. Harris, H. "The Principles of Human Biochemical Genetics," North-Holland-American Elsevier, New York, 1971.
12. Harris, H. and Whittaker, M. Differential response of human serum cholinesterase types to an inhibitor in potato. *Nature* 183:1808, 1959.
13. Harris, O. D., Cooke, W. T., Thompson, H., and Waterhouse, J.A.H. Malignancy in adult celiac disease and idiopathic steatorrhea. *Am. J. Med.* 42:899, 1967.
14. Hillman, R. E. Genetic aspects of nutrient absorption and transport. *In* this volume, 1982.
15. Holmes, G.K.T., Cooper, B. T., and Cooper, W. T. Malignant lymphoma in coeliac disease. *In* "Perspectives in Coeliac Disease" (B. McNicholl, C. F. McCarthy, and P. F. Fottrell, eds.), pp. 301-309. MTP Press, Lancaster, England, 1978.
16. Holmes, G.K.T., Stokes, P. L., Sorahan, T. M., et al. Coeliac disease, gluten-free diet, and malignancy. *Gut* 17:612, 1976.
17. Hu, H. Advances in anther culture investigations in China. *In* "Proceedings of Symposium on Plant Tissue Culture, May 25-30, 1978," pp. 3-10. *Science Press,* Peking, 1978.
18. Jacobi, A. Milk-sugar in infant feeding. *Trans. Am. Pediatr. Soc.* 13:150, 1901.
19. Jefferson, J. W. and Griest, J. H. "Primer of Lithium Therapy." The Williams and Wilkins Co., Baltimore, 1977.
20. Johnson, J. D., Kretchmer, N., and Simoons, F. J. Lactose malabsorption: Its biology and history. *Advances in Pediatrics* 21:197, 1974.
21. Kingsbury, J. M. "Poisonous Plants of the United States and Canada." Prentice-Hall, Inc., Englewood Cliffs, N.J., 1974.
22. Kitchener, W. "The Art of Invigorating and Prolonging Life." Hurst, Robinson and Co., London, 1822.
23. Liener, I. E. Miscellaneous toxic factors. *In* Toxic Constituents of Plant Foodstuffs" (I. E. Liener, ed.), pp. 429-467, Second Edition. Academic Press, New York, 1980.
24. Lisker, R. Lactase deficiency. *In* this volume, 1982.
25. Maga, J. A. Potato glycoalkaloids. *CRC Critical Reviews in Food Science and Nutrition* 12:371, 1979.
26. Mendelwicz, J., Fieve, R. R., Stallone, F., et al. Genetic history as a predictor of lithium response in manic-depressive illness. *Lancet* i:599, 1972.
27. Ouyang, T. W., Hu, H., Chuang, G. G., and Tseng, C. C. Induction of pollen plants from anther of *Triticum aestivum L.* in culture in vitro. *Scientia Sinica* 16:79, 1973.

28. Pandey, G. N., Ostrow, D. G., Haas, M., Dorus, E., Casper, R. C., Davis, J. M., and Toteson, D. C. Abnormal lithium and sodium transport in erythrocytes of a manic patient and some members of his family. *Proc. Natl. Acad. Sci.* 74:3607, 1977.
29. Payne, P. R. Variability of nutrient requirements. *In* this volume, 1982.
30. Rosenberg, L. E. Inborn errors of metabolism as methodological tools. *In* this volume, 1982.
31. Salaman, R. N. "The History and Social Influence of the Potato." University Press, Cambridge, 1949.
32. Schull, W. J. Food, water, and genes. *Fukuoka Acta Medica* 71:47, 1980.
33. Schull, W. J. and Rothhammer, F. A multinational Andean genetic and health programme: A study of adaptation to the hypoxia of altitude. *In* "Genetic and Nongenetic Components in Physiological Variability" (J. S. Weiner, ed.), pp. 139-139. Society for the Study of Human Biology, London, 1977.
34. Sun, C. S. Study of the cell biology of male pollen development in Triticum triticale. *Botanical Reports* 15:163, 1973.
35. Vargas, D. "Plantas Andinas." Universitaria, Santiago, 1972.
36. Weijers, H. A., Van de Kamer, J. H., Mossell, D.A.A., and Dicke, W. K. Diarrhoea caused by deficiency of sugar splitting enzymes. *Lancet* ii:296, 1960.
37. Wilson, G. S. A small outbreak of solanine poisoning. *Monthly Bulletin Minister of Health* (London) 18:207, 1959.
38. Wostmann, B. S. Intestinal flora and nutrient requirements. *In* this volume, 1982.

DISCUSSION[1]

According to Motulsky, Schull's talk raised a very important topic which is often overlooked. The frequency distribution of different alleles of a number of enzymes could be explained by a sort of "plant mechanism" in the past.

One of these enzymes is serum cholinesterase which is inhibited by solanine from potatoes. Testing for frequency of this enzyme, he found 3% heterozygotes in European population, but practically none in African black and Oriental populations, which is difficult to explain in terms of selection.

There is a very interesting serum enzyme, called paraoxonase, which has recently received much attention. The natural substrate of this enzyme is unknown, but it happens to work on an artificial substance, paraoxon, a poison which is a very potent cholinesterase inhibitor. Paraoxon is the first product of parathion —a widely used insecticide— and the enzyme breaks it down to nontoxic substances. Half the European population are homozygotes for the low-activity allele of paraoxonase and the gene frequency in the population is 0.7. In African and Oriental populations as well as in 300 recently examined Mexicans, it has not been possible to find the same allele as in Europeans. It is conceivable that some plant poisons might have led to selection of this particular polimorphism; there are other enzymes with unknown substrates probably selected in the past by plant factors we do not currently understand.

[1]*Summary of the discussion prepared by H. Bourges*

Cohen called the attention to a particular genetic anomaly. A Japanese agricultural scientist from Kobi studied ornithine transcarbamilase in chicken kidneys and, through 20 or 30 crossbreeds, obtained enzyme variants from low to high activity in what may be considered as an amazing documentation of the genetic impact on enzyme level. Ornithine transcarbamilase is apparently out of place in the kidney and in the chicken; it has no known function and one must ask, why this metabolic burden? This bizarre situation —Cohen stressed— leads to the question of how much vestigial genetic information is carried on, that is perhaps expressed under unusual circumstances. Why is the DNA of the chicken doing that? Are there comparable examples in the human, nor yet uncovered because we do not know how to look for these vestigial potential activities?.

Cerderbaum then expressed his opinion that we should not use the term vestigial but "beyond our comprehension ability" and referred to the case of red blood cell arginase. This enzyme is very abundant in human RBC as well as in the erythrocytes of all higher primates, except the baboon, but it is not present in lower mammals. This enzyme is able to lower arginine levels in the RBC, from high to undetectable amounts; although its function is not know, it works, it is not just sitting there. One has to think that evolutionary pressures selected this enzyme.

Velázquez added that pyruvate carboxylase, an enzyme he and others have studied in human fibroblast cultures, may be in the same situation. There is no known function for this enzyme in these cells, which lack the gluconeogenetic pathway and have a negligible tricarboxilic acid cycle.

PART III

NUTRIENT REQUIREMENTS AND METABOLISM

VARIABILITY OF NUTRIENT REQUIREMENTS

Philip R. Payne

Department of Human Nutrition
London School of Hygiene and Tropical Medicine
Keppel Street
London, United Kingdom

INTRODUCTION

The object of this paper is to discuss the significance of the general pheno-menon of variability with respect to establishing and applyng nutritional re-quirements. Although this Workshop is mainly concerned with genetic factors, it will be necessary to take a broad view of variability including adaptive res-ponses to environmental factors as well as the kinds of individual variability which are commonly assumed to be constitutional in nature. In fact, I shall ar-gue that the real challenge for experimental nutrition in the future will be to study the variability between individuals of their capacity to adapt to environ-mental changes without an unacceptable loss of function. Up to now, many, if not most, nutritionists have tended to overlook this problem area, partly be-cause of the quite severe experimental problems and restrictions involved in studying it, but partly also because the models most commonly used to describe the interaction of requirements and nutrient intake, implicitly assume that un-der normal conditions adaptations is a relatively minor component of total variability: if adaptation does occur, the situation must be abnormal and, failing proof to the contrary, the adapted state is presumed to confer some dis-advantage.

The Concept of Nutritional Requirement

It would be well to begin with a statement that reflects my own perspective of the subject. This is not offered as a new definition in the hopes of universal acceptance, but simply to convey some understanding of why I see the subject in the way that I do.

GENETIC FACTORS IN NUTRITION

177

For me, the statement of a nutrient requirements level is essentially a prediction on the basis of past knowledge, about what is likely to happen in the future to a member of a particular class of individual. The scientific value of such statements is essentially that they summarise in quantitative terms our total current knowledge of the functional significance and metabolism of the nutrient concerned, and of the capacity of the particular class of individuals to make an effective adaptive response.

It has to be admitted that few satisfactory statements of this kind are possible, e.g. that there is a probability of 0.1 ± 0.01 that 15 year old non-pregnant females will develop night blindness if they sustain an intake of less than 400 RE of vitamin A per day' (needless to say, I do not know if this is in fact true). Ideally, the probability should be established within confidence limits, and the dysfunction to which it refers must be spcecified and measurable. Other kinds of dysfunction related to vitamin A status may be known to exist, and their probabilities could also be stated for that same level of intake. Some other departures from health may only be suspected, but with respect to these, no true requirement figure can or should be stated.

Something which is specifically excluded from this definition is the notion of an "optimum" state of nutritional health, the achievement of which might be the criterion for a requirement level. Adherence to the idealistic notion that there should exist some preferred or optimum state of the body has probably done much to inhibit the growth of understanding in this subject.

There seem to be two kinds of attitude which sustain the concept of optimum health. One is a view which reacts against minimum prescriptions, and would prefer to see emphasis placed on the need for the complete fulfilment of human potential. This feeling, of course, demands respect. However, I believe it should be directed more towards objecting to the misapplication of requirements than towards distorting the figures themselves.

The other attitude is essentially mystical in origin, and is thus perhaps more difficult to deal with: it is that optimum states are somehow inherent in "natural" systems, and given the right environment, that these will be expressed. A common explanation for this is that natural selection will have maximised "fitness", and that therefore there should exist a state of nutrition in the individual which will be a reflection of that fitness. However, unless we are prepared to take the Panglossian view that (by definition) "everything is for the best in the best of all possible worlds" we will have to concede that natural selection acts so as to maximise fitness in the genotype, and that we somatotypes, by contrast, may value aspects of function which have never been subjected to selection pressure, or indeed may even have been selected against: we have no reason whatever to believe that there is some preferred state of metabolism or physiology in the individual which brings to a maximum simultaneously all qualities that we happen to consider desirable.

In practice, therefore, in nutrition as in economics, we cannot rely on a "hidden guiding hand", but must agree about and list those attributes of health and function that we regard as important, and agree, too, upon how they should be measured. Even then, we may have to make choices. Probably the best example of a problem of choice will be that of early growth versus ageing. There is now much evidence in support of the theory of accumulating transciption errors as the main cause of ageing. Kirkwood [8] has argued that an evolutionary stable strategy could be the result of a minimum investment (of energy and nutrients) in error correcting systems, consistent with survival to reproductive maturity. This would suggest that the inverse relationship between early growth rate and longevity found in rats has a genetic basis and will be common to all species including Man. Ross, Lustbader and Bras [13] have shown that this relationship holds for individual animals: self selection of diets by young rats results in a range of individual variation in food energy consumption and growth rate, which are negatively correlated with lifespan, to the extent that 50% of the variance in lifespan is explained on the basis of dietary history during the first 100 days of life.

Diet restriction imposed on a group of young rats acts so as to restrain the intake and growth of the most vigorous individuals, and lifespan on average increase. In this instance at least, it is clear that energy requirements for the young could be based either on the criterion of achieving the full genetic potential for early growth, or on subsequent longevity, but not both.

Models of Individual Variability

The model which has most commonly been assumed to describe individual variability or requirements is that adopted by the 1973 Joint FAO/WHO Committee of Energy and Protein Requirements [3]. This assumes that each individual in a population has his or her own specific requirement level (in theory for any nutrient, but specifically for protein), and that this is in some way fixed and unalterable. The distribution of these values is assumed to conform to a normal Gaussian curve, and this in turn implies that we could specify an intake which will reduce the probability of deficiency to a low level such as 0.025 by making an additional allowance of twice the standard deviation above the mean value for the group.

An alternative model has been proposed by Sukhatme and Margen [14], who offer evidence that nitrogen equilibrium is not fixed, but can and usually does vary over time. This variation is due to the operation of an autoregulatory system, which confines the nutritional balance and hence the requirements of the body to within a certain range, but within those limits is not fixed. If this model is the more correct one then the probability of deficiency in a individual might be less than 0.025 for intakes down to the mean value minus two standard deviations if we assume that the range of variation observed is a measure of the range permissable adaptation. The choice of model obviously affects the result very substantially: in the case of protein, the 1973 UN report [3] suggests a value of 15% for the coefficient of variance of individual variability. If we accept this, the alternative models predict a 0.025 probability of deficiency for intakes of, respectively, average plus 30% (FAO) and average minus 30% (Sukhatme): a discrepancy which is probably much greater than the degree of uncertainty attached to the average requirement itself.

Despite the practical importance, little has been done in a systematic way to test the validity of either model. A major difficulty is that adult human protein requirements are almost entirely based on experiments in which the objective was to maintain nitrogen balance. In practice these involve selecting individuals from an apparently healthy population (*i.e.* people who exhibit no discernable ill health) and establishing levels of intake which are sufficient to maintain them at their existing level of body nitrogen. It is often said that N balance is the criterion of adequacy for these estimates of protein requirements: in fact it is not, but is simply an indicator of whether the subject's equilibrium state is changing or not. The presumption behind these tests is that the subjects will be at or close to their "preferred" states of nitrogen metabolism. In some studies, for example Yoshimura [16] and Garza, Scrimshaw and Young [5], measurements have been also made of a number of biochemical and physiological parameters such as urinary steroid levels, blood levels of various proteins and amino transfer enzymes. Departures of these from "normal" levels is variously quoted by these authors as evidence of inadequacy, however, the health significance of such changes is not known.

Clearly, the "fixed individual requirement" model stands or falls on whether or not autoregulation takes place, and whether or not adaptive metabolic or physiological responses to changes in protein status carry any risk of functional impairment.

Sukhatme and Margen [14], and Durkin, Ogar, Tilve and Margen [2] have demonstrated the existence of autoregulation by applying time series analysis to the results of long term N balance studies. Durkin *et al.* also showed that some subjects on low protein intakes showed an inicital negative balance, followed by a return to a new equilibrium.

It would indeed be surprising if this were not the case. Homeostatic mechanisms are likely to operate body protein content, and generally such mechanisms are dynamic in their operation, producing continual "hunting" over a range rather than a rigidly maintained set point. In additon, we know that adaptation does take place in response to changes in diet: Individuals respond to changes in level by gradually coming to a new equilibrium either above or below their initial state. The crucial question is still how large can such a response be without producing an unacceptable loss of some specific aspect of function?

Evidently, we are a long way from being able to make the kinds of statement about requirements exemplified earlier, when in the case of protein, which has arguably received by far the most attention and resources for research during the last century.

Even if we accept Sukhatme's model as being closer to reality than that currently advocated by the UN committees, this still does not provide us with an

adequate basis for prediction. Variability evidently has a number of components. If we consider measurements made there will be at least the following
sources of variance apart from technical measurements errors:

i)   Differences in adpative response. These might be further subdivided into
      those reflecting the primary expression of genetic factors, and those which
      are the outcome of more or less irreversible modifications of those primary
      differences arising through the effects of diet and environment during
      growth and development (*e.g* the varying rates of ageing of rats program-
      med by early feeding behaviour).
ii)   Differences due to the extent and nature of continuous autoregulatory ad-
      justments.
iii) A "noise" component due to random, unrelated fluctuations in the envi-
      ronment, the diet, measurement errors, etc.

   If we are to conduct experiments in order to established the safe limits of
adaptive response to different intake of some nutrients, we would need to distinguish between these sources of variability. Assuming that in general we
would find both upper and lower limits to the range, with some risk of dysfunction attached to high levels of intake as well as low levels, the situation
would be as shown in the diagram, Figure 1.

   Instead of a single figure for the safe level for the particular nutrient, we
would have a "safe range", with upper and lower limits bounded by points for
which the probability of dysfunction rises above an acceptable level.

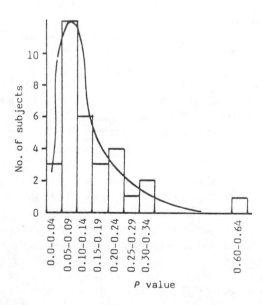

Figure 1. Safe limits of adaptive response to different intake of some nutrients.

The Range of Adaptation

The mechanism involved in adaptation are themselves of a very varied nature. Since adaptation means that the system changes from one internal state to another in response to some change in inputs or outputs, all the various mechanisms must have in common is that they will involve some type of negative feedback response by which the body is able in part to cancel out the change in inputs or outputs, and maintain the internal state near its original condition. Quite apart from the complexity of the system, another complicating factor is that the feedback paths return to different points, so that establishing effects are sometimes confined to various sub-systems. In the particular case of energy, one feedback loop even extends outside the body, so that an individual may adapt by modifying his interaction with the environment, and hence changing his requirement for energy of bring it into line with intake.

Other feedback mechanisms will act so as to protect organs and tissues which are more important for survival, whilst others change in size and metabolic rate. Thus the whole strategy of adaptive responses for energy ranges from individuals and social changes in behaviour to changes in body weight, body composition and metabolic regulation. It may well be that individuals differ in the relative balance of these components. Figure 2, which is taken from Dugdale and Payne [1] shows data ion subjects subjected to semi-starvation in the experiments of Keys, Brozek, Honschel, Michelson and Taylor [6]. These men showed a wide variation in the way they responded to a negative energy balance. Although on average 15% of energy was lost from lean tissue stores, and 85% from fat. This ratio spanned a ten-fold range, with some losing 3% from protein and some as much as 39%.

We do not know the extent to which this propensity to store and utilise protein as opposed to fat is a result of genetic differences, and how much is a result of patterns stablished during early growth. We do know that under some circumstances a tendency to use fat as an energy store might be a good survival strategy, whereas in other circumstances it could lead to obesity. The nature of responses to increased energy intakes may be similarly varied. The data of Miller and Mumford [9] showed considerable variations between individuals in respect of degree of weight gain during overfeeding. Besides the possibility that the capacity for thermogenesis varies from one person to another, it seems entirely likely that individuals with a propensity for fat storage will gain more weight before their increased resting metabolism balances out the higher intake, than will individuals who store metabolically active lean tissue.

As we know so little about this complex strategy of adaptation, and have at the moment no reliable indicators to predict how a given individual will respond to changes in intake-either by body weight, composition or behaviour, we have almost no basis for defining energy requirements. If we could isolate and predict changes in body weight, or better still perhaps, body mass index (weight $\div$ height^2) as a component of adaptation, we might move forward a little, since

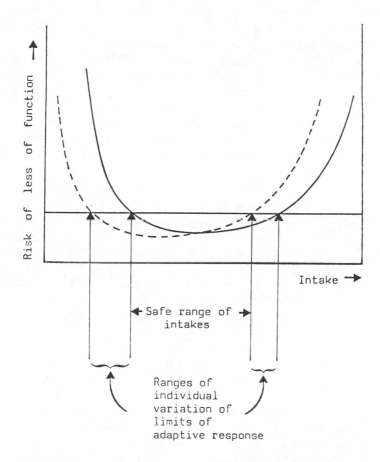

Figure 2 Variation in response to a negative energy balance. Subjects subjected to semi-starvation. From Dugdale and Payne (1).

we know from Keys [7] that changes in body mass index beyond both lower and upper limits of a range are associated with increased mortality risk.

In respect to protein, we are hardly better off. Obsession with nitrogen balance as a "criterion" of adequacy has led to a neglect for the study of adaptive changes and mechanisms. Nonetheless, it is well established that such mechanisms exist. Waterlow [15] reviewed the evidence for adaptive responses in nitrogen metabolism and concludes that the body possesses powerful mechanisms for economising nitrogen. Current estimates of ranges of interindividual variation are simply those differences found to exist in groups of experimental subjects for whom little information is available regarding previous patterns of diet or life style. Even if we accepted these as true estimates of individual differences, *i.e* if we continue to ignore the work of Sukhatme and Margen, we cannot regard them even as measures of the range of adaptability: they are even less acceptable as measures of variation of adaptive capacity.

Some elements of those mechanisms will be related to those involved in energy regulation. Durkin *et al.* [2] show that in most cases, adaptation to reduced levels of nitrogen intake was accompanied by loss of body weight, and it seems not unreasonable that this should be so. Nicol and Phillips [10] showed that Nigerian farmers habituated to diets relatively low in protein as compared to those common in the USA, utilised protein more efficiently than do American subjects, and could maintain balance on about 30% less, *i.e.* these subjects were adapted to low intakes.

Enough has been said about the subject of individual variability to underline the extent to which our knowledge and understanging of this factor limits our ability to make quantitative statements about nutrient requirements.

I began by suggesting that the nature and precision (in a statistical sense) of requirements is best regarded as a measure of the progress of epidemiological and laboratory research towards understanding the causes of a range of health related problems, and predicting the conditions which will give rise to them in the future. This suggests almost that requirements statements are simply the outcome of successful research rather than a primary objective. Obviously this is not a view which is generally held: government and international agency appointed committees have produced over the years a stream of reports listing figures of requirements, safe levels and recommended dietary allowances. These are consulted by an audience which is much broader than nutritional physiologists, as indeed it is intended they should be. The problem is that there are many who tend to apply these numbers as if they possessed the precision and the authority of tables of physical constants. It is outside the scope and intention of this workshop to review the aplications of requirement estimates. Broadly, however, they can be classified as either analytical, *i.e* used as part of the process of trying to assess the extent to which problems of manifest ill health in populations can be attributed to dietary causes. Alternatively as prescriptive, *i.e.* as the basis for advice to individuals or guidelines for policies aimed at curing those problems.

As regards problem analysis, if we cannot predict in quantitative terms the connection between leveles of intake under controlled conditions, and the emergence of specific dysfunctions, and if we do not know the extent to which individual variability in response limits the confidence of those predictions, then we should place very little if any reliance on a comparison of intake data with requirements at the individual level as a means of assessing causes of problems in population even if the intake data itself were reliable which is almost never the case. Attempts to analyse country or global problems by comparing requirements with average food supply, *e.g.* FAO [14] and Reutlinger and Alderman [11] which are the basis for statements such as that 400 million people in the world, or that 60 to 70% of some third world country populations are in energy deficit, involve additional uncertainties, and entail assumptions about manipulations of data that can only be described as "heroic"!

As far as prescription is concerned, advice intended to have an effect on individual choice or behaviour obviously must be based on a sound understanding of the probability not only of causes, but of the likelihood of benefits to individuals. At the national level, it seems probable that the constraints and limitations on the possibilities for administrators to influence food production, especially, in "free market" economies have been considerably underestimated. If this is true, a careful examination of what kinds of information planners need and can use might show that even the very large uncertainties underlying current estimates are less than those inherent in the data on production, input costs and effective demand levels which are the subject of policy decisions.

If this proves to be the case, then we can perhaps draw some comfort from the broad consistency to advice offered at least with respect to energy over the years: there is in fact no significant difference between the thirteen or so estimates of the average energy needs of moderately active male subjects endorsed by such famous names as Playfair, Voit, Rubner, Chittenden, etc., over the period 1885 to 1909 (see Table I), and values endorsed as applying to their own populations by the governments of thirteen different countries at the present time [12] (Table II). Perhaps we would do well to reassure the food planners that we have gained no far-reaching insights lately about how much food people are likely to be eating during the next 70 years.

TABLE I *Some estimates of energy requirements made by physiologists before 1914. Values are for adult males in Europe on the USA. Average body weights are assumed, where stated values range from 60—70 kg.*

| Source | Energy requirement [b] | | |
	Light activity	Moderate activity	Hard Work
Moleschott 1859		3160	
Lyon Playfair 1865 [a]	3029	3146	4060
Ranke 1876		3195	3574
Studemund 1878		3229	
Voit 1881		3055	3370
Hultegren & Landegren 1891		3436	4726
Atwater 1885	3000	3500	
Rubner 1902 [a]	2631	3121	3644
Lichtenfelt 1903		2700	3088
Schmidt 1901		3235	
Gautier 1907		2830	4247
Chittenden 1907		2800	
Lusk 1909		3000	

Philip R. Payne

TABLE II

Country		Energy requirement [a] Sedentary	(kcal/day) Moderately active
Australia		2800	—
Canada		2650	—
Colombia	(f)	2850	—
Czechoslovakia	(f)	2700	—
Denmark		(b)	(b)
Eire		(c)	(c)
Finland	(f)	2400	3000
France	(f)	—	3000
German Democratic Republic	(f)	2700	3000
German Democratic Federal Republic	(f)	2550	—
Hungary	(f)	2400	2700
India	(f)	2400	—
Indonesia	(f)	2600	—
Italy		2700	3000
Japan	(f)	2500	—
Jugoslavia		(d)	(d)
Malaysia	(f)	2500	—
Netherlands	(e)	2600	2900
Norway	(e)	2800	3000
Philippines	(f)	2500	—
Poland	(f)	2600	3200
Romania	(f)	2500	3500
Spain		2700	3000
Sweden	(e)	—	2800
Thailand	(f)	2550	—
Turkey	(f)	3000	—
UK		2700	3000
USA	(e)	2800	—
USSR	(e)	—	3000

REFERENCES

1. Dugdale, A.E. and Payne, P.R. Pattern of Lean and Fat Deposition in Adults, *Nature,* 266: 349, 1977.
2. Durkin, N., Ogar, D.A., Tilve, S.G. and Margen, S. Human Protein Requirements: Auto-correlation and Adaptation to a Low Protein Diet. Joint FAO/WHO/UNU Expert Consultation on Energy and Protein Requirements, October, 1981.
3. FAO. Joint FAO/WHO Ad-Hoc Expert Committee Report on Protein and Energy Requirements. FAO Nutrition Meetings Report Series No. 52. Rome, 1973.
4. FAO. The Fourth World Food Survey FAO Statistics Series No. 11. Food and Agriculture Organization of the United Nations Rome, 1977.

5. Garza C. Scrimshaw, N.S. and Young, V.R. Human Protein Requirements a long-term metabolic nitrogen balance study in young men to evaluate the 1973 FAO/WHO safe level of egg protein intake. *J. Nutr.* 107:335, 1976.
6. Keys, A., Brozek, J., Henschel, A., Michelson, O. and Taylor, H.L. "The Biology of Human Starvation". University of Minnesota Press, Minneapolis, Minn., 1950.
7. Keys, A. Overweight, obesity, coronary heart disease and mortality. *Nutrition Reviews.* 38: 297, 1980.
8. Kirkwood, T.B.L. Evolution of Ageing. *Nature* 270:301, 1977.
9. Miller, D.S. and Mumford, P. Gluttony I. An experimental study of over-eating low or high protein diets. *Amer. J. Clin. Nutr.* 20:1212, 1967.
10. Nicol, B.M. and Phillips, P.G. Endogenous nitrogen excretion and utilisation of dietary protein. *Brit. J. Nutr.,* 35:181, 1976.
11. Reutlinger, S. and Alderman, H. The prevalence of calorie deficient diets in developing countries. World Bank Staff Working Paper No. 374, 1980.
12. Rivers, J.P.W. and Payne, P.R. The comparison of energy supply and energy need: A critique of energy requirements. Proceedings of a symposium on Energy and Effort. Taylor & Francis, 1982. (in press).
13. Ross, M.H., Lustbader, E. and Bras, G. Dietary Practices and Growth Responses as Predictors of Longevity. *Nature* 262:548, 1976.
14. Sukhatme, P.V. and Margen, S. Models for Protein Deficiency. *Amer. J. Clin. Nutr.* 31: 1237, 1978.
15. Waterlow, J.C. Adaptation to Different Intakes and Environments. Joint FAO/WHO/UNU Expert Consultation on Energy and Protein Requirements, October, 1981.
16. Yoshimura, H. Physiological Effect of Protein Deficiency with Special Reference to Evaluation of Protein Nutrition and Protein Requirement. *World Rev. Nutr. Dietet.,* 14:100, 1972.

DISCUSSION[1]

Scrimshaw took issue with some examples of genetic differences in the population ability to use nutrients presented by Payne. Actually, long-term nitrogen balances carried out in numerous healthy subjects have shown that the phenomenon described as autocorrelation by Jukhatme and Margen, is most likely due to an unmeasured loss of lean body mass and occurs only exceptionally; it probably is of little or no relevance for the definition of nutritional requirements.

[1]*Summary of the discussion prepared by S. Frenk.*

VARIABILITY OF NUTRIENT REQUIREMENTS IN THE HUMAN

George H. Beaton

Department of Nutritional Sciences
Faculty of Medicine, University of Toronto
Toronto, Ontario, Canada

INTRODUCTION

The present paper will discuss the variability of human nutritional requirements and in the process attempt to differentiate the genetic and environmental sources of variation. It will focus in particular upon true interindividual variability of requirement which is believed to include a major component of genetic origin as well as of phenotypic expression. Other contributions to observed differences in requirements will be illustrated. Finally, the paper will return to the question of adaptation in nutrient requirement at the level of the individual and at the level of the population, and to the possibility of evolutionary differences in nutrient requirements between subpopulations.

Meaning of "Requirement"

Before proceeding further it is germane to clarify the meaning of the term *requirement*. In essence, this is a term that is applicable to an individual. It may be defined as the lowest level of habitual intake of a nutrient that serves to maintain a predetermined level of nutritional health in the individual. There are three important dimensions in this definition. First, we are talking about the level of *habitual* intake; we are talking about something continuing over time although as a convenience we express this as a rate of intake (intake per day). Second, we are talking about the *maintenance* of health; this presupposes that the individual is already healthy and eliminates from consideration the disease state. Finally, the definition refers to a *predetermined level of nutritional health*. The important point is that today nutritional requirements are not set on the basis of preventing disease but rather on the basis of achieving an index of nutritional adequacy. This will be specific to the nutrient. For protein, the usual criterion relates to nitrogen balance in adults or nitrogen accretion during growth [12]. For iron, the presence of nutritionally significant storage is expected [13]. For ascorbic acid, there is a movement toward the use of metabolic turnover rates as an index of suitable intake [21]. For all of these nutrients, requirements judged against these criteria are undoubtedly much higher than would be the case if need were judged against the prevention of the clinically apparent deficiency disease, a level that has sometimes been termed the minimal requirement [13].

Interindividual Variability

If requirement is a term applicable to an individual, can we assume that all individuals have the same requirement? The answer is clearly no! When the investigator sets out to measure nutritional requirement in human subjects he will study a group of generally similar subjects, for example, young healthy adult males. He will then attempt to estimate the *average requirement* for that group of subjects. In early studies the usual approach was to monitor group behaviour as intake was varied. For example when the mean nitrogen balance in a group of men approximated 0, the average requirement was approximated. More recently the approach has been to estimate the requirements of each of the individuals in the group and then to estimate the group average [4, 12, 23]. When individual data are obtained in this manner, it is clear that there is major variability in requirements. Thus, for example, in United Nations University sponsored studies of protein requirement, the coefficient of variation was estimated to be about 17.5% after adjustment for body weight [23]. This CV includes both true individual differences and "experimental error". Recently an FAO/WHO/UNU group has suggested that about half of the observed variance might be methodologic and concluded that a reasonable estimate of the CV of requirement under these standardized conditions might be about 12.5% (unpublished). Earlier, using indirect measures such as the interindividual variability of urinary nitrogen excretion with very low nitrogen intake, the variability of adult protein requirement had been estimated to be about 15% [12]. Although the available data base is too limited to test the normality of the distribution of measured requirement, there does not appear to be any marked deviation from a Gaussian distribution.

On these assumptions, the range of protein requirement encompassing 95% of the population would be the average ± 25-30%, indeed a wide range.

How then should requirements be described? Again we fall back to a convention that has been adopted but not always understood. The convention is to describe the *Recommended Intake* or *Safe Level of Intake* of a nutrient as the amount (of nutrient) considered necessary to meet the physiological needs and maintain health of nearly all persons in a specified group [12]. Where there is an estimate of the variability of requirement and where this can be assumed to approximate the Gaussian distribution, the *Recommended Intake* has been set at the average + 2 standard deviations to cover 97.5% of the population. This approach is portrayed in Figure 1.

Current conventions, then, explicitly recognize the existence of individual variability of requirement among seemingly similar individuals. Unfortunately this is not always recognized when the published requirement estimates are used. The published numerical values represent single points on distributions of requirements. The distribution is sometimes forgotten and the assumption is made that the single numbers apply to all individuals!

Beaton [2] presented this issue in 1972 and argued for a probability approach to the interpretation of observed nutrient intake. That is, it was argued that since there is a variability of requirement among otherwise similar individuals, one should use a knowledge of this variability, or assumption about this variability, in generating statements about the probable adequacy or inadequacy of the observed intake of an individual. This is also portrayed in Figure 1. For a nutrient for which the requirement distribution is assumed to be normal, an intake 2 standard deviations above the average, that is the *Recommended Intake,* implies a probability of inadequacy for the randomly chosen individual of only

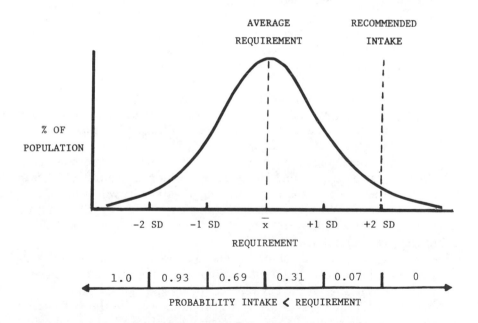

Fig. 1. The Variability of Nutrient Requirement. Portrayed is a distribution of individual requirements for a homogeneous class of individuals. The average requirement is shown. The convention of stipulating the recommended intake as the average + 2 standard deviations is shown. Given the assumption of a Gaussian distribution, the probabilities of inadequacy of intake for a randomly selected individual may be derived from standard tables of the area under the normal curve. Probabilities so derived are shown on the lower scale. (Based on Anderson et al (1)).

0.025. At the level of the average requirement, the probability of inadequacy rises to 0.5 and at the average − 2 standard deviations it rises to 0.975, almost certainty. He argued that for a population of individuals, the expected prevalence of inadequate intakes could be estimated by application of the probability distributions to the individuals, summing the results for the group. Recently Anderson et al [1] have applied this approach to dietary data interpretation for a Canadian population.

The probability approach does not demand the assumption of a normal distribution. It demands only that the nature of the distribution be known or reasonably assumed. A classical example of a non-Gaussian distribution is that of iron requirements of menstruating women. When data from two large total community studies are examined it appears that menstrual iron loss follows a logarithmic distribution in adult women [3]. The distribution curve still can be described. This still serves to define the probability that any given intake is or is not adequate for the randomly selected individual [2].

Gradually these concepts are gaining acceptance. They were set forth in a recent U.S. National Academy of Sciences report [22] and are expected to be given prominence in the soon to be published "Recommended Nutrient Intakes for Canadians" and in a forthcoming FAO/WHO/UNU report on Energy and Protein requirements. Two points must be emphasized. The simple approach described is not applicable to energy [12]. Although variability in energy requirement is recognized, there exist also mechanisms of intake regulation that give rise to correlation between intake and requirement. This correlation imposes additional considerations in the application of a probability approach. Second, the approach that has been set forth refers to the examination of habitual or usual intakes. Because there is wide day-to-day variation in intakes within free-living subjects (intraindividual variation of intake) major misinterpretation can result from comparisons of estimates of "habitual" requirement with observations of one day intake [4, 5, 8].

It is certain, then, that individual variability of nutrient requirement is attracting increased interest, and increased recognition. It is probable that in coming years the data base and understanding of variability will improve. It is to be hoped that this Workshop will accelerate this process since there are still many fundamental questions to be addressed. For example, is the variability of nutrient requirement truly genetic or is it the result of environmental influences that have conditioned the expression of genetic potential? If the latter, is an individual's position on the distribution of requirements fixed over time or does this change as the environment of the individual changes?

In the case of iron requirements of menstruating women, the evidence on the latter point seems quite strong. The magnitude of iron loss of individual women in successive menstrual periods is quite consistent; this is in contrast to the wide differences between women in their characteristic menstrual loss [7, 14]. Conversely, Sukhatme and Margen [19, 20] have argued that protein, and more particularly energy, requirements as currently measured may not recognize the effect of long term fluctuations in requirements of individual. That is, they argue that the position of an individual in the requirement distribution is not necessarily fixed over time and that in fact current estimates of the variability of requirements between individuals may be overestimated. The data base available to either support or refute this argument is extremely limited. There would be need for estimations of requirements repeated in the same individuals over extended intervals of time if their hypothesis was to be adequately tested. These authors tangentially address the question of the real source of observed interindividual variability, their work has both theoretical and practical implication in the setting of this Workshop.

Other Sources of Variation

In free-living populations, the range of nutrient requirements is larger than is implied by the discussion to this point. Figure 2 presents a framework in which a perspective of interindividual variation, as discussed above, can be presented. It should serve also as a reminder of the need to ensure a common understanding of terms and concepts when discussing the variability of requirements.

In the centre of the figure are portrayed the processes of digestion, absorption and utilization of the nutrient to satiate body needs.

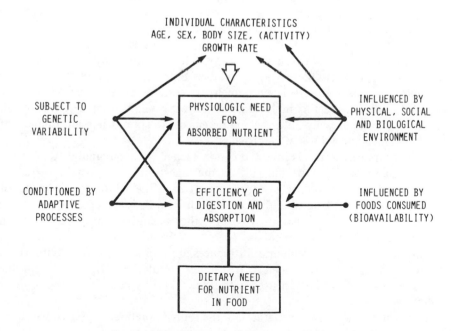

Fig. 2. Some Sources of Differences in Human Nutrient Requirements.

At the top of the figure are portrayed the type of variables that are conventionally used to classify individuals in describing nutrient requirements. Thus, all discussion of variability of requirement refers to variability within such classes of individuals rather than between classes.

On the left of the diagram are portrayed the endogenous traits of individuals that might affect his or her particular requirement. These are subdivided into two groups. Those which *seem* to be subject to genetic variability and those that may be conditioned by adaptive processes. On the right side of the diagram are portrayed the exogenous, or environmental, factors that may affect the individual's need for nutrients in food.

Up to this point we have been discussing the interindividual variability of requirement under relatively controlled conditions. This is portrayed in the figure as the variation attributable to genetic differences or, as mentioned earlier to differences in the expression of genetic potential. It is assumed that this is fixed for any particular individual, at least after maturity. These genetic factors are recognized as influencing digestion and absorption, metabolic and physiologic utilization, and even such recognized classification variables as growth rate in children and mature size in adults.

On the opposite side of the diagram is portrayed the potential effect of the environment. A few examples will suffice to illustrate this type of effect. The physical environment, for example temperature, can influence the loss of nutrients through sweat [9]. The social environment can influence expected activity levels both in work and in leisure and hence the requirement for energy (and for nutrients for which the requirement depends upon total food intake) [12]. The social and biological environments interact to affect disease. In turn, this can influence nutrient absorption or utilization [17] or, in children, growth rates both during and after illness [6, 12]. In recognition of these types of variables, nutrient requirements are customarily stated in terms of specified environmental conditions and for "the maintenance of health in already healthy individuals". Where it is known that the environment (e.g. temperature, activity) influences requirement, an approach to adjustement of the requirement estimate is often provided.

The nature of the foods ingested can influence the bioavailability of minerals such as iron [3] and zinc [18] or the digestibility of protein [12]. The amount of food ingested or its constituents can influence the requirement for other nutrients. For example, the need for vitamin B_6 is affected by the intake of protein. Again it is customary to take these variables into account when describing nutrient requirements.

Although these environmental influences are real and do contribute to the range of nutritional needs seen in free-living populations, they are separable from, and should not be confused with, the variability inherent in the subjects themselves.

It may not be as easy to separate out the fourth potential source of variation in human nutrient requirements, that which has been termed "adaptation". If the body is capable of adjusting its metabolic and physiologic processes in a manner that reduces the need for a nutrient in short supply, then adaptation is said to have occurred.

In the framework of the present discussion it is necesary to take this concept a bit further if the implications are to be understood and potential confusion minimized. It is clear that the homeostatic mechanisms of the body to regulate absorption, turnover rates, excretion and other aspects of metabolism of nutrients such that equilibria are established between intake and utilization. This is appropriately described as an adaptive process, and is one of considerable importance to life. However, it is not necessarily an adaptation of requirement. That is, since requirement is defined as the *lowest* level of intake of the nutrient at which the body can maintain its functional characteristics, this homeostatic adaptation takes place at levels *above* requirement. In effect we are defining the lower limit of this type of adaptability when we speak of an individual's requirement.

The critical question is whether subjects who are maintained for long periods on intakes below the requirements estimated for the reference study populations undergo a further adaptation which indeed lowers their requirement. At first consideration the answer would seem to be yes, such adaptation must be possible. If population groups continue to live with intakes below estimated requirements, there would seem to be prime facie evidence of adaptation. This conclusion may be erroneous. "Adaptation" may have been accomplished by an alteration in body size or body composition with an associated reduction in the amount of nutrient required to maintain the new equilibrium. Thus, for example, the amount of iron needed to maintain a stable hemoglobin level in the anemic range would be expected to be much less than required to maintain "desirable" levels of iron stores. There has not been a true adaptation of iron requirement. Rather, there has been a forfeiture of the definition of health upon which the original requirement estimate was based! A similar situation may be described with regard to energy. The famous studies of Keys and co-workers on The Biology of Human Starvation [15] suggest that when healthy young men were faced with a reduction in food intake they reestablished energy balance through a series of adjustments: voluntary activity was reduced, body weight and lean body weight were reduced, there was an associated fall in BMR, and BMR exhibited a further fall not accounted for by the reduction in lean body weight. Only the last of these could be termed a true adaptation and then only if it could be demonstrated that the BMR adjustment took place without compromise of activity or body composition, and that it acted to systematically change energy need rather than being a part of the apparent homeostatic day to day variation of energy metabolism.

When "adaptation of requirement" is considered within the confines of these considerations, and after having taken into account the environmental variables, it is difficult to find clear evidence that adaptation does occur in the human. One exception may be calcium [10, 16]. It was noted long ago that in populations with chronic low intake, calcium absorptions were increased relative to those seen in North America or Britain. When calcium intake was reduced in persons habituated to generous intakes, there was evidence that some subjects adjusted absorption rapidly while some remained in negative calcium balance for extended periods. Since bone calcium levels were not measured in these studies, and since expected adult stature was an uncontrolled variable in the children, it is difficult to be sure whether these adjustments represent adaptations in the sense implied in this paper.

In studies recently conducted under the auspices of the United Nations University, there was little or no evidence of systematic differences in protein requirement between population [23]. Conversely, it cannot be stated with assurance that the subjects studied had been chronically exposed to low protein intakes.

The absence of clear evidence of adaptation of requirements across population groups is interesting in another regard. There is clear evidence that variability of nutrient requirement among comparable individuals does exist. This is a phenotypic expression of a genotype, presumably influenced by many factors during development.

Given the concepts of evolution and of selection for advantage, one might have expected that either the genotype itself, or at least the phenotypic expression, would differ across population subgroups historically exposed to low intakes. This may suggest either that habitual intakes are not sufficiently low to provide the type of challenge needed to evoke these alterations in nutrient requirement or that the other influences of phenotypic expression are so great that they override any systematic effects. Recognize that in this discussion, requirement is described in terms of existing body size. That is, a major alteration of phenotypic expression, presented as lower growth rates and lower adult stature would serve to reduce the need for all nutrients *per day* without needing to evoke any change in the requirement per unit body size. Perhaps this has been a more dominant component of the adjustment of populations to chronic low intakes.

SUMMARY

An attempt has been made to separate the components of variation in human nutrient requirements and to isolate what has been termed the true interindividual variability of requirement. It has been suggested that this is of considerable magnitude, perhaps having a coefficient of variation of the order of 15% for many nutrients. It can be accepted that this variability represents both genotypic variation and variability of phenotypic expression. However there is very limited evidence of any systematic adaptation of the requirement in situations of low intake. There may be other bodily adjustments that compensate for low intake; these may or may not have functional significance but they do represent a change from the conditions of health that are used to define requirement and hence should not be considered true adaptations.

Although uncertainty remains about the variability of human nutrient requirements, and hence about the parameters of the distributions of requirements, it is argued that these distributions cannot be ignored in interpreting requirement estimates or in assessing the adequacy of observed intakes. A probability approach to dietary assessment, based upon assumptions about the expected distribution of requirements has been described and is recommended.

REFERENCES

1. Anderson, G.H., Peterson, R.D., and Beaton, G.H. Estimating Nutrient Deficiencies in a Population from Dietary Records: The Use of Probability Analysis. *Nutr. Res.,* in press, 1982.
2. Beaton, G.H. The Use of Nutritional Requirements and Allowances. *In* "Proceedings of the Western Hemisphere Nutrition Congress III" (P.L. White and N. Selvey, eds.), pp. 356-363, Futura Publishing Co., Mount Kisko, 1971.
3. Beaton, G.H. Epidemiology of Iron Deficiency. *In* "Iron in Biochemistry and Medicine" (A. Jacobs and M. Worwood, eds), pp 477-528, Academic Press, London, 1974.
4. Beaton, G.H. What Do We Think We Are Estimating? *In* "Proceedings of the Symposium on Dietary Data Collection, Analysis and Significance" (V.A. Beal and M.J. Laus, eds.) *Univ. of Massachusetts Research Bull.* No. 675, 1982.
5. Beaton, G.H. Evaluation of Dietary Intake of the Elderly. *In* "Assessing Nutritional Status of the Elderly: State of the Art" (D.E. Redfern, ed.) Third Ross Roundtable on Medical Issues, Ross Laboratories, in press, 1982.
6. Beaton, G.H., Calloway, D., and Waterlow, J. Protein and Energy Requirements: A Joint FAO/WHO Memorandum. *Bull. World Hlth Org.* 57: 65, 1979.
7. Beaton, G.H., Myo Thein, Milne, H. and Veen, M. Iron Requirements of Menstruating Women. *Am. J. Clin. Nutrit.* 23: 275, 1970.
8. Beaton, G.H., *et al.* Sources of Variance in 24-hour Dietary Recall Data: Implications for Nutrition Study Design and Interpretation. *Am. J. Clin. Nutrit.* 32: 2546, 1979.
9. Consolazio, C.F., Matoush, L.O., Nelson, R.A., Harding, R.S., and Canham, J.E. Excretion of Sodium, Potassium, Magnesium and Iron in Human Sweat and the Relation of Each to Balance and Requirements. *J. Nutrit.* 79: 407, 1963.
10. FAO/WHO Expert Group Calcium Requirements. *FAO Nutrit. Meetings Rept. Ser.* No. 30, Rome, 1962.
11. FAO/WHO Joint Expert Committee Eight Report. *World Hlth. Org. Tech. Rept. Ser.* No. 477, Geneva, 1971.
12. FAO/WHO Joint Ad Hoc Expert Committee "Energy and Protein Requirements" *World Hlth. Org. Tech. Rept. Ser.* No. 522, Geneva, 1973.
13. FAO/WHO Joint Expert Group "Requirements of Ascorbic Acid., Vitamin D, Vitamin B_{12}, Folate and Iron" *World Helth. Org. Tech. Rept. Ser.* No. 452, Geneva, 1970.
14. Hallberg, L. and Nilsson, L. Constancy of Individual Menstrual Blood Loss. *Acta Obstet. Gynecol. Scand.* 43: 352. 1965.
15. Keys, A., Bruzek, J., Hanschel, A., Mickelson, O. and Taylor, H.L. The Biology of Human Starvation, 2 volumes. University of Minnesota Press, Minneapolis, 1950.
16. Leitch, I. Calcium and Phosphorous. In "Nutrition: A Comprehensive Treatise". (G.H. Beaton and E.W. McHenry, eds.) Vol. I, pp 261-307. Academic Press, New York, 1964.
17. Scrimshaw, N.S. et al. Interactions of Nutrition and Infection. *World Hlth. Org. Monograph Ser.* No. 57. Geneva. 1968.
18. Solomons, N. Biological Availability of Zinc in Humans. *Am. J. Clin. Nutrit.* 35: 1048, 1982.
19. Sukhatme, P.V. and Margen, S. Models for Protein Deficiency. *Am. J. Clin. Nutrit.* 31: 1237, 1978.

20. Sukhatme, P.V. and Margen, S. Autoregulatory Homeostatic Nature of Energy Balance. *Am. J. Clin. Nutrit.* 35: 355, 1982.
21. U.S. Food and Nutrition Board Committee on Dietary Allowances "Recommended Dietary Allowances" Ninth Edition, National Academy of Sciences, Washington, 1980.
22. U.S. Food and Nutrition Board Committee on Food Consumption Patterns "Assessing Changing Food Consumption Patterns" National Academy of Sciences, Washington, 1981.
23. United Nations University World Hunger Programme "Protein-Energy Requirements of Developing Countries: Evaluation of New Data" B. Torun, V.R. Young and W.M. Rand (Editors) The United Nations University Food and Nutrition Bulletin Supplement 5, Tokyo, 1981. "Protein-Energy Requirements in Developing Countries: Results of Internationally Coordinated Research" W.M. Rand, R. Uauy and N.S. Scimshaw (Editors), ibid, in preparation.

DISCUSSION[1]

Payne pointed out that initially he had thought that the differences between his and Beaton's points of view were mostly semantic, but as it turns out, they are of a conceptual order. If one defines individual nutritional requirements as the intake that will maintain nutritional health, this implies on one hand a knowledge on how to measure the nutritional health status but on the other that the adequacy of a series of health functions have been assessed in that individual in terms of appropriate standards. For Payne, requirements may be defined as the intake which prevents the appearance of inadequate health functions and in this, there is no discrepancy with Beatons's view. However if one takes balance studies as indicators of requirements, the latter may be defined as those intakes which maintain the subjects in the same state as at the beginning of the balance. This has little to do with the essence of the maintenance of health. As for the phenomenon of autocorrelation, it disappears on very low or very high nutrient intakes. In other words, the adaptive mechanisms to individual changes act only within certain ranges. The classical model has still to stand the test of showing whether or not individuals are always maintained in the same nitrogen equilibrium.

[1]*Summary of the discussion prepared by S. Frenk.*

GENETICS AND INTESTINAL ABSORPTION

Richard E. Hillman

Division of Medical Genetics
Washington University Medical School
St. Louis, Missouri

INTRODUCTION

Transport processes for small molecules in the intestine and the kidney have been studied extensively over the past several decades. In this period of time, several specific inherited defects in transport have been described and, in some instances, heterozygote carriers have been detected. Thus far all of these specific transport defects have been quite rare. However, transport defects have always been considered in a digital fashion, either present or absent, and very little is known about the effects of partial defects in specific transport systems under conditions of decreased substrate availability, e.g., in undernutrition or during infestation with intestinal parasites, or under conditions of increased need, e.g., during periods of rapid growth. In addition, since the organ which controls absorption is the brush border membrane, transport defects which are inapparent in healthy individuals might well produce significant deficiency when the brush border is damaged. This damage might be environmental or possibly inherited as in patients with sprue.

Transport processes for small molecules may be specific, that is, mediated by a stereospecific carrier process, or nonspecific, that is, mediated by simple diffusion or by differential solubility in lipid or water. Specific transport processes may be concentrative, i.e., able to transport against an electrical or chemical gradient, and energy requiring. In many cases the transport of one substance requires the contransport of another. Sodium is transported in conjunction with the tranport of both neutral amino acids and glucose [1]. For most active and concentrative transport systems the kinetics of the transport process can be analyzed by assuming that the carrier molecule behaves in a manner analagous to an enzyme which obeys Michaelis-Menten kinetics. Thus most transport systems can be thought of as having an affinity constant and a maximal rate of transport. The affinity constant is expressed as the Km, the concentration of substrate which produces one half the maximal transport rate. The maximal rate of transport is usually called the Vmax. These terms may be compared to the terms used in studies of renal tubular transport.

Although measured in quite a different way, the Vmax may be compared to the Tmax, the maximal rate of tubular reabsorption, and alterations in the Km for a substrate would be expected to change the Tmin, the minimal substrate concentration at which a substance is not totally reabsorbed. The kinetics of transport have additional levels of complexity in both kidney and gut because the same substrate may be transported by several different transport systems. For example, proline has been shown to be carried by at least three different transport systems with markedly different affinities and maximal transport rates [2]. Thus even the total loss of a single transport system may not totally prevent the uptake of a particular substrate.

As complex as transport is in the kidney, still additional factors must be considered when dealing with the intestine. Dr. Robert K. Crane several years ago [3] wrote of the digestive-absorptive unit. He reminded us that transport through the brush border cannot be considered in isolation. Each substrate that is ingested must pass through at least four sequential phases; luminal, brush border, intracellular, and basal membrane. Thus, an alteration in any one of these four phases may affect the apparent movement of a substrate through any of the other compartments. Deficiency of a substance could be caused by decreased intake, by poor digestion of complex molecules to simple ones, by decreased transport by the brush border membrane, or by decreased transport from the intestinal cells into the blood stream. What is not clear is the effect of concurrent partial deficiencies in two or more of these phases. For example, we know very little about the effect of a partial decrease in brush border transport in the face of markedly reduced intake during malnutrition. Since both the affinity for a particular substance and its maximal rate of transport may be genetically determined, it should be expected that the impact of malnutrition in specific individuals and in specific populations may well be determined by inherited differences in the intestinal transport systems.

The following review can only skim the surface of this exciting field of study. To bring some order to the mass of available material, I shall divide my presentation into short discussions of the transport of carbohydrates, amino acids, water soluble vitamins, and fat soluble vitamins. Thus I shall deal with the transport of small organic molecules and leave discussion of metal ion transport to others.

Carbohydrate Absorption

Carbohydrate absorption procedes in three general stages: digestion of complex carbohydrates, hydrolysis of di-and tri-saccharides, and specific transport of monosaccharides across the intestine. It is clear that genetic alteration of any of these factors will influence the effectiveness of a particular source of carbohydrate in providing calories. Very little data are available on the genetics of complex carbohydrate digestion and particularly about variability in the time of development and substrate specificity of the various amylases.

However, there are suggestions from other studies that genetic variations may occur. There has been intense interest in recent years in the use of complex carbohydrates in the treatment of disorders of carbohydrate metabolism, particularly diabetes, and in early infant nutrition. These studies have shown great center to center variability which might be as well explained by population differences as by differences in technique. Recent studies of glucose and insulin responses to carbohydrate loading have shown marked differences which depend on the carbohydrate source [6].

Similary, DeVizia [7], in infants, demonstrated differences in the utilization of starch from rice, corn, wheat, and tapioca. Additional evidence of genetic variation can be found in the 'allergy' literature. Families which are intolerant of specific carbohydrate sources such as corn have been documented [8]. Since complex carbohydrates represent the major source of sugars for the majority of the world's population, these data suggest that genetic as well as cultural factors may have to be considered in providing nutritional sources to a particular population.

The disaccharidases have long been a subject of intense interest to nutritionists and geneticists. They have already been discussed elsewhere in this volume. I would like here to make only two comments. First, I would remind you that the dissacharidases are closely associated physically with the brush border where transport occurs. Secondly, it is important to note that the rate limiting step in the uptake of carbohydrates is the transport process except in the case of lactose where the rate of hydrolysis to glucose and galactose is far less than the Vmax of the transport system [9].

Glucose and galactose are actively absorbed by the brush border of the intestine by a well characterized and highly specific transport system [10]. This transport system is concentrative, saturable, and sodium and energy dependent. Kinetic studies of transport of glucose and its analogues have suggested the additional active transport systems may also participate in glucose uptake [11]. Fructose, on the other hand, is probably transported by a single, sodium independent system which is not concentrative. An inherited disorder of glucose-galactose malabsorption was first delineated by Lindquist and Meeuwisse [12] in a large Swedish pedigree. They demonstrated most of the criteria for recessive inheritance, consanguinity, evidence of affected siblings, and absence of vertical transmission. Perhaps the best evidence for the inheritance of this disorder comes from the studies of Dr. L.J. Elsas and Dr. L.E. Rosenberg [13] in a Georgian family. That laboratory demonstrated convincingly that the parents and a half sibling of a child with total absence of glucose transport had a partial transport defect. Specifically, kinetic analysis showed that the obligate heterozygotes had a reduced capacity, but a normal affinity for glucose transport. More than 20 patients with this disorder have now been described. Although the family studied by Elsas had a normal affinity for glucose by the intestinal transport system, by analogy with the similar disorder of the kidney, renal glycosuria, other families who are carriers for this disorder may be expected to have decreased affinity as well as capacity for glucose transport. Harking back to Dr. Crane's model of the digestive-absorptive unit, it is not clear what effect a decreased affinity might have in the face of otherwise compromised intestinal function. For example, we would expect that decreased disaccharidase activity in a person with decreased affinity for glucose might produce a clinical picture similar to complete loss of enzyme or transport system.

Absorption of Amino Acids

The nutritional use of free amino acids will be dealt with later and only a brief description of some of the genetic aspects of amino acid transport will be discussed here. Amino acids are transported across the intestinal brush border membrane by several different and highly specific transport systems. The relationship of the inheritance of these transport systems to the comparable systems in the kidney is not entirely clear. Although numerous examples of concurrent transport abnormalities in gut and kidney have been reported, in other individuals and families normal transport in the intestine has been reported in the face of striking renal tubular defects. One of the best documented examples of this inconsistent association of renal and intestinal transport defects comes from the studies of the disease cystinuria by Rosenberg, Segal, and their colleagues [14]. In 10 of 12 cystinuric patients with indistinguishable renal defects in cystine and dibasic amino acid clearance, mediated uptake of cystine, lysine, and arginine by jejunal mucosa was absent. However, in the other two, transport was only somewhat impaired. Extension of these studies to the obligate heterozygotes for this disorder demonstrated that at least three distinct, allelic mutations in this transport system were present. Although none of the patients or carriers of this disorder are known to have nutritional disorders, a disorder of another dibasic amino acid transport system presumably under separate genetic control has produced clinical deficiencies [15]. This condition which has variously been described as lysinuria, lysinuric protein intolerance, and hyperlysinuria with hyperammonemia is now known to be related to a renal and intestinal transport defect in a system used by the dibasic amino acids but not by cystine. This defect appears to be quite common in Finland and also to be present in other populations [16]. The hyperammonemia is probably a consequence of deficiency of two of the substrates needed in the urea cycle, arginine and ornithine. Another intestinal transport defect of major clinical significance is known as Hartnup disease [17]. In this disorder of one of the neutral amino acid transport systems tryptophan is among the amino acids malabsorbed. Because tryptophan is a major precursor of niacin in humans, some of the consequences of this disorder may be caused by niacin deficiency.

Similar to my discussion of partial defects in carboydrate transport, very little is known of the effects of partial defects in amino acid transport in an intestine already compromised by other disease. Again we must wonder about the effects of substate limitations in persons who have decreased affinity for a specific amino acid. In this instance there is clinical evidence that problems can occur. Heterozygotes for Hartnup disease often get pellegra when their nutrition is marginal [18]. Here too the limitations of the transport systems may alter the usefulness of specific sources of protein in particular populations. Dr. Cavalli-Sforza [19] has suggested that the coefficient of selection for lactose digestion would be sufficient to give rise to the high frequency of this ability among dairying peoples today. It is equally possible that other peoples have been selected on the basis of their amino acid transport systems by efficient utilization of proteins poor in a particular amino acid.

Absorption of the Water Soluble Vitamins

The water soluble vitamins are a diverse group of compounds. Most are part of the so-called B-complex. Besides the common characteristic of being relatively hydrophilic (when compared to the fat soluble vitamins), these compounds share other properties as well. Unlike the fat soluble vitamins, only small amounts of these compounds are retained in the body and catabolism and the daily losses in urine and stool dictate frequent dietary intake to avoid deficiency. In addition, deficiencies can occur due to increased needs during periods of increased metabolic activity, for example, during pregnancy, or during periods of rapid growth. Water soluble vitamins function in intermediary metabolism primarily as precursors of cofactors important for a wide variety of enzymatic processes, but do not themselves fill any caloric or nitrogen requirements. In their absence, enzymes which require cofactors cannot function, and the resultant deficiencies are often indistinguishable from known inborn errors where an inactive or absent protein produces blockage in a necessary metabolic pathway. In many cases the particular enzymatic disturbance which produces the clinical picture seen in a deficiency state is not known. For example, we do not know for sure why patients with niacin deficiency have pellegra or why patients with B-12 deficiency have anemia. Another characteristic of these compounds is that only very minute amounts are necessary to maintain adequate concentrations of cofactors in the body. It would be anticipated that compounds present in food in such small amounts and so necessary for normal function would be absorbed by highly selective processes rather that by simple diffusion or mass action. In every case where data is available, selective transport of the water soluble vitamins has been found. However, the best evidence, as always, is genetic. For at least three of these vitamins, folic acid, B-12 and biotin, genetic defects in specific transport processes in the intestine have been described which produce clinical disease. Although the transport of vitamin B-12 is the best understood of all of the transport processes known for the water soluble vitamins, it is not within the scope of this article to give adequate justice to this complex subject.

A specific defect in the absorption of folic acid was first described by Luhby and his coworkers in 1961 [20]. These workers described a child who had recurrent megaloblastic anemia starting at age three months. Investigation of the intestinal tract revealed no other abnormalities, suggesting that the defect was quite specific for folic acid. Because the child's sibling was found to have the same disorder [21], they suggested that the defect in folate absorption was inherited as an autosomal recessive trait. In addition to the anemia the children had ataxia, mental retardation, and a seizure disorder. A specific defect in folate transport was found not only in the intestine, but also in the spinal cord membranes. Other similar cases have been described [22]. Studies of the heterozygote carriers have not yet determined the mechanism of the defect. It is possible that the same defect might produce the clinical picture of homocystinuria of the folate responsive form, [23] although one would expect to also have megaloblastic anemia in this situation.

Biotin deficiency was believed not to occur naturally in man because gastrointestinal bacteria produce biotin and it is present in virtually all natural foods. Previously biotin deficiency has been produced in man only by feeding large amounts of raw egg whites which contain a protein which binds biotin tightly, avidin. Recently biotin deficiency has been observed in infants receiving total parenteral alimentation [24]. Because no deficiency states are normally encountered, few if any studies of the intestinal transport of this vitamin have been done. In fact a computer search of the medical literature failed to reveal any studies in the last 5 years until the recent papers described below. The new interest in biotin has resulted from the description of children with an inherited disorder of several different biotin requiring enzymes, multiple carboxylase deficiency. The carboxylases requiring biotin as a cofactor include those for the coenzyme A thioesters of acetate, beta-methylcrotonate, propionate, and pyruvate. The first children described with this condition were believed to have biotin responsive forms of either propionic acidemia [25] or beta-methylcrotonyl glycinuria [26]. It was then found that these patients had disorders of all of their carboxylases which were measured [27]. The initial patients were found by Sweetman's laboratory to have a defect in the lygase or synthetase which covalently binds biotin to the carboxylases [28]. Subsequently however, patients have been described who have low levels of biotin in their blood and urine and who appear to have a selective defect in biotin absorption from the intestine [29, 30]. Thus the first genetic evidence has been provided that biotin has a specific transport system. Further studies will be required to define the kinetics of the transport system and to evaluate the obligate heterozygote state. Recently we have evaluated a multiple carboxylase deficiency in an older child with a history of non-specific diarrhea. This child had a history of ataxia, fragile hair, and acidosis, all features of multicarboxylase deficiency. However, the organic acids present in his serum and urine, though typical of this disease, were only two to three fold elevated, less than has been reported. Because GI disease is not part of the known symptoms of this condition, we assume that his biotin problems resulted from, rather then caused, his intestinal problem. It would not be surprising to find that children with non-specific or infectious diarrhea, particularly during periods of rapid growth, suffer from similar problems.

Thiamine in its phosphorylated form is an integral part of the enzyme complexes required for at least two major groups of reactions; decarboxylation of alpha-keto acids (e.g., pyruvate, alpha-keto glutarate, and the branched chain keto acids), and transketolase reactions involved in the metabolism of glucose. Thiamine deficiency results in one of the three forms of beriberi, dry, wet and acute. Thiamine is known to be trasported by the intestine selectively [31] although at high concentrations it can be absorbed passively. No specific inherited transport defects have been described, but children with thiamine responsive disorders have been documented. Some of these might possibly represent thiamine transport defects. Scriver et al [32] described an infant with a thiamine responsive form of maple syrup urine disease, branched chain keto-acid dehydrogenase deficiency. In addition children have been described who have thiamine responsive megaloblastic anemias, [33] and chronic lactic acidosis [34].

Thiamine deficiency may also occur during periods of apparently adequate intake. Thiamine is another water soluble vitamin whose requirements are believed to increse during periods of rapid growth and especially during conditions giving rise to increased catabolic states including heavy labor. In our laboratory we have begun to investigate the thiamine status of infants during periods of rapid growth spurred on by the discovery of an infant with a three-fold elevation of the branched chain amino acids and keto acids and a several fold increase in lactic acid. This child responded to modest increases in his thiamine intake, 10 mg QD. His branched chain dehydrogenase was normal and we are waiting expectantly for him to become old enough to do thiamine transport studies. Thiamine deficiency has been commonly associated with alcoholism and alcohol is known to interfere with thiamine absorption from the bowel [35]. Certain foods, such as raw shellfish and even raw scaled fish such as carp contain thaiminases which can catabolize thiamine in the intestine [36]. It is less clear whether thiamine deficiency occurs commonly with other forms of bowel disease. Most patients with these problems receive multiple vitamin preparations. It would be anticipated that during periods of rapid growth, absorption in children with intestinal disturbances might very well be inadequate.

If space permitted, riboflavin, pyridoxine, and niacin could all be discussed similarly to my treatment of the other water soluble vitamins. Although no specific transport deficiencies for these vitamins have been described, multiple dependency syndromes for pyridoxine [37] are known and it should be anticipated that at least some of these patients may prove to have absorptive problems of a hereditary derivation. Like the other water soluble vitamins, greatly exaggerated claims have been made in the popular press for their usefulness in a variety of disorders. However, we should not dismiss all of this natural medicine movement out of hand despite its adoption by medical charlatans. If I may have the liberty of quoting one of my forebearers. If we are only wise enough to find it, there is much truth in tradition.

Absorption of the Fat Soluble Vitamins

The four fat soluble vitamins, A, E, D, and K, have quite different chemical structures and entirely different biological functions in the body. They are grouped together by unifying chemical characteristic, solubility in lipids and insolubility in aqueous solutions. Far more than the water soluble vitamins, their absorption is linked to all accessory organs of the gastrointestinal tract. Malabsorption can occur in any circumstance in which general lipid malabsorption occurs including malfunction of the liver and biliary system, the pancreas, or the intestine itself. In fact any condition which effects the emulsification of lipids can profoundly change the adsorptive pattern. These factors include pH and particularly the presence of other lipids in the diet. Only vitamins A and Kl in this group are known to have specific brush border membrane transport systems. However, the serum transport of all of these compounds is highly dependent on the binding proteins required to keep them soluble and these proteins also appear to be important in their transfer across the basal membrane of the intestinal cells. These vitamins are all stored in the body, primarily in the liver. Therefore, ingestion need not be as frequent as is necessary for the water soluble vitamins and several weeks or months of a deficient diet are usually required before deficiency occurs in the human. Storage, however produces the potential for intoxication. Hypervitaminosis A and D are frequently encountered in populations prone to taking large amounts of proprietory vitamines. Vitamin E is ingested in even larger quantities, but no toxic state has been described.

Vitamin A deficiency in common is most areas of the world and is a major cause of blindness. Vitamin A alcohol, retinol, is transported by a specific, saturable process when present in the intestine in the concentrations normally released from dietary sources [38]. However, as the concentration of A is further increased, it is absorbed by an unsaturable process. This secondary absorption is part of the nonspecific absorption of lipids and Vitamin A absorbed by this route circulates initially in the serum in the lipoprotein fraction [39]. The concentrations of Vitamin A in the serum under normal circumstances are highly regulated by a specific binding protein, retinol binding protein, RBP [40]. The concentration of RBP is under the control of at least growth hormone [41] and requires the presence of zinc [42]. Thus, zinc deficiency and hereditary problems with zinc absorption both lead to low circulating concentrations of RBP and vitamin A. We have recently confirmed in our own patients that total serum vitamin A is reduced in growth hormone deficiency, but the significance of this observation remains obscure. Provitamin A's, beta-carotenes, are absorbed by the intestinal mucosa by a nonsaturable process. However, the conversion of the provitamins to vitamin A is highly regulated. This enzymatic process is stimulated by thyroid hormones [43] and is largely inactive in hypothyroid states. One child has been reported who could not convert beta-carotene to retinol and who had clinical vitamin A deficiency, [44] but no specific inherited transport deficiencies for vitamin A have yet been described.

There are two major forms of vitamin K of importance to people, vitamin Kl derived from vegetable sources and vitamin K2 which is produced by bacteria in the large intestine. The absorption of these two compounds is quite different [45]. Vitamin Kl is absorbed in the proximal small intestine by a saturable and energy requiring process. On the other hand, vitamin K2 is absorbed largely from the distal intestine because of its source. Its uptake is passive and nonsaturable. At higher concentrations even Kl is taken up nonspecifically and appears in the chylomicron fraction of the thoracic duct lymph [46]. No inherited forms of vitamin K malabsorption have been described. The newborn infant, particulary when premature, is subject to vitamin K deficiency, but it is assumed that this is due to the limited secretion of bile salts, to the undeveloped intestinal flora, and perhaps to an immaturity of the vitamin K related enzymes in the liver.

Both vitamin D and vitamin E appear to be absorbed non-specifically [47]. Although deficiency states occur for both of these compounds and dependency is well described for vitamin D, none of these conditions have been related to specific transport problems.

SUMMARY

Small organic molecules are usually absorbed from the intestine by highly specific transport systems. Although total absence of some of these systems has been described and usually produces significant disease, the effects of partial defects are unknown. Although partial defects would not be expected to lead to malabsorption in the face of substrate excess in individuals with normal intestinal function, they might well produce deficiencies in instances where there is limited substrate available or in which intestinal function is hampered by disease. Molecular transport which is sufficient under normal circumstances may also be insufficient during periods of metabolic stress. Genetic variation in the affinities or capacities of transport systems may effect the usefulness of specific foodstuffs in feeding populations prone to deficiency diseases. At this time too little data is available to assess the role of the genetic control of intestinal transport in the control of malnutrition in large populations.

MONOSACCHARIDE TRANSPORT SYSTEMS

Specific

   1) Glucose - Galactose
      —sodium and energy dependent
      —concentrative
   2) Fructose
      —sodium and energy independent
      —non-concentrative
      —may depend on conversion to glucose in cell

Non-Specific

   3) Xylose

AMINO ACID TRANSPORT SYSTEMS

   1. Neutral
      —leucine preferring
      —alanine preferring
   2. Imino-glycine
   3. Dibasic
      —Ornithine, arginine, lysine, + cystine
   4. Acidic

MONOSACCHARIDE TRANSPORT SYSTEMS

Specific

   1) Glucose - Galactose
      —sodium and energy dependent
      —concentrative
   2) Fructose
      —sodium and energy independent
      —non-concentrative
      —may depend on conversion to glucose in cell

Non-Specific

   3) Xylose

AMINO ACID TRANSPORT SYSTEMS

1. Neutral
   —leucine preferring
   —alanine preferring
2. Imino-glycine
3. Dibasic
   —ornithine, arginine, lysine, + cystine
4. Acidic

WATER-SOLUBLE VITAMINS

Thiamine	—specific active transport
	—sodium dependent
Riboflavin	—specific transport system
	—saturable
Pyridoxine	—transport probably specific
Niacin	but not studied
Biotin	—s p e c i f i c
	—defect causes multiple carboxylase deficiencies

FAT-SOLUBLE VITAMINS

Vitamin A (Retinol)

—specific saturable process at physiological
  concentrations
—non-specific process at high concentrations

Carotene

—non-specific uptake - passive diffusion
—specific conversion to vitamin A

Vitamin K₁ (vegatable sources)

—saturable
—energy requiring

Vitamin K₂ (bacterial)

—passive diffusion

Vitamins D and E

—probably passive diffusion

REFERENCES

1. Curran, P.F., Hajjar, J.J., and Glynn, I.M. J. *Gen. Physiol.* 217:1261-1286 (1970).
2. Hillman, R.E., and Rosenberg, L.E. *J. Biol. Chem.* 244:4494-4498 (1969).
3. Crane, R.K *Amer. J. Clin. Nutrition* 22:242-249 (1969).
6. Collier, G. and O' Dea, K *Amer. J. Clin. Nutrition* 36:10-14 (1982).
7. DeVizia, B., Cicimerra, F., DeCicco, N., and Auricchio, S. *J. Pediatr.* 86:50-55 (1975).
9. Alpers, D.H., and Seetharam, B. *N. Engl. J. Med.* 296:1047-1052 (1977).
10. Faust, R.G., Leadbetter, M.G., Plenge, R.K., and McCaslin, A.J. *J. Gen. Physio.* 52:482-494 (1968).
11. Kimmich, G.A. and Randles, J. *J. Membrane Biol.* 27:363-379 (1976).
12. Meeuwisse, G.W., and Lindquist, B. *Acta Paediat. Scand.* 59:74-79 (1970).
13. Elsas, L.J., Hillman, R.E., Patterson, J.H., and Rosenberg, L.E. *J. Clin. Invest.* 49:576-585 (1970).
14. Rosenberg, L.E., Downing, S.J., Durant, J.L., and Segal, S. *J. Clin. Invest.* 45:365-371 (1966).
15. Simell, O., Perheentupa, J., Rapola, J., Visakorpi, J.K., and Eskelin, L.E. *Amer. J. Med.* 59:229 (1975).
16. Whelan, D.T., and Scriver, C.R.. *Pediatr. Res.* 2:525-534 (1968).
17. Baron, D.N., Dent, C.E., Harris, H., Hart, E.W., and Jepson, J.B. *Lancet* I:421-428 (1956).
18. Jepson, J.B. in ' The Metabolic basis of inherited disease' Fourth ed. J.B. Stanbury, J.B. Wyngaarden, and D.S. Fredrickson, editors. McGraw Hill, New York (1978).
19. Cavalli-Sforza, L.L. *Amer. J. Hum. Genet.* 25:82-89 (1973).
20. Luhby, A.L., Eagle, F.J., Roth, E., and Cooperman, J.M. *Amer. J. Dis. Child.* 102:482-484 (1961).
21. Luhby, A.L., and Cooperman, J.M. (abstract) *American Pediatr. Soc.* (1967).
22. Lanzkowsky, P. *Amer. J. Med.* 48:580-583 (1970).
23. Freeman, J.M., Finkelstein, M.D., and Mudd, S.H. *N. Engl. J. Med.* 292:491-496 (1975).
24. Mock, D.M., Delorimer, A.A., Liebman, W.M., Sweetman, L., and Baker, H. *N. Engl. J. Med.* 304:820-823 (1981).
25. Barnes, N.D., Hull, D., Balgobin, L., and Gompertz, D. *Lancet* II:244-245 (1970).
26. Weyler, W., Sweetman, L., Maggio, D.C. and Nyhan, W.C. *Clin. Chim. Acta* 76:321 (1977).
27. Packman, S., Sweetman, L., Baker, H. and Wall, S. *J. Pediatr.* 99:418-420 (1981).
28. Sweetman, L. *J. Inherited Metab. Dis.* 4:53-54 (1981).
29. Munnich, A., Saudubray, J.M., Carre, G., *et al Lancet* II:263 (1981).
30. Thoene, J.G., Sanghvi, R.S. and Lemons, R. (abstract) *Soc. Ped. Res.* (1982).
31. Rindi, R.S. and Ventura, U. *Physiol. Rev.* 52:821-827 (1972).
32. Scriver, C.R., MacKenzie, S., Clow, C.L., and Lelvin, E. *Lancet* I:310-312 (1971).
33. Porter, F.S., Rogers, L.E., and Sidbury, J.B., Jr. *J. Pediatr.* 74:494-504 (1969).
34. Brunette, M.G. Delvin, E., Hazel, B., and Scriver, C.R. *Pediatrics* 50:702-711 (1972).
35. Baker, H., Frank, O. Zettalman, R.K., *et al Amer. J. Clin. Nutr.* 28:1377-1383 (1975).
36. Greene, H.L. in ' Pediatric Nutrition' R.M. Suskind ed. Raven, New York (1981).
37. Scriver, C.R., and Rosenberg, L.E. in ' Metabolic Control and Disease' P.K. Bondy and L.E. Rosenberg, ed. Saunders, Philadelphia (1980).
38. Hollander, D. *J. Lab. Clin. Med.* 97:449-462 (1981).
39. Blomstrand, R., and Werner, B. Scand. *J. Clin. Lab. Invest.* 19:339-345 (1967).
40. Goodman, D.S. *Vitam. Horm.* 32:167-180 (1974).
41. Mohan, P.S. and Rao, K.S.J. *Clin. Chim. Acta* 96:241-246 (1979).
42. Smith, J.C., Jr. *Ann. N.Y. Acad. Sci.* 355:62-75 (1980).
43. Hillman, R.W., and Nerb, L. *Amer. J. Digest. Dis.* 18:185-189 (1952).
44. McLaren, D.S. and Zekian, B. *Amer. J. Dis. Child.* 121:278-280 (1971).
45. Hollander, D. *Amer. J. Physiol.* 225:360-369 (1973).
46. Forsgren, L. *Acta Chir. Scand.* 399:1-29 (1969).
47. Hollander, D., Rim, E., and Muralidhara, K.S. *Gastroenterology* 68:1492-1497 (1975).

INTESTINAL MICROFLORA AND NUTRIENT REQUIREMENTS

Bernard S. Wostmann
Margaret H. Beaver

Department of Microbiology/Lobund Laboratory
University of Notre Dame
Notre Dame, Indiana

INTRODUCTION

' Souvent, dans nos causeries du laboratoire, depuis bien des années, j'ai parlé, aux jeunes savants qui m'entouraient, de l'intérêt qu'il y aurait à nourrir un jeune animal (lapin, cobaye, chien, poulet), dés sa naissance avec des matières nutritives pures. Par cette dernière expression, j'entends désigner des produits alimentaires qu'on priverait artificiellement et complètement des microbes communs. Sans vouloir rien affirmer, je ne cache pas que j'entreprendrais cette étude, si j'en avais le temps, avec la pensée préconcue que la vie, dans ces conditions, deviendrait impossible.''
Louis Pasteur, 1885

When Pasteur made this well known statement [43] he implied that microorganisms may affect nutrition by otherwise "pure nutrients". To my knowledge he never elaborated on his statement, at least not in writing, but the impetus of his ideas led, within 10 years, to the first germfree study. Nuttal and Thierfelder in 1895 reported caesarian derivation on the first germfree guinea pig that managed to survive for 13 days [40]. Even this short survival is surprising, since lack of knowledge of the nutritional consequences of sterilization of the cow's milk used to nurse the newborn animal may well have led to a very inadequate dietary intake.

As work with germfree animals expanded, uncertainty about the nutritional consequences of the absence of a microflora grew [66]. It had become increasingly obvious that the intestinal flora might produce a number of vitamins, and possibly other essential nutrients. Studies by Lih and Baumann [36],

Sauberlich [58] and Jones and Baumann [27], in which various antibiotics were added to diets deficient in B vitamins had suggested a role of the microflora in vitamin metabolism. Work by Wostmann *et al* [65] demonstrated that the "vitamin-sparing action" of antibiotics was not found under germfree conditions (Fig. 1), and was probably caused either by increased microflora production, or by an enhanced availability of that production. Somewhat later Gustafsson [21], Wostmann [69], Daft [8] and Sacquet and coworkers [62] showed that in the rat intestinal microflora production would largely cover requirements of vitamin K, biotin, folic acid and vitamin B_{12}, respectively. Thiamin production on the other hand, although sufficient to almost cover daily requirements, proved to be hardly available to the animal [69].

A few years later Dubos and Schaedler, in a classic experiment, showed that ex-germfree mice repopulated with a controlled non-pathogenic microflora could survive, and even grow, on corns as the sole source of nutrients, whereas mice harboring a "normal" microflora would loose weight on such a regime, and eventually die [9]. Even when the diet contained protein of more adequate quality, but marginal quantity (e.g. 15% casein), growth of the "clean" mice was always much better than that of the conventional "dirty" mice. Thus, although the investigations mentioned earlier pointed to the intestinal microflora as a potential source of essential nutrients, the latter study suggests that this flora will, to a considerable extent, actually determine nutritional requirements of the host-microflora complex.

Although most of the studies in this field were performed with germfree, gnotobiotic and conventional rats, mice, rabbits and chickens, an approximation to the human condition is possible. In underdeveloped countries hygienic conditions may be worse than in the average experimental animal quarters of our universities, and prevent the most efficient utilization of nutrients even in the absence of overt disease. And even in developed countries relatively little is known about composition and stability of the human intestinal microflora and its effects on nutrient requirements and utilization.

EFFECTS OF THE INTESTINAL MICROFLORA ON FUNCTION AND METABOLISM

Gastro-intestinal function

Although lactobaccili and yeasts populate distinct sites of the stomach lining, little is known about the possible consequences of their presence. In the small intestine, however, the presence of a microflora affects many aspects of function and metabolism. Administration of penicillin with the diet will, through changes in microbial population that are ill understood, lead to a substantial reduction in the weight of the intestinal tissue [16]. Peristalsis of small and large intestine will be affected by the bacterial population [1, 54].

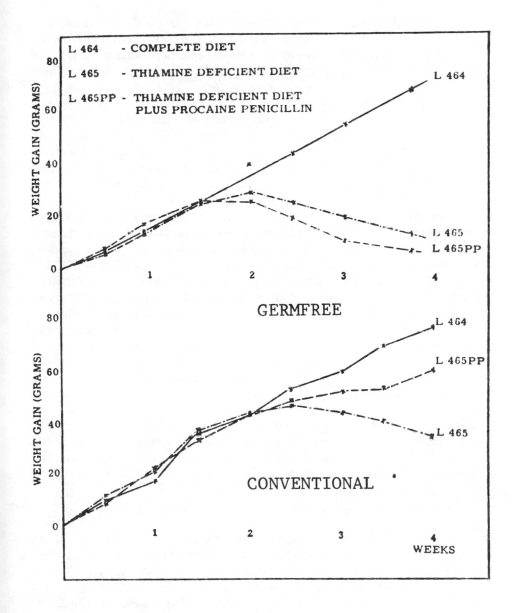

Fig. 1. "Vitamin-sparing action" of antibiotics under conventional and germ free conditions.

Of special importance will be the influence of the gut flora on local bile acid concentration and composition [29, 37] which in turn will affect enzyme action, absorption of lipid materials, and possibly enterocyte kinetics [56]. In the absence of a microflora, enterohepatic bile acids pools may be 2-4 times normal size.

The presence of bacteria will reduce the concentration of the various digestive enzymes in the lumen of the gut [32, 48], and will have a profound effect on the oxidation-reduction potential of gut contents [70]. Size and form of the villi will be affected [17, 23, 38]. Enterocyte kinetics may be affected both directly and indirectly, and with it the average age of the mucosal cell [58a]. This in turn may influence the activity of the various brush borden enzymes like lactase, maltase, sucrase and alkaline phosphatase [47, 63]. Presumably a lower turnover rate (found in germfree and certain gnotobiotic animals) will lead, on the average, to an "older" mucosal cell with higher enzyme concentrations [47]. Less obvious is the cause for the increased activity of Ca^{++}-, Mg^{2+}- dependent and (Na^+ + K^+)- stimulated ATPase in the absence of an intestinal flora [52, 76].

The size of the rodent cecum depends on the composition of the local microflora. In germfree rodents, rabbits and guinea pigs the cecum may be enlarged to 10 times its "normal" size. Upon population a gradual reduction in size occurs. Combinations of 4 to 6 organisms often reduce the cecum to approximately twice its normal size [4, 74]. Beyond that, a more complex flora is needed to achieve further reduction [13, 29]. Clostridia and fusiform bacteria appear important in determining the size and biochemical activity of the cecum.

Under especially unfavorable conditions, enterotoxic enteropathies may occur, due to enterotoxins elaborated by certain *E. colis* and vibrios. These toxins activate adenyl cyclases, and the resulting cAMP leads to secretory diarrheas with extensive loss of K^+, bicarbonate ions and Cl^-. Other diarrheas of microbial origin may lead to considerable fluid loss and interfere with the uptake of nutrients.

The growth-depressing factor

Earlier, we mentioned the nutrient sparing action of antibiotics. When Coates *et al* compared the growth of chickens fed penicillin with that of germfree chickens, it became obvious that the antibiotic actually counteracted a growth-depressing effect of the prevailing microflora [5a]. Eyssen and DeSomer found that growth of germfree chickens could be depressed by association with *Streptococcus faecalis,* in addition to the administration of a cell-free fecal filtrate [10]. This resulted in a thickening of the intestinal wall and increased fecal excretion of lipids, a syndrome that could be reversed to a large extent by the oral administration of antibiotics. The authors concluded that the cell-free filtrate contained a viral agent. A similar conclusion was reached by Lee and Dubos, who reported a lasting depression of body weights in SPF mice that had been inoculated at 2 days of age with an intestinal filtrate of "dirty" mice [31].

However, no viral agent was ever found. Recently, Fuller *et al* reported that *Streptococcus faecium* effectively depressed growth in associated chicks. Again, a fecal filtrate fed soon after hatching produced additional growth depression, but the authors categorically state that "so far our efforts to demonstrate a virus by tissue culture or electron microscope have been unsuccessful" [14]. Thus, growth depression by fecal filtrates appears to be a reproducible phenomenon, but the actual causative factor(s) remain to be elucidated.

Lifespan, resting oxygen consumption, and thyroid function

In the absence of the challenge of potentially pathogenic microorganisms, germfree rats and mice live much longer than their conventional counterparts [19, 44]. They grow old in obviously good health, but with increasing age, tumors become more and more prevalent. The male germfree Lobund Wistar rat maintained on natural ingredient colony diet has a median lifespan of approximately 1000 days. Spontaneous liver tumors were observed in 87% of germfree rats that were over 30 months of age, 10% of which were classified as hepatocellular carcinomas. Ten percent of germfree male rats in that age group also developed adenocarcinomas of the prostate gland. In conventional Lobund Wistar rats malignancy is observed only sporadically, since the animals usually succomb to infectious disease before malignancy may become manifest [44].

The extended lifespan of the germfree rodent may also be caused in part by other factors which are indirectly related to the absence of a microflora. Germfree rats and mice have smaller hearts, a smaller cardiac output, and a lower resting O_2 consumption [3, 71]. They do, however, show normal concentrations of circulating thyroid hormones (T3 and T4), and a normal half life of the main hormone produced by the thyroid, T4 [59, 75]. Surprisingly, T3 and T4 levels of aging germfree rats and mice do not decrease, as is the case in the conventional rodents, but remain at "young adult" levels well past the animal's middle age [75].

Association of germfree rats with *Escherichia coli* increased resting O_2 consumption to almost normal levels. Association with *Clostridium perfringens* or *Bacteroides sp*, on the other hand, did not increase O_2 consumption, suggesting that indirect, possibly species-specific microbial effects may influence the resting O_2 consumption of rats and mice [35].

MICROFLORA AND NUTRIENT REQUIREMENTS

Intestinal microfloras may produce vitamins, amino acids and lipids. The extent and emphasis of the microbial production will depend on the host species, and its hygienic and nutritional condition. On the other hand, intestinal microorganisms may require certain nutrients, and as such may compete with the host. A third possibility is an effect to the microflora on the host which changes the host's requirement for a certain nutrient. A prime example is the reduced requirement for vitamin A of the germfree rat that is needed for survival. Germfree Sprague-Dawley rats were able to maintain life on diets containing only traces of this vitamin, although typical symptoms of deficiency were obvious, and growth was arrested at approximately 200 g. Conventional rats would survive for only 8-10 weeks under those conditions [55].

Energy requirements

Although the feeding of low levels of antibiotics may lead to increased efficiency of feed utilization with diets that are considered nutritionally adequate, little specific information seems available on the effect of microorganisms on energy requirements. Studies comparing germfree and conventional chickens suggested a slightly higher energy extraction by the conventional animals [7]. Gordon established that germfree mice ate more than conventional mice, but also excreted more fecal material [20]. More recent experiments revealed that adult GF rats of stable body weight excreted twice the fecal dry matter voided by their conventional counterparts of similar body weight. However, dietary intake of the germfree rats was 18% higher, and as such compensated for the increased caloric losses in the feces. Both germfree and conventional rats retained approximately 607 kJ/kg/day (481 kJ/kg$^{.75}$/day) from their total caloric intake. This amounted to 71% of intake for the germfree, and 80% of intake for the conventional rat (Wostmann, B.S., unpublished data). Since the increase in fecal matter voided by the germfree rat occured almost totally in the form of water soluble material containing both proteins and hexuronic acids, one might speculate that microbial breakdown of these materials might have made them, at least in part, available to a conventional host, thereby increasing the efficiency of extraction of dietary energy.

But our data suggest that some fiber material may even be digested by the conventional rat, presumably producing energy in the form of volatile fatty acids which may be at least partially absorbed. It is known that in the rabbit this process can supply up to 30-40% of energy requirements. Recently, Wolin has intimated that similar processes may make at least some energy available via fermentation in the human large intestine [64].

Protein and amino acids

The study of Dubos and Schaedler, mentioned earlier, showed that ex-germfree mice harboring a controlled, nonpathogenic microflora could sustain themselves on diets containing low quality proteins which in conventional mice would have prevented weight gain and eventually would have resulted in death. Even when fed a diet containing limited amounts (15%) of casein, weight gain of the "clean" mice was always much better than of the conventional "dirty" mice [9]. Chawla *et al* administered antibiotics to rats fed diets suboptimal in casein and, in valine, threonine or tryptophane. Under these conditions they were able to demonstrate substantial increases in body weight gain by administering a mixture of neomycin, bacitracin and polymixin B with the drinking water. The authors state that while the concentration of microorganisms in the small intestine remained the same, a shift in population occurred with yeasts or *Proteus* replacing the anaerobic species [5]. This does not, however, explain the mechanisms behind this "sparing effect", since valine, threonine and tryptophane follow different metabolic pathways, but are spared to approximately the same degree. Similarly, Stoewsand *et al*, who fed defined diets containing increasing amounts of lysine to conventional mice, to mice harboring a defined, nonpathogenic microflora, and to germfree mice, found that the gnotobiotic and germfree mice grew maximally on 2/3 of the lysine content required by the conventional mice.

Gustafsson has reported acceptable growth in germfree rats on diets containing 6-8% protein [22] and Reddy *et al* found a slightly higher nitrogen retention in young germfree rats, in agreement with data obtained by others [51]. On the other hand, data by Salter *et al* on germfree chicks [57], and other studies with germfree rats [25, 34], including our own, point to increased fecal N losses in the germfree animal, presumably of endogenous origin.

In the absence of an intestinal flora, little decomposition of amino acids occurs, and absorption may even be somewhat faster than in the conventional animal [24], though the latter fact may be of little practical importance. In the presence of a microflora, extensive release of amino-N may take place. The resulting NH_3 can be reincorporated into microbially produced protein, incorporated into non-essential amino acids (also nucleotides, etc.) in the liver, or leave the body as urea or uric acid. It appears that, depending on protein nutrition and the size of the microbial reservoir (in monogastric mammals particularly the cecum), the microflora may act to the advantage or disadvantage of its host. In the rat and mouse, protein and amino acids appear to be generally more efficiently utilized in the absence of certain, as yet unknown elements of the conventional microflora. Increased fecal losses seem to be of endogeneous origin and the animal appears to compensate, at least in part, by the somewhat increased dietary intake dictated by its caloric requirements (see Energy requirements). In the rabbit [77], and possibly in the chicken [42] it would seem that the host may profit from its microflora, especially when dietary protein is marginal in quality or quantity. Comparison of the protein quality of the socalled "soft feces" of germfree and conventional rabbits (soft feces are the cecal contents of the rabbit which are voided several times a day and directly eaten by the conventional animal) shows that in case of the conventional rabbit, protein quality es definitely enhanced over that of the diet, while in the germfree animal it remains approximately the same [77].

Lipid requirements

The influence of the microflora on lipid nutrition does not seem to be of primary importance, except for the fact that the microflora will determine to a large extent the quality and quantity of the enterohepatic bile acid pool [37], and as such may influence lipase action and intestinal absorption of lipids. Most intestinal microfloras of any diversity will deconjugate biliary bile acids extensively. Other microorganisms (lactobacilli, *E.coli,* bacteroides, clostridia, etc.), will 7α-dehydroxylate and form keto-acids, thereby leading to a relative decrease in ileal bile acid reabsorption, an enhanced excretion and a lowering of the enterohepatic bile acid pool [11, 73].

Accordingly, no substantial effect of the microflora on fatty acid absorption has been reported, although the uptake of cholesterol is somewhat enhanced under germfree conditions (72). And while normal rat feces will contain a quantity of branched fatty acid and odd C number fatty acids of microbial origin, it will also contain less of the 18:1 and 18:2 fatty acids than in the absence of the microflora. Eyssen *et al* have described *Eubacterium lentum* as the organism responsible for this biohydrogenation of unsatured fatty acids which seems to take place exclusively in the cecum [11]. It remains to be established whether this phenomenon may affect PUFA requirements in any significant way.

Vitamin requirements

During the 1950s it became clear that, even in monogastric animals, the microflora could produce vitamin K [21] and most, if not all, of the B vitamins [6, 8] in significant amounts. What was less clear was the extent to which this production was available to the host, and whether, under certain conditions, a microflora might utilize more of a B factor than it potentially produced. In addition the question had to be asked to what extent an intestinal microflora could alter the systemic requirements of the host.

The B vitamins

Under conventional conditions the various B vitamins are produced by the microflora in amounts that could cover a significant part of the systemic requirement of the host. In the case of thiamine it has been estimated the under usual laboratory conditions the flora of the Wistar rat produces 60 to 80% of its systemic thiamin requirement (68). It could also be shown, however, that under those conditions, less than 10% of this intestinal production was available, even if coprophagy was not prevented (67). Further study suggested that systemic requirements in the presence or absence of a microflora might be different, since the thiamin concentration in the liver (but not in heart on other tissues) of the conventional rat was 50% higher than in the comparable germfree animal. It was presumed that this difference is related to the lower metabolic rate in the germfree murine rodents (see under Function and Metabolism). However, maximal growth of both germfree and conventional rats was obtained with diets containing 1.1 μg of thiamin/g diet [68]. In the presence of a conventional microflora a potential small benefit from flora-derived thiamine could be offset by a slightly higher requierement because of the presence of that microflora.

Although true vitamin B_6 deficiences occur in rats fed vitamin B_6 deficient diets, there are signs that the microflora may make some slight contribution to the vitamin B_6 status of the host [26]. On the other hand, in the case of biotin, folic acid and possibly pantothenic acid it appears that the microflora production is usually sufficient to cover systemic requirements [8]. In the case of vitamin B_{12}, most animal experiments suggest the substantial amounts are being synthesized by the microflora [2, 41]. Although its availability is still a matter of debate, it is speculated that, especially in developing countries, microflora production may make a significant contribution to vitamin B_{12} nutriture [39]. At the same time, as in the case of vitamin B_1, Oace and Abbot claim that systemic requirements of vitamin B_{12} may be reduced in the germfree state [41], and a similar statement has been made for pantothenic acid [30].

Ascorbic acid

No microflora production of ascorbic acid has been reported. However, as in the case of some of the B vitamins, studies with germfree guinea pigs fed an ascorbic acid deficient diet indicated that in the absence of a microflora, the animals lived longer and showed less severe signs of deficiency [33].

Fat soluble vitamins

The germfree rat was found to survive on extremely low levels of vitamin A, although growth of these Sprague-Dawley rats was arrested at approximately 200 g, and typical symptoms of vitamin A deficiency were obvious. Conventional rats maintained under these conditions survived at best for 8-10 weeks [55]. These data seem to imply a requirement for vitamin A to mantain epithelial integrity in the face of microbial challenge. However, studies with germfree chicken could not confirm the vitamin A sparing action of the germfree state [7].

Requirements for vitamins D and E seem independent of microbial status. On the other hand, while conventional animals usually do not have a requirement for vitamin K after the first early period of life, germfree animals have very distinct vitamin K requirements [69].

Mineral requirements

The absence of an intestinal microflora appears to enhance the absorption of Ca and Mg (15, 49). It is surprising that in the germfree rodent homeostatic mechanisms do not appear to compensate for this increased uptake. Instead, heavier skeletons are found and, under certain dietary conditions, a tendency to soft tissue calcification [50]. To prevent this, Ca levels in diets for germfree rats and mice are often reduced. There is no indication that the absence of specific elements of the microflora is involved in this phenomenon, but the generally increased size of the enterohepatic bile acid pool found in germfree animals may play a role here. Another possibility may lie in the greater activity of Ca^{++} and Mg^{++} dependent ATPases in the gut wall of the germfree rodent [52], which in turn may relate to the fact that in the absence of a microflora, cells of the intestinal epithelium may be older and show higher activities of a number of enzymes (See under Function and Metabolism).

Zn requirements were also found to be influenced by the presence or absence of a microflora. However, it is not clear whether systemic requirements are reduced in the absence of a flora, or if a microflora may sequester some of the available dietary Zn [60]. These observations are importante because of the crucial role of Zn in cell-mediated immunity, including anti-bacterial and anti-cancer defense [12].

The data on Fe and Cu metabolism are conflicting. On the one hand they suggest a generally slower rate of metabolism in the germfree state [45]. But on the other hand severe Fe-dependend anemia occurred in germfree rabbits (not in germfree rats) when dietary iron intake was considered normal, but consisted largely of inorganic Fe. Parameters of Cu metabolism were not effected. Either conventionalization of the germfree rabbits by exposure to a "normal" microflora, or replacement of "inorganic" by "natural ingredient" Fe (e.g. soy bean meal) alleviated all symptoms of Fe deficiency in a matter of weeks. It is presumed that in the germfree state the oxidation-reduction potential in the small intestine was not low enough to allow the absorption of the non-complexed Fe ion [46].

Queuine, a nutrient of possibly microbial origin?

Queuosine is a hypermodified purine nucleoside found in the wobble position of the tRNAs for asparagine, aspartic acid, histidine and tyrosine, where its base, queuine, has replaced a guanine residue [28]. When germfree mice are fed a chemically-defined amino acid-glucose diet, these tRNAs appear to lose their queuine content, and after approximately one year become totally queuine-negative. Upon dietary administration of queuine, reincorporation into these 4 tRNAs was rapid and proportional to the amount administered [53]. It is as yet not clear what advantage the incorporation of queuine imparts to these 4 tRNAs. At the Lobund Laboratory we have observed a decrease in reproductive performance in the later litters of germfree C3H mice maintained on the aforementioned glucose-amino acids diet. But other parameters of function and metabolism appeared to be all within a range normal for the germfree C3H mouse.

It has been speculated that insertion of the queuine moiety in these tRNAs reduces the potential for "reading errors" during protein formation. Further study will be needed to be establish if queuine is indeed an essential nutrient, and whether the presence of an intestinal microflora will guarantee its availability to the host at all times in sufficient amounts.

CONCLUSIONS

The fact that the efficacy of subtherapeutic levels of antimicrobials in animal feeds is strongly related to the hygienic conditions of the animal quarters points to a major effect of the intestinal microflora on nutrient availability and nutrient utilization. Especially, this can be demonstrated by the "sparing action" of antimicrobials on certain B vitamins and amino acids. Gnotobiotic, non-pathogenic microfloras reduce "conventional" requirement in a similar way.

This implicates certain, as yet largely unknown, members of a conventional microflora which, in some way, prevent the most effective use of at least a number of nutrients. In addition, enterotoxins may affect gut physiology, and have negative effects on nutrient uptake. Certain materials of bacterial origin may also affect the well-being of the host in more indirect, as yet unknown ways.

On the positive side, the microflora is known to produce a number of nutrients and the administration of antimicrobials may well enhance either the production of these nutrients or their availability to the host. The often undefinable changes in intestinal ecology that are produced by these antimicrobials suggest that with good hygienic conditions, a certain management of the intestinal microflora may be possible, which would not only improve the host's nutritional status, but which could also lead to a more or less effective exclusion of non-indigenous pathogens [29].

REFERENCES

1. Abrams, G.D. and Bishop, J.E. Effect of the normal microbial flora on gastrointestinal motility. *Proc. Soc. Exp. Biol. Med.* 126:301, 1967.
2. Albert, M.J., Mathan, V.I. and Baker, S.J. Vitamin B_{12} synthesis by human intestinal bacteria. *Nature* 283:781, 1980.
3. Bruckner-Kardoss, E. and Wostmann, B.S. Oxygen consumption of germfree and conventional mice. *Lab. Anim. Sci.* 28:282, 1978.
4. Celesk, R.A., Asano, T. and Wagner, M. The size, pH and redox potential of the cecum in mice associated with various microbial floras. *Proc. Soc. Exp. Biol. Med.* 151:260, 1976.
5. Chawla, R.K., Hersh, T., Lambe, D.W., Wadsworth, A.D. and Rudman, D. Effect of antibiotics on growth of the immature reat. *J. Nutr.* 106:1737, 1976.
5a. Coates, M.E., Fuller, R., Harrison, D.F., Lev, M. and Suffolk, S.F. A comparison of the growth of chicks in the Gustafsson germ-free apparatus and in a conventional environment, with and without dietary supplements of penicillin. *Br. J. Nutr.* 17:141, 1963.
6. Coates, M.E., Ford, J.F., Harrison, G.F. Intestinal synthesis of vitamins of the B complex in chicks. *Br. J. Nutr.* 22:493, 1968.

7. Coates, M.E. Nutrition and metabolism in the gnotobiotic state. *In* "Clinical and Experimental Gnotobiotics" (T. Fliedner, ed.), pp. 29-37. Gustav Fisher Verlag, Stuttgart, 1979.
8. Daft, F.S., McDaniel, E.G., Harman, L.G., Romine, M.K., Hegner, J.R. Role of coprophagy in utilization of B-vitamins synthesized by intestinal bacteria. *Fed. Proc.* 22:129, 1963.
9. Dubos, R.J. and Schaedler, R.W. The effect of intestinal flora on the growth rate of mice and on their susceptibility to experimental infection. *J. Exp. Med.* 111:407, 1960.
10. Eyssen, H. and DeSomer, P. Effects of *Streptococcus faecalis* and a filtrable agent on growth and nutrient absorption in gnotobiotic chicks. *Poultry Sci.* 46:323, 1967.
11. Eyssen, H.J. and Parmentier, G.G. Influence of the microflora of the rat on metabolism of fatty acids, sterols and bile salts in the intestinal tract. *In* "Clinical and Experimental Gnotobiotics" (T. Fliedner, ed.), pp. 39-44. Gustav Fisher Verlag, Stuttgart, 1979.
12. Fernandes, G., Nair,M., Onoe, K., Tanaka, T., Floyd R. and Good, R.A. Impairment of cell-mediated immunity functions by dietary zinc deficiency in mice. *Proc. Natl. Acad. Sci. USA* 76:457, 1979.
13. Freter, R. and Abrams, C.D. Function of various intestinal bacteria in converting germfree mice to the normal state. *Infect. Immun.* 6:119, 1972.
14. Fuller, R., Coates, M.E. and Harrison, G.F. The influence of specific bacteria and a filtrable agent on the growth of gnotobiotic chicks. *J. Appl. Bacteriol.* 46:335, 1979.
15. Garnier, H. and Sacquet, E. Absorption apparente et rétention du sodium, du potassium, du calcium et du phosphore chez le rat axénique et chez le rat haloxénique. *CR Acad. Sci. Paris* 269:370, 1969.
16. Gordon, H.A. Wagner, M. and Wostmann, B.S. Studies of conventional and germfree chickens treated orally with antibiotics. *Antibiotics Annual* 1957-58:248, 1958.
17. Gordon, H.A. and Bruckner-Kardoss, E. Effect of normal microbial flora on intestinal surface area. *Am. J. Physiol.* 201:175, 1961.
18. Gordon, H.A., Bruckner-Kardoss, E., Staley, T.E., Wagner, M., and Wostmann, B.S. Characteristics of the germfree rat. *Acta Anat.* 64:301, 1966.
19. Gordon, H.A., Bruckner-Kardoss, E. and Wostmann, B.S. Aging in germfree mice: life tables and lesions observed at natural death. *J. Gerontol.* 21:380, 1966.
20. Gordon, H.A. Is the germfree animal normal? A review of its anomalies in young and old age. *In* "The Germfree Animal in Research" (M.E. coates, H.A. Gordon, and B.S. Wostmann, eds.), pp. 127-150; Academic Press, New York, 1968.
21. Gustafsson, B.E., Daft, F.S., McDaniel, E.G., Smith, J.C., and Fitzgerald, R.J. Effects of vitamin K-active compounds and intestinal microorganisms in vitamin K-deficient germfree rats. *J. Nutr.* 78:461, 1962.
22. Gustafsson, B.E. Introduction of specific microorganisms into germfree animals. *In* "Nutrition and Infection. Ciba Study Group No. 31" (G.E.W. Wolstenholme and M. O'Connor, eds.), p. 16. Little Brown, Boston, 1967.
23. Heneghan, J.B. Enterocyte kinetics, mucosal surface area and mucus in gnotobiotics. *In* "Clinical and Experimental Gnotobiotics" (T. Fliedner, ed.), pp. 19-27. Gustav Fisher Verlag, Stuttgart, 1979.
24. Herskovic, T., Katz, J., Floch, M.H., Spencer, R.D., and Spiro, H.M. Small intestinal absorption and morphology in germfree, monocontaminated and conventional mice. *Gastroenterology* 52:1136 (Abstr.), 1967.
25. Hoskins, L.C. and Zamcher, N. Bacterial degradation of gastrointestinal mucins. 1 Comparison of mucous constituents in the stools of germfree and conventional rats. *Gastroenterology* 54:210, 1968.
26. Ikeda, M., Hosotani, T., Kurimoto, K., Mori, T., Ueda, T., Kotake, Y., and Sakakibara, B. The differences of the metabolism related to vitamin B6-dependent enzymes among vitamin B6-deficient germfree and conventional rats. *J. Nutr. Sci. Vitaminol.* 28:131, 1979.
27. Jones, J.D. and Baumann, C.A. Relative effectiveness of antibiotics in rats given limiting B vitamins by mouth or by injection. *J. Nutr* 57:61, 1955.

28. Katze, J.R. and Farkas, W.R. A factor in serum and amniotic fluid is a substrate for the RNA-modifying enzyme tRNA-guanine transferase. *Proc. Natl. Acad. Sci. U.S.A.* 76:3271, 1979.
29. Koopman, J.P., Welling, G.W., Huybregts, A.W., Mullink, J.W. and Prins, R.A. Association of germfree mice with intestinal microfloras. *Z. Versuchstierk* 23:145, 1981.
30. Latymer, E.A. Factors affecting pantothenic acid requirements of the chick. Ph. D. thesis. Univ. Reading, England.
31. Lee, C.J. and Dubos, R. Lasting biological effects or early environmental influences. III. Metabolic responses of mice to neonatal infection with a filterable weight-depressing agnet. *J. Exp. Med.* 128:153, 1968.
32. Lepkovsky, S., Wagner, M., Furuta, F., Ozone, K., and Koike, T. The proteases, amylase and lipase of the intestinal contents of germfree and conventional chickens. *Poultry Sci.* 43:722, 1964.
33. Levenson, S.M., Tennant, B., Geever, E., Laundy, R., and Doft, F. Influence of microorganisms on scurvy. *Arch. Intern. Med.* 110:693, 1962.
34. Levenson, S.M. and Tennant, B. Some metabolic and nutritional studies with germfree animals. *Fed. Proc.* 22:109, 1963.
35. Levenson, S.M., Doft, F., Lev, M., and Kan, D. Influence of mircroorganisms on oxigen consumption, carbon dioxide production and calonic temperature in rats. *J. Nutr.* 97:542, 1969.
36. Lih, H. and Baumann, C.A. Effects of certain antibiotics on the growth of rats fed diets limiting in thiamine, riboflavin or pantothenic acid. *J. Nutr.* 45:143, 1951.
37. Madsen, D.C., Beaver,M.H., Chang, L., Bruckner-Kardoss, E., and Wostmann, B.S. Analysis of bile acids in conventional and germfree rats. *J. Lip. Res.* 117:107, 1976.
38. Meslin, J.C., Sacquet, E., and Guenet, J.L. Action de la flore bacterienne sur la morphologie et la surface de la muguese de l'intestine grele du rat. *Ann. Biol. Anim. Biochim. Biophys.* 113:203, 1973.
39. Nutrition Foundation. Contribution of the microflora of the small intestine to the vitamin B_{12} nutriture of man. *Nutr. Rev.* 38:214, 1980.
40. Nuttal, G.H.F. and Thierfelder, H. Thierisches Leben ohne Bacterien Im Verdauungskanal. *Z. Physiol. Chem.* 21:109, 1895-1896.
41. Oace, S.M. and Abbot, J.M. Methylmalonate-, formino-glutamate and amino imidazole carboxamide excretion of vitamin B_{12}-deficient germfree and conventional rats. *J. Nutr.* 102:17, 1972.
42. Okumura, J., Hewitt, D., Salter, D.N., and Coates, M.E. The role of the gut microflora in the utilization of dietary urea by the chick. *Br. J. Nutr.* 36:265, 1976.
43. Pasteur, L. Observations relatives à la note précédente de M. Duclaux. *CR Acad. Sci., Paris* 100:68, 1885.
44. Pollard, M. and Luckert, P.H. Spontaneous liver tumors in aged germfree Wistar rats. *Lab. Anim. Sci.* 29:74, 1979.
45. Reddy, B.S., Wostmann, B.S., and Pleasants, J.R. Iron, copper and manganese in germfree and conventional rats. *J. Nutr.* 86-159, 1965.
46. Reddy, B.S., Pleasants, J.R., Zimmerman, D.R., and Wostmann, B.S. Iron and copper utilization in rabbits as affected by diet and germfree status. *J. Nutr.* 87:189, 1965.
47. Reddy, B.S. and Wostmann, B.S. Intestinal disaccharidase activities in growing germfree and conventional rats. *Arch. Biochem. Biophys.* 113:609, 1966.
48. Reddy, B.S., Pleasants, JR., and Wostmann, B.S. Pancreatic enzymes in germfree and conventional rats fed chemically-defined water-soluble diet free from natural substrates. *J. Nutr.* 97:327, 1969.
49. Reddy, B.S., Pleasants, J.R. and Wostmann, B.S. Effect of intestinal microflora on calcium phosphorus and magnesium metabolism in rats. *J. Nutr.* 99:353, 1969.
50. Reddy, B.S., Pleasants, J.R. and Wostmann, B.S. Studies on calcium phosphorus and magnesium metabolism in rats: effect of intestinal microflora. Proc. 8th Int. Cong. Nutr., Prague Czechoslovakia, Excerpta Medica Intern. Cong. Ser. 213:418, 1969.

51. Reddy, B.S., Wostmann, B.S. and Pleasants, J.R. Protein metabolism in germfree rats fed chemically defined, water-soluble and semi-synthetic diet. *Adv. Exp. Med. Biol.* 3:301, 1969.

52. Reddy, B.S. Calcium and magnesium absorption: role of intestinal microflora. *Fed. Proc.* 30:1815, 1971.

53. Reyniers, J.P., Pleasants, J.R., Wostmann, B.S., Katze, J.R., and Farkas, W.R. Administration of exogenous queuine is essential for the biosynthesis of queuosine-containing transfer RNAs in the mouse. *J. Biol. Chem.* 256:11591, 1981.

54. Riottot, M., Sacquet, E., Vila, J.P. and LePrince, C. Relationship between small intestine trans and bile acid metabolism in axenic and hoxoxenic rats fed different diets. *Reprod. Nutr. Develop.* 20:163, 1980.

55. Rogers, W.E., Bieri, J.G., and McDaniel, E.G. Vitamin A deficiency in the germfree state. *Fed. Proc.* 30:1773, 1971.

56. Roy, C.C., Laurendeau, G., Doyon, G., Chartrand, L. and Rivest, M.R. The effect of bile and sodium taurocholate on the epithelial cell dynamics of the rat small intestine. *Proc. Soc. Exp. Biol. Med.* 149:1000, 1975.

57. Salter, D.N., Hewitt, D. and Coates, M.E. The utilization of protein and excretion of uric acid in germfree and conventional chicks. *Br. J. Nutr.* 31:307, 1974.

58. Sauberlich, H.E. Effect of aureomycin and penicillin upon the vitamin requirements of the rat. *J. Nutr.* 46:99, 1952.

58a Savage, D.C., Siegel, J.E., Snellen, J.E. and Whitt, D.D. Transit time of epithelial cells in the small intestine of germfree mice and ex-germfree mice associated with indigenous microorganisms. *Appl. Environ, Microbiol.* 42:996, 1981.

59. Sewell, D.L. and Wostmann, B.S. Thyroid function and related hepatic enzymes in the germfree rat. *Metabolism* 24:695, 1975.

60. Smith, J.C., McDaniel, E.G., McBean, L.D., Doft, F.S., and Halsted, J.A. Effect of microorganisms upon zinc metabolism using germfree and conventional rats. *J. Nutr.* 102:711, 1972.

61. Stoewsand, G.S., Dynsza, H.A., Ament, D., and Trexler, P.C. Lysine requirement of the growing gnotobiotic mouse. *Life Sci.* 7:689, 1968.

62. Valencia, R., Sacquet, E. and Jacquot, R. Les charactères de l'avitaminose B_{12} chez le rat axénique et le rat normal. *J. Physiol.,* Paris 60:561, 1968.

63 Whitt, D.D. and Savage, D.C. Kinectic changes induced by indigenous microbiota in the activity levels of alkaline phosphatase and disaccharidases in small intestinal enterocytes in mice. *Infect. Immun.* 29:144, 1980.

64. Wolin, M.J. Fermentation in the rumen and human large intestine. *Science* 213:1463, 1981.

65. Wostmann, B.S., Knight, P.L., and Reyniers, J.A. The influence of orally administered penicillin upon growth and liver thiamine of growing germfree and normal stock rats fed a thiamine-deficient diet. *J. Nutr.* 66:577, 1958.

66. Wostmann, B.S. Nutrition of the germfree mammal. *Ann. NY Acad. Sci.* 78:175, 1959.

67. Wostmann, B.S. and Knight, P.L. Synthesis of thiamine in the digestive tract of the rat. *J. Nutr.* 74:103, 1961.

68. Wostmann, B.S., Knight, P.L., and Kan, D.F. Thiamine in germfree and conventional animals: effect of the intestinal microflora on thiamine metabolism of the rat. *Ann. NY Acad. Sci.* 98:516, 1962.

NUTRITION AND PARASITISM

Noel W. Solomons

Department of Nutrition and Food Science,
Massachusetts Institute of Technology,
Cambridge, Massachusetts

Division of Human Nutrition and Biology,
Institute of Nutrition of Central America and Panama,
Guatemala City, Guatemala.

INTRODUCTION

> *The possibility of contact between*
> *parasite and host is regulated by*
> *ecological and behavioral factors,*
> *but once contact is made, the*
> *outcome of infection is governed*
> *by factors arising from the*
> *innate and acquired*
> *characteristics of the host.*
> *D. Wakelin*

Dr. Wakelin's comment [1] is incisive in its characterization of the evolution of parasitic disease. The term "innate" characteristics referes to the genetic constitution of the host. To a nutritionist like myself, "acquired" characteristics immediately brought to mind dietary intake and nutritional status of the host. It is estimated that over one billion people are infected with the common roundworm, *Ascaris lumbricoides* [2]. An even greater number of individuals, perhaps a quarter of the world's population, is infected with hookworm [3]. The incidence of malaria is approximately 100 million cases per year resulting in nearly one million deaths, mostly in children under 14 years of age [4].

A consideration of the present topic is also important by virtue of years of neglect by research scientists. Keusch [5] has commented:

GENETIC FACTORS IN NUTRITION
225

"Although an enormous proportion of the world's population is infected by parasitic agents (frecuently by several at the same time), parasitic diseases have often been left out of the picture in favor of the acute bacterial and viral diarrheas and respiratory disease. Quantitative data that demonstrate the importance of these latter diseases in the malnutrition-infection complex have been obtained, and programs of intervention have been developed. However, a similar formulation for the various parasitic diesease has not been undertaken, even though modern chemotherapeutic agents offer the possibility of successful mass control for some infections (those caused by *Ascaris lumbricoides,* for example), and insecticides can be effectively used for others (malaria), . . . , primarily quantitative data linking parasites and nutrition are lacking. In such a vacuum, governmental decisions may be made on *a priori* grounds and valuable resources wasted on ill-conceived or low-priority programs."

Finally, this topic appears to be a fruitful focus for the discussion of several important biological issues that highlight the workings of genetic factors in the expression of human disease.

Taxonomy of Parasites

Prior to our discussing issues of interaction, however, it is important to provide a brief orientation to the classification to the classification of human parasites. A parasite can be defined as an "organism that lives on or in another and draws its nourishment therefrom." [6]. They can be classified first by their location, as *ectoparasites* or *endoparasites*. Ectoparasites live in the integumentary regions of the body, e.g. mites, lice, ticks, and affliction with these organisms is termed *infestation*. Endoparasites are found on mucosal surfaces or within the body itself, e.g. malarial organisms, intestinal protozoa, and cause *infection*. Our discussion will be confined to a consideration of endoparasites.

Endoparasites can be further subdived taxonomically into two sub-kingdoms within the animal kingdom: the unicellular organisms or *protozoa;* and the multicellular organisms or *metazoa*. These are further subdivided into phyla, classes and finally into individual species. Examples are listed in Table I [7]. A comprehensive listing of metazoan endoparasites (worms) with proven or suspected pathogenicity has been compiled recently by Mata [8]; it included 72 different species.

Finally, on a biological basis related to the location of the infection within the host, parasites can be classified as visceral or *blood-borne* (those that circulate in the bloodstream or take up primary residence in deep internal organs) and *intestinal* (those that live in the alimentary tract or in the mesenteric circulation). Malaria, Changa' s disease, onchoceriasis, and African sleeping sickness are parasitoses caused by blood-borne parasites while amebiasis, giardiasis, schistosomiasis (mansoni) and hookworm disease are intestinal parasitoses [7].

TABLE I *Classification of Pathogens*

Subkingdom	Phylum	Class	Representative genera
PROTOZOA (Unicellular)	Protozoa	Sarcodina (amebas)	Entameba
		Mastigophora (flagellates)	Trichomonis Giardia Leishmania
		Ciliata (ciliates)	Balantidium
		Sporozoa (Sporozoans)	Plasmodium Toxoplasma
METAZOA (Multicellular)	Platyhelminthes (flatworms)	Trematoda (flukes)	Fasciolopsis Schistosoma
		Cestoidea (tapeworms)	Diphyllobothrium Taenia
	Nemathelminthes (roundworms)	Nematoda (roundworms)	Ancylostoma Ascaris Strongyloides Onchocerca

The Two-Dimensional Nature of the Interaction of Nutrition and Parasitism with Genetic Factors

The present topic provides us with a potentially more *dynamic* exploration of the exercise of genetic factors in human biology because of the inherently two-dimensional nature of the concepts under discussion. This is illustrated schematically in Figure 1. It emphasizes fundamental assumption in genetics that neither nutrition nor parasitism can influence the gene (at least in any given generation). Genetic variation can, however, affect the demand for and/or the utilization of nutrients. Genetic variation can also affect the course of an exposure to parasites.

Examples for limb A of our scheme (Fig. 1) have been discussed eloquently elsewhere in this Workshop. Dr. Jackson discussed evidence for a change in the utilization of glycine in sickle cell anemia while Prof. Rosenberg describes the mechanism for increased demand for vitamin B_{12} in certain forms of methylmalonicaciduria. These are both examples with clearly defined genetic markers. The discussion of individual variation in nitrogen metabolism by Profs. Scrimshaw, Payne and Beaton suggest that genetic factors might also be operative in defining protein requirements; as yet, however, no genetic markers have been defined.

Some classical illustrations of limb B of our scheme - genetic influence on parasite: host interaction - have been described with respect to malaria. Most

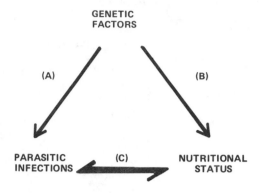

Figure 1. Schematic representation of interactions among genetic factors, parasitic infection and nutritional status. Genetic influences affect both susceptibility to parasitic infection and the nutritional status. Parasitoses and nutritional status have reciprocal interactions of both synergistic and antagonistic natures. Beisel [18] with permission of the copyright holder. The University of Chicago Press.

famous, perhaps, was the demonstration by Allison [9] that individuals heterozygous for the sickle hemoglobin gene (sickle trait) had lower levels of parasitemia with one form of malaria organism, *Plasmodium falciparum*. This protection did not extend to *P. malariae* infections. The classical molecular explanations for this phenomenon relate to the *in vitro* demonstration of lower invasion rates, the reduced intraerythrocytic multiplications, and the increased sickling of red cells with SA hemoglobin, all under conditions of low oxygen tension analogous to the venous beds of the human circulation where *in vivo* replication of plasmodia usually proceeds [10]. Epidemiological observation of a higher gene frequency of two other inherited human hemolytic diseases -glucose-6-phosphate dehydrogenase and thalassemia - in areas originally endemic for *P. falciparum* malaria led to the speculation that these disorders might also provide protection against parasitemia [11]; the evidence, however, is less conclusive [12].

Another example for limb B of the scheme is the documentation in Dr. Louis Miller's laboratory that the Duffy blood group (FyFy) determinants govern susceptibility to invasion of human red cells by the simian malarial parasite, *P. knowlesi*. The erythrocytes of individuals who are Duffy group-negative are resistant to invasion [13]. A similar finding was seen with the human pathogen, *P. vivax.,* in Duffy-negative individuals [14]. Since most black Africans are Duffy negative, a natural resistance to *P. vivax* due to this genetic factor operates to the advantage of the indigenous populations [15].

The most intriguing aspect of the scheme illustrated in Figure 1, however, is the interaction between nutrition and parasitism (limb C). Nutritional status can influence the susceptibility to parasitoses, and parasitic infection can affect nutritional status. Since, as discussed, genetic factors can influence both parasitic infection and host nutriture, the bidirectional nature of the interaction between the latter two conditions sets stage for a truly two-dimensional character for the total interaction. This two directional interaction of nutrition and parasitism is discussed in detail in the subsequent section.

Synergism and Antagonism in the Interaction of Nutrition and Infection

An important concept in the biology of communicable (infectious) diseases was developed in 1959 by Scrimshaw, Taylor and Gordon in a paper entitled "Interactions of nutrition and infection" [16]. This was later expanded and embellished in a WHO Monograph 9 years thereafter [17]. In these treatises, they compiled the available evidence from animal experiments and observations in human studies, and expounded a principle which, simply stated, dictated that malnutrition and exposure to pathogens often *interact* in a given host such that the simultaneous effect of both conditions together is not equivalent to the sum of the effects of each occurring separately (Table II). This interaction could be *synergistic*, such that malnutrition increased the susceptibility to and/or the disease burden of a given infection, or, conversely, infection causes a deterioration in nutritional status; alternatively, the interaction could be *antagonistic*, such malnutrition decreased the susceptibilite to and/or morbidity from a pathogenic organism (see footnote in Table II). Examples of each of the potential reactions are illustrated in Table II. Concepts of synergism and antagonism have been discussed recently in detail, specifically for parasitic diseases and malnutrition, by Beisel [18].

Parasitic Infections on Nutritional Status

Synergism: Falciparum malaria in childhood produces growth retardation and stunting [19-21]. Parasites that produce intestinal bleeding, e.g. amebas, hookworm, can obviously impair iron nutriture [22, 23]. *Diphyllobothrium latum,* the fish tapeworm, competes with the host for intraluminal vitamin B_{12}; frank vitamin B_{12} deficiency with anemia and neurological degeneration have been observed [24, 25].

Nutritional Status on Parasitic Infections

Synergism: Protein-energy malnutrition (PEM) seems to aggravate infection with certain parasites. Studies in severely malnourished, hospitalized children in Costa Rica by Lopez et al. [26] showed a high rate of colonization with *G. lamblia.* Malnutrition reduces gastric acid secretion, and in the Costa Rican study, giardial prevalence was directly correlated with achlorhydria. Observations both in South African children with kwashiorkor and in North American children with hematological malignancies, suggest that PEM conditions the expression of *Pneumocystis carinii* pneumonia [27].

TABLE II

EXAMPLES OF SYNERGISM AND ANTAGONISM IN THE INTERACTION OF NUTRITION AND PARASITIC INFECTION

SYNERGISTIC INTERACTION
AND
ANTAGONISTIC INTERACTION

PARASITIC INFECTION ON NUTRITIONAL STATE	NUTRITIONAL STATE ON PARASITIC INFECTION

SYNERGISTIC INTERACTION

Malaria on growth	Protein-energy on giardiasis malnutrition
Amebiasis on iron status Hookworm	Protein-energy on pneumocystosis malnutrition
Diphyllobothrium latum infection on vitamin B_{12}	Protein deficiency on schistosomiasis Calorie deficiency

ANTAGONISTIC INTERACTION

	malaria Iron deficiency on parasitemia
	Vitamin E on rodent malaria deficiency
(see footnote)	Protein-energy schistosomal on malnutrition granulomata

Note: In an experimental mouse model of schistosomiasis, severe caloric restriction ameliorated the hypoalbuminemia (ref. 29), but it is unclear whether this is a nutritional phenomenon or a change in intravascular fluid distribution.

Severe protein deficiency as severe energy restriction in an experimental animal (mouse) model causes excessive morbidity and tissue changes, as compared to controls, after a challenge with *S. mansoni* [28, 29].

Antagonism: Of the 474 studies of nutrient deficiency involving all types of pathogenic microorganisms reviewed by Scrimshaw et al [17], 93 [20%] showed antagonism; i.e. a *less* severe infection in the presence of malnutrition. Beisel [18] has emphasized instances of this form of interaction with parasitic organisms. Examples in human subjects are rare. Murray et al. [30] treated iron-deficient Somalian refugees with therapeutic dosages of iron; malaria parasitemia appeared rapidly in some members of the iron-treatment cohort. Vitamin E deficiency has been found to confer protection against *Plasmodium berghei* infection in a rodent model of malaria [31, 32]. The decreased survival of the parasitized vitamin E-deficient red cells apparently retards the development of parasitemia; this may represent the acquired, nutritional analogue of the inborn, hemolytic disorders discussed above. Its relevance to human malaria has yet to be demonstrated, however. Finally, also from rodent models, has come evidence that PEM will reduce the development of granulomas in experimental *S. mansoni* infection [28, 29]. Since the inflammatory granuloma response is the pathogenetic basis of illness in schistosomiasis, malnutrition may contribute to less severe manifestations of infection. Once again, conclusive evidence for the operation of antagonism in humans remains to be developed [33].

Mechanistic Considerations

There are large gaps in our understanding of the interaction of parasitism and nutrition, but certain facts and speculations about the biological mechanisms involved are worth considering. That parasitic infection of the intestine can cause deterioration in nutritional status is not difficult to understand given the central role of the alimentary tract in the uptake of nutrients from the diet. The mechanism of nutritional impairment in gastrointestinal parasitoses are listed in Table III. Of note is the fact that nutrients can be lost in significant quantities through the intestine, and that febrile complications can cause catabolic losses. It has been claimed that giardiasis produces some of its antinutritional effects by favoring upper intestinal colonization by fecal bacteria [34].

TABLE III Mechanisms of Nutritional Impairment in Gastrointestinal Parasitoses

---

Impairment of enzymatic digestion
Impairment of mucosal absorption
Competition for host's nutrients
Gastrointestinal loss of nutrients
Catabolic loss of nutrients
Conditioning of bacterial overgrowth (?)

The facts that many types of nutritional deficits impair the functioning of the host immune defenses, and that parasites themselves can influence the immunological processes of the host are believed to be instrumental in the mediation of both synergistic and antagonistic interactions. The interrelationships are illustrated in Figure 2. Wakelin [1] has dissected various processes in the mammalian antiparasite immune response (Figure 3). It becomes obvious that the same processes are also sensitive to alteration by nutritional factors. Moreover, as pointed out by Keusch [35], in the host: parasite interaction, the parasite often uses disguise to outwit the host's immune defenses. Secondary to either nutritional or genetic factors, however, the host may unwittingly retaliate. If the characteristics of intestinal mucus are instrumental in the establishment of amebic infection in the colon, then genetic changes or nutritional factors that alter the composition of mucus, may reduce the susceptibility of the host to invasion.

The infectivity of *Leishmania donovani* in a mouse model seems to be linked to a specific genetic locus mapped to chromsome 1 [36]. If the protein alteration which dictates resistance or susceptibility represents a cellular receptor site for the protozoa, then a mechanism by which both genetic factors and nutritional deficiencies could determine the virulence of *L. donovani* in the host could be conceived of. Investigations to determine whether or not an analagous situation obtains with human leishmaniasis are currently underway.

Models for the Genetic Modulation of the Parasite: Nutrition Interaction in Humans

The purpose of the foregoing background biology was to set the stage for the understanding of the two-dimensional interaction with genetic factors provided under our topic. Let us now explore some hypothetical, but plausible, cases of interaction between parasitic infections and nutrition.

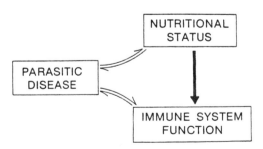

Figure 2. A schematic representation of the factors that cause synergistic or antagonistic changes in the serverity of parasitic diseases. Malnutrition in its various forms typically interferes with functions of the immune system, while the nutritional status and immune system competence of the host have reciprocal influences on parasitic disease [18]. Reproduced with permission.

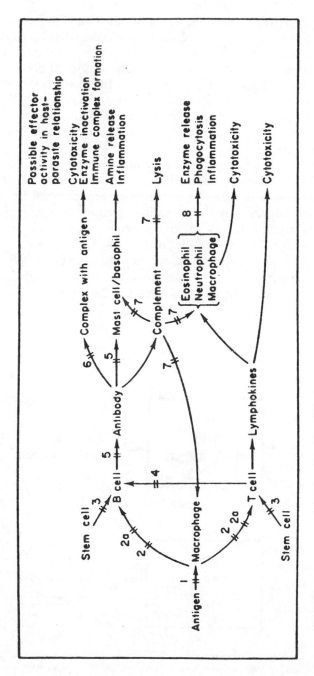

Figure 3. Diagram showing points at which genetic control may be exerted during the development and expression of anti-parasite immune responses. 1) Antigen handling by macrophage; 2) antigen presentation by macrophage; 2a) antigen recognition by lymphocyte; 3) stem cell deficiency; 4) T-B cell interaction (helper/suppresor function); 5) control of antibody production (class/level/specificity); 6) antibody affinity; 7) defects in complement components affecting lysis, chemotaxis, opsonization; 8) defective population or activity [1]. Reproduced with permission.

CASE # 1: Hookworm disease and iron nutrition

The first involves hookworm infection and iron nutrition. We know that there is variation in the population with respect to iron requirements; we shall assume that this is dictated primarily by genetic factors. If a fixed stress is superimposed uniformly on the population in the form of a constant hookworm infection of moderate proportions in all subjects, then the factor determining whether there be overt expression of deficiency manifestations or accomodation with complete preservation of iron-dependent physiological functions could be high intrinsic iron requirements (former) and low intrinsic iron requirements (latter). (Figure 4).

Another scenario involving the same parasite and nutrient could also be envisioned. In this case, a free-living population is assessed in a survey fashion using the determination of iron turnover as the index of individual iron requirements, and a distribution of individuals along a continuum of requirements is established (Figure 5). If, in fact, certain portion of that population had graded infections with hookworm, the differential worm loads, themselves, could have been responsible for the apparent (observed) distribution of iron requirements. If then mass chemotherapy were applied to this population and the hookworm eradicated, a subsequent survey might reveal a narrower

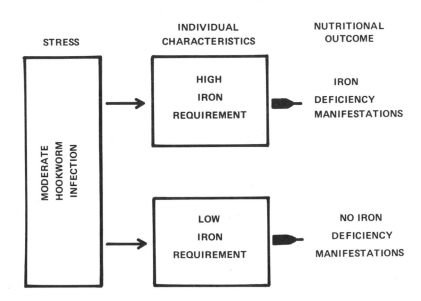

Figure 4. Schematic representation of the potentially differential nutritional outcome from a moderate hookworm infection. Individuals with high intrinsic (genetic) iron requirements would be more likely to manifest anemia than individuals with low intrinsic (genetic) iron requirements.

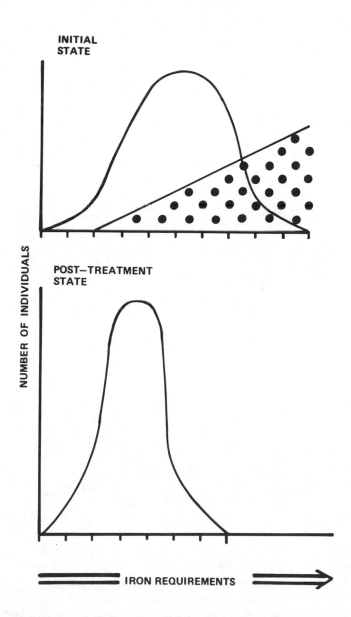

Figure 5. Hypothetical situation in which the distribution of iron requirements of a population was determined (initial state) without cognizance of a graded level of hookworm infection ranging from none to severe (dotter area). The distribution was again determined after chemotherapeutic eradication of hookworm infection in the population (post-treatment state). The distribution would be narrowed and shifted to the left. The individual ranking within the population might have changed as well.

range of variation in iron requirements and the individual ranking along the distribution might be substantially realigned (Figure 5).

CASE #2: Amebiasis and iron nutrition

Even more complex consequences of the interplay among genetic factors, parasitism and nutrition can be envisioned. For a second case, let us consider special issues involving iron status and infection with *Entamoeba histolytica* (amebiasis). It has been observed that individuals vary in their resistance to the clinical evolution of symptomatic amebiasis after exposure to *E. histolytica;* we shall assume that this represents genetic variation in host: parasite interaction along the lines discussed by Wakelin [1], although the details are not yet understood.

A curious biological aspect of the ameba has been recognized: its remarkable requirement for iron [37]. This has been explored in a golden hamster model in the laboratory of Dr. Louis Diamond [38]. These workers demonstrated a greater susceptibility to severe hepatic lesions in hamsters overloaded with iron that were challenged with cultured amebae. Elsdon-Dew [39, 40] in Durban, South Africa, had suggested that diet might play a role in the differential expression of amebiasis in local citizens whereby the European whites rarely had amebic dysentery or any other form of infection whereas in the black population (Zulus) fulminating amebic dysentery and severe extraintestinal infection were common. Reanalyzing the South African experience, Diamond et al. [38] have suggested that iron overload (nutritional siderosis) from consuming the iron-rich native (kaffir) beer might explain the excess morbidity and mortality from amebiasis among the Zulus of Durban. Murray et al. [41] lend additional support to the association in a controlled, prospective iron-supplementation trial among the Masai of Kenya. They reported a greater prevalence of seropositivity and of stools positive for amebic cysts and trophozoites in iron-treated subjects as compared to untreated controls. Thus, total-body iron status will be assumed to represent a nutritional factor influencing the resistance to amebic infections.

Genetic factors influencing iron storage in humans are identifiable. Iron depletion would be favored by a tendency to heavier menstrual bleeding or by hemophilia. Iron overload is seen in hemochromatosis and in treated thalassemia.

We are now in a position to construct a model in which a human population group could be distributed along two genetically-determined axes simultaneously: one representing gradations in susceptibility to amebiasis determined by non-nutritional genetic factors; the other representing iron storage tendencies in the population (Figure 6). The latter, by extension of the previously developed argument, should represent a distribution of amebiasis susceptibility/resistance. Given two presumably independent, genetically-influenced schemes, random assortment would provide for individuals: 1) with a combination of nutritional and non-nutritional resistance factors; 2) with a combination of nutritional and non-nutritional susceptibility factors; and 3) many individuals in whom the non-nutritional and nutritional genetic influences would act in opposite directions.

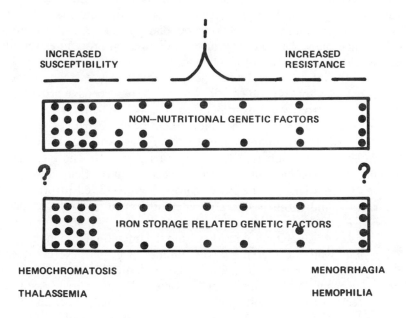

Figure 6. Interplay of non-nutritional genetic factors and specific genetic factors related to iron-storage in the development of increased resistance (right-hand direction) or increased susceptibility (left-hand direction) to severe amebiasis in humans. The non-nutritional factors remain to be defined (? . . . ?) (above), but the tendency toward iron overload and iron depletion (below) are suggested as nutritional determinants.

Limitations to the Study of the Parasitism-Nutrition Interaction

It is important to point out the various barriers, limitations and pitfalls in the investigation of human genetics and human nutrition. Progress in understanding of the interaction of nutrition and parasitism has been hampered not only by its lack of recognition, but also by conceptual and technical limitations.

The diagnosis of human parasitic infections is often elusive. There are, for instance, three species of *Entamoeba* capable of forming four-nucleated cysts: *E. histolytica, E. hartmanni* (small race), and *E. histolytica*-like ameba (low temperature strains) [42]. Only *E. histolytica* is virulent, capable of causing disease in man. Serological diagnosis is notably unreliable for identifying active cases of amebiasis [18]. The only reliable diagnosis rests on the identification of the motile *trophozoite* by an experienced morphologist.

The diagnosis of giardiasis by examination of fecal specimens has a low sensitivity. Alternative, and more reliable, techniques involve a peroral intubation procedure of one form or another: 1) intestinal biopsy; 2) duodenal aspiration; 3) string test. Fecal analyses often miss up to 50% of the cases of giardiasis identified by means of one or the other techniques for sampling the contents of the upper small intestine. Field studies that rely on stool diagnosis alone, suffer from poor sensitivity, while the widepread application of intubation procedures for survey purposes would face problems of compliance.

Even when the infection can be detected, *quantitative* assessment of the parasitic burden of the host is problematic. Too often, reports have provided only *qualitative* results from stool examinations [43, 44]. Whenever possible, the reporting of protozoa or ova in the stool should be expressed per gram of feces. In the case of *Ascaris* quantitative egg counts based on a 24 h fecal output can be related to the number of female worms present in the intestine; the practical problems in obtaining 24-h stool collections in the field, however, are formidable. Alternatively, some investigators have collected information on the number of roundworms passed after chemotherapeutic purging to develop a retrospective estimation of the original worm burden [45, 46]. For parasites such as *S.mansoni,* which do not reside within the interstinal lumen, but rather in the intestinal wall and mesentery, the number of eggs in excreta does not necessarily reflect the burden of mating pairs within the host.

Sound approaches to the nutritional assessment that accompanies studies of parasitic effects are important. This has been especially prominent when growth has been the index criterion. One study of the effect of treatment for ascariasis on nutritional status [47] used an observation period of only 6 weeks; this is hardly sufficient time for marked divergences in growth curves to become manifest. Another such investigation employed an adequate observation interval, one year, but the criterion for improvement or deterioration of nutritional status was a change of only one per cent from the initial height-for-weight classification [48]. If a more generous margin, e.g. two per cent, is applied to the data in the Gupta study [48], all apparent statistically significant differences due to treatment disappear.

Finally, the framework of the concepts of synergism and antagonism in nutrition: infection interactions are based on infections with a single strain of organism [16, 17]. This can be established in a laboratory model, but the reality in free-living human populations is one of polyparasitism. Infected individuals most often have multiple parasites [44, 49], and often both intestinal and blood-borne species are present. Keusch and Migasena [50] have characterized the situation in the following way:

"Polyparasitism appears to be the rule, rather than the exception, both in populations and in individuals in developing countries of the world. Thus, polyparasitism represents coendemicity in the epidemiological sense and simultaneous infections in individual patients in the clinical sense."

Theoretically, the behavior of a given parasite when present alone may be quite different from its impact when the host has other parasitic infections. Accounting for the influence of accompanying parasites on both the clinical and epidemiological aspects of the nutrition: parasitism interaction is a severe challenge for future research. To date there are preliminary indications of interactions *between* parasites that might have nutritional consequences. Murray *et al* [51] suggest that *Ascaris* infection tends to *suppress* the expression of *Falciparum* malaria, and speculate that this is mediated through an effect on one or more nutrients essential both to the host and the *Plasmodium*.

Thus, it is important that investigators be able to identify with certainty the presence of parasites, to determine how many parasites, and measure the nutritional status in reliable and precise terms. It is not inconceivable that the biological relationships between nutritional variables and pathogen variables involve *thresholds* of parasite loads, below which no adverse nutritional consequences are to be expected. And finally, the reorientation of research to include more holistic perspectives of the zootic environment of the subjects under study will be important for the interpretation of those former studies which have purported to study single strains of parasites.

CONCLUSION

There are a host of identifiable genetic factors in the expression of nutritional requirements and in the susceptibility to and resistance to parasitic infections. Many more relationships with genetic factors remain to be uncovered. The genetic implications become all the more intriguing in this area because of the complex, bidirectional synergistic and antagonistic interactions between nutritional status and parasitic infection. As illustrated by two simple hypothetical examples presented in this paper, the fact of a triangular interaction matrix among genetic, nutritional and parasite factors makes for rich, conceptual possibilities in scientific investigation. However, profound public health consequences may also be discovered. The investigation of human parasitic infection and its relationship to nutrition is fraught with pitfalls and technical limitations, but careful attention to detail and interpretation of the quasi-experimental designs should allow major new advances in our understanding of the interaction of genetic factors with infectious and nutritional variables in human population that will benefit both scientific knowledge and the quality of life in developing countries.

REFERENCES

1. Wakelin D: Genetic control of susceptibility and resistance to parasitic infection. *In:* Advances in Parasitology, vol 16, WHR Lumsden, R Muller, JR Baker, eds., pp 219-308, London, Academic Press, 1978.
2. Peters W: Medical aspects-comments and discussion. II. *In:* Symposia of the British Society for Parasitology, vol 16, pp 25-40, Oxford, Blackwell, 1968.
3. Stoll NR: On endemic hookworm, where do we stand today? *Exp Parasitol 12:* 241-252, 1962.
4. Anonymous: Epitaph for global malaria eradication? *Lancet* 2:15-16, 1975.

5. Keusch GT: Introduction to the Workshop on interaction of nutrition and parasitic diseases. *Rev. Inf Dis 4:* 735, 1982.

6. *Stedman's Medical Dictionary,* Twenty-first Edition, Baltimore, The Williams & Wilkins Co., 1966, p. 1178.

7. Solomons NW, Keusch GT: Nutritional implications of parasitic infections. *Nutr Rev 39:* 149-161, 1981.

8. Mata L: Sociocultural factors in the control and prevention of parasitic diseases. *Rev Inf Dis 4:* 871-879, 1982.

9. Allison AC: Protection afforded by sickle-cell trait against subtertian malarial infection. *Br Med J 1:* 290-294, 1954.

10. Wyler DJ: Malaria: Host-pathogen biology. *Rev Inf Dis 4:* 785-797, 1982.

11. Motulsky AG: Hereditary red cell traits and malaria. *Am J Trop Med Hyg 13:* 147-158, 1964.

12. Luzzatto L: Genetics of red cells and susceptibility to malaria. *Blood 54:* 961-976, 1979.

13. Miller LH, Mason SJ, Dvorak JA, McGinniss MH, Rothman IK: Erythrocyte receptors for (Plasmodium knowlesi) malaria: Duffy blood group determinants. *Science 189:* 561-563, 1975.

14. Mason SJ, Miller LH, Shiroishi T, Dvorak JA, McGinniss MH. The Duffy blood group determinants: their role in the susceptibility of human and animal erythrocytes to *Plasmodium knowlesi* malaria. *Br J Haematol 36:* 327-335, 1977.

15. Miller LH, Mason SJ, Clyde DF, McGinniss MH: The resistance factor to *Plasmodium vivax* in blacks: The Duffy-blood-group genotype, FyFy. *N Engl J Med 295:* 302-304, 1976.

16. Scrimshaw NS, Taylor CE, Gordon JE: Interactions of nutrition and infection. *Am J Med Sci 237:* 567-403, 1959.

17. Scrimshaw NS, Taylor CE, Gordon JE: *Interactions of nutrition and infection.* WHO Monograph 57. Geneva: World Health Organization, 1968.

18. Beisel WR: Synergism and antagonism of parasitic disease and malnutrition. *Rev Inf Dis 4:* 746-750, 1982.

19. Marsden PD: The Sukuta project. A longitudinal study of health in Gambian children from birth to 18 months of age. *Trans R Soc Trop Med Hyg 58:* 455-489, 1964.

20. Rowland MGM, Cole TJ, Whitehead RGA: A quantitative study into the role of infection in determining nutritional status of Gambian village children. *Br J. Nutr 37:* 441-450, 1977.

21. McGregor IA, Gilles HM, Walters JH, Davies AH, Pearson FA: Effects of heavy and repeated malaria infections on Gambian infants and children: Effects of erythrocytic parasitization. *Br Med J 2:* 686-692, 1956.

22. Roche M, Perez-Gimenez ME, Layrisse M, DiPrisco E. Study-of the urinary and fecal excretion of radioactive chromium Cr^{51} in man. Its use in the measurement of intestinal blood loss associated with hookworm infection. *J Clin Invest 36:* 1183-1192, 1957.

23. Foy H, Nelson GS: Helminths in the etiology of anemia in the tropics with special reference to hookworms and schistosomes. *Expt Parasit 14:* 240-262, 1963.

24. von Bonsdorff B, Gordin R: *In* which part of the intestinal canal is fish tapeworm found. *D. latum* and pernicious anemia. IX. *Acta Med Scand 129:* 142-155, 1947.

25. Nyberg W, Saarni M: Calculations on the dynamics of vitamin B_{12} in fish tapeworm carriers spontaneously recovering from vitamin B_{12} deficiency. *Acta Med Scand 175* (Suppl 412): 65-71, 1964.

26. Lopez ME, Mata L, Lizano C, Gamboa F: Duodeno-jejunal infection in the child with protein-energy malnutrition. *Rev. Med. Hosp. Natl. Ninos 13:* 53-62, 1978.

27. Hughes WT, Price RA, Price RA, Sisko F, Havron WS, Kafatos AG, Schonland M, Smythe PM: Protein-calorie malnutrition: A host determinant for *Pneumocystic carinii* infection. *Am J Dis Child 128:* 44-52, 1974.

28. Akpom CA, Warren KS: Calorie and protein malnutrition in chronic murine schistosomiasis mansoni: effect on the parasite and the host. *J Infect Dis 132:* 6-14, 1975.

29. Knauft RF, Warren KS: The effect of calorie and protein malnutrition on both the parasite and the host in acute murine schistosomiasis mansoni. *J Inf Dis 120:* 560-575, 1969.

30. Murray MJ, Murray AB, Murray MB , Murray CJ: The adverse effect of iron repletion on the course of certain infections. *Br Med J 2:* 1113-1115, 1978.

31. Eaton JW, Eckman JR, Berger E, Jacob HS: Suppression of malaria infection by oxidant-sensitive host erythrocytes. *Nature 264:* 758-760, 1976.

32. Eckman JR, Eaton JW, Berger E, Jacob HS: Role of vitamin E in regulating malaria expression. *Trans Assoc Am Physicians 89:* 105-115, 1976.

33. DeWitt WB, Oliver-Gonzalez J, Medina E: Effects of improving the nutrition of malnourished people infected with *Schistosoma mansoni. Am J Trop Med Hyg 13:* 25-35, 1964.

34. Leon-Barua R, Lumbreras-Cruz YH: The possible role of intestinal bacterial flora in the genesis of diarrhea and malabsorption associated with parasitosis. *Gastroenterology 55:* 559, 1966.

35. Keusch GT: Immune responses in parasitic diseases. Part A: General concepts. *Rev. Inf Dis 4:* 751-755, 1982.

36. Bradley DJ, Taylor BA, Blackwell J, Evans EP, Freeman J: Regulation of leishmania populations within the hast III mapping of the locus controlling susceptibility to visceral leischmaniasis in the mouse *Clin Exp Immunol 37,* 7-14, 1979.

37. Latour NG, Reeves RE: An iron-requirement for growth of *Entamoeba histolytica* in culture and the antiamebal activity of 7-iodo-8-hydroxyquinoline-5-sulfonic acid. *Exp Parasitol 17:* 203-209, 1965.

38. Diamond LS, Harlow DR, Phillips BP, Keister DB: *Entamoeba histolytica:* iron and nutritional immunity. *Arch Invest Med* (Mex) *9* (Suppl 1): 329-338, 1978.

39. Elsdon-Dew R: Some aspects of amoebiasis in Africans. *S Afr Med J 20:* 580-587 and 620-626, 1946.

40. Elsdon-Dew R: Endemic fulminating amebic dysentery. *Am J Trop Med Hyg 29:* 337-340, 1949.

41. Murray MJ, Murray AB, Murray CJ. The salutary effect of milk on amoebiasis and its reversal by iron. *Br Med J 280:* 1351-1352, 1980.

42. Diamond LS: Amebiasis: Nutritional implications. *Rev Inf Dis 4:* 843-850, 1982.

43. Schneider RE, Torun B, Shiffman M, Anderson C, Helms R: Absorptive capacity of adult Guatemalan rural males living under different conditions of sanitation. *Food and Nutrition Bulletin* (Supplement 5) 139-149, 1981.

44. Blumenthal DS, Schultz MG: Effect of *Ascaris* infection on nutritional status in children. *Am J Trop Med Hyg 25:* 682-690, 1976.

45. Stephenson LS, Crompton DWT, Latham MC, Schulpen TWJ, Nesheim MC, Jansen AAJ: Relationship between *Ascaris* infection and growth of malnourished preschool children in Kenya. *Am J Clin Nutr 33* 1165-1172, 1980.

46. Brown KH, Gilman RH, Khatun M, Ahmed MG: Absorption of macronutrients from a rice-vegetable diet before and after treatment of ascariasis in children. *Am J Clin Nutr 33:* 1975-1982, 1980.

47. Freij L, Meeuwisse GW, Berg NO, Wall S, Gebre-Mehdin M: Ascariasis and malnutrition. A study in urban Ethiopian children. *Am J Clin Nutr 32:* 1545-1553, 1979.

48. Gupta MC, Mithal S, Arora KL, Tandon BN: Effects of periodic deworming on nutritional status of *Ascaris*-infected preschool children receiving supplementary food. *Lancet 2:* 108-110, 1977.

49. Mata LJ: *The children of Santa Maria Cauque: A Prospective Field Study of Health and Growth.* Cambridge, MA: The MIT Press, 1978, pp. 395.

50. Keusch GT, Migasena P: Biological implications of polyparasitism. *Rev Inf Dis 4:* 880-882, 1982.

51. Murray J, Murray A, Murray M, Murray C: The biological suppression of malaria: an ecological and nutritional interrelationship of a host and two parasites. *Am J Clin Nutr 31:* 1363-1366, 1978.

DISCUSSION[1]

Lisker asked if iron stores are a factor in susceptibility to amebiasis, is there a discrepancy between the incidence in males and females, especially after puberty? Solomons replied that the data necessary to answer that question were not available. Scrimshaw thought Solomons may have oversimplified the relationship between iron intake and parasitic infestation. The effects of iron supplementation have been seen primarily in hosts immunocompromised as a result of malnutrition. In this case, iron may facilitate replication of a parasite or microbe prior to the hosts regaining immunocompetence. Parasitic disease is hard to look at separately from bacterial or viral disease, since both are prevalent in the same individuals.

[1]*Summary of the discussion prepared by S. Cederbaum.*

BIOLOGICAL FACTORS INFLUENCING THE UTILIZATION OF AMINO ACIDS

Alfred E. Harper

Department of Biochemistry
Department of Nutritional Sciences
University of Wisconsin-Madison
Madison, Wisconsin

INTRODUCTION

Amino acids are the building blocks of tissue proteins. They are also precursors of many physiologically important nitrogenous molecules such as nucleic acids; heme; neurotransmitters, e.g., serotonin and norepinephrine; and hormones, e.g., thyroxine and epinephrine. Nine of the amino acids in food proteins cannot be synthesized by mammals. They are, therefore, essential nutrients that must be obtained from foods. A continuous supply of these amino acids is required for growth of the young, for reproduction and lactation, and for maintenance of the adult. A lack of any one of them for more than a few hours results in growth failure of the infant and loss of tissue protein by the adult.

Although amino acids are needed primarily for synthesis of tissue proteins, they are also important as sources of energy. Amino acids consumed in excess of the amounts needed as building blocks are degraded; the nitrogen they contain is converted to urea and excreted in the urine; the α-keto acids remaining can be used for synthesis of glucose or fatty acids or can be oxidized directly.

One of the end products of amino acid catabolism, ammonia, is toxic. Also, high concentrations of many of the individual essential amino acids in body fluids lead to adverse effects and even toxicity [16]. In infants with genetic defects of amino acid metabolism, the concentration of the amino acid that cannot be degraded rises abnormally in blood and body fluids. This rise is frequently associated with the development of mental retardation [34]. A low phenylalanine diet has been used to reduce blood phenylalanine concentration in patients with phenylketonuria— a disease resulting from the inability to convert phenylalanine to tyrosine. It also reduces the degree of mental retardation [2]. The success of this treatment, and of analogous treatments for other metabolic defects of amino acid metabolism, indicates that the adverse effects of such diseases are attributable specifically to accumulation of the amino acid that cannot be degraded normally or to a metabolic product formed in an alternative metabolic pathway. Adverse, and even toxic, effects have also been observed in animals that have been fed excessive amounts of individual amino acids in an effort to mimic effects of genetic defects of amino acid metabolism [6].

A discussion of biological factors that influence the utilization of amino acids can be separated logically into two parts: one dealing with nutritional aspects of the subject; the other with metabolic aspects. *From a nutritional viewpoint,* major concern is with dietary factors that influence the efficiency with which amino acids in a diet or a protein are used for protein synthesis; rarely is much attention given, other than in a general way, to the utilization of amino acids as sources of energy. *From a metabolic viewpoint,* major concern is with factors that influence the regulation of amino acid metabolism, including synthesis of tissue proteins, catabolism of amino acids and interactions between these two processes. The relative importance of the different regulatory systems depends upon the nutritional state of the organism which, in turn, determines the extent to which amino acids are used as sources of energy and the likelihood of adverse effects from the accumulation of amino acids in body fluids.

Dietary Aspects of Amino Acid Utilization

Much attention has been given over the years in studies of protein nutrition to what is usually termed "efficiency of protein utilization". This term is defined in a very specific way as the proportion of either the ingested or the absorbed nitrogen that is retained by the body. It is accepted as a measure of the proportion of the dietary amino acids that are used for tissue protein synthesis and the synthesis of other biologically important nitrogenous compounds. The underlying assumption is that the proportion of nitrogen not retained represents a measure of amino acid wastage. No credit is given for the portion of amino acids as sources of energy [6]. The main biological factors that influence amino acid utilization, defined in this way, are: one, the relative proportions of amino acids present in the diet; and, two, the total quantity of amino acids consumed.

The influence of these two factors is determined by amino acid requirements. The requirement represents the minimum amount of amino acid that must be ingested to support the maximum rate of growth of the young or to prevent nitrogen loss in the adult. The requirement should, thus, be a measure of the minimum amount of amino acid required for the maximum rate of tissue protein synthesis together with the minimum amount of amino acid that is unavoidably oxidized under these conditions. If the pattern of essential amino acids present in a dietary protein resembles closely the pattern of amino acid requirements, and the quantity consumed is just sufficient to meet the total nitrogen requirement, efficiency of utilization of each of the essential amino acids in that protein should be the maximum attainable for the adequately nourished organism. The pattern of essential amino acids in cow's milk proteins resembles closely the pattern of amino acid requirements of the human infant (6 months) as shown in Figure 1. Such proteins should be used with close to the maximum possible efficiency, in the nutritional sense of this term, for normal growth when they are fed in an amount that will just meet the total nitrogen requirement. Efficiency of nitrogen retention will fall if the quantity consumed exceeds the amount needed to meet the requirements. It will also fall if the proportions of amino acids in the dietary protein deviate from the proportions of the requirements [15] as all amino acids must be present together in the correct proportions for synthesis of proteins.

These situations are illustrated for human adults in Figure 2. The amino acid requirements are expressed as mg per gm of protein required. Each gram of cow's milk protein consumed provides considerable excess of each of the es-

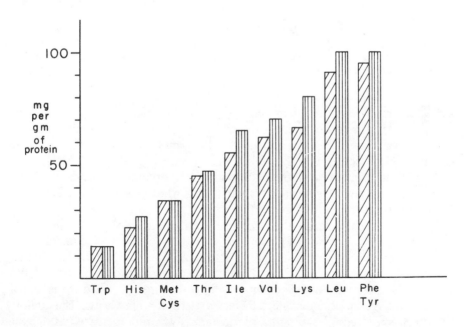

Figure 1. Amino acid patterns of human infant (6 mo.) requirements and cow's milk proteins. Requirements are expressed as mg of amino acid required per gm of protein required, assuming requirement = 2 gm protein per kg body wt. ▨ Requirements of infants (mg/gm protein) ▥ Content of cow's milk (mg/gm protein).

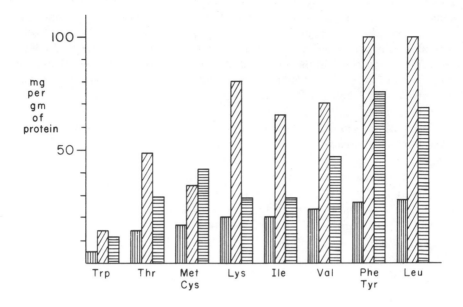

Figure 2. Amino acid patterns of human adult requirements and cow's milk and wheat proteins. Requirements are expressed as mg of amino acid required per gm of protein required, assuming requirement = 0.5 gm. protein per kg body wt. ⦀ Requirements of adults (mg/gm protein) ▨ Content of milk proteins (mg/gm protein) ▤ Content of wheat proteins (mg/gm protein).

sential amino acids over the amount required. Although the amino acid pattern of wheat proteins differs considerably from that for cow's milk proteins, each gram of wheat proteins consumed will provide surpluses of most of the essential amino acids, with the exception of lysine and possibly of isoleucine. The implication of these comparisons is that essential amino acids of dietary proteins are not used highly efficiently by adults when proteins are fed at a level that meets the nitrogen requirement.

Figures 3 and 4 illustrate the effects of both amino acid pattern and intake on efficiency of utilization of protein for growth by rats that were fed different quantities of a variety of proteins or mixtures of proteins which differed considerably in amino acid pattern. In Figure 3 the wide spread of protein intakes required by different animals to support a particular rate or growth is indicative of the effect of an unbalanced dietary pattern of amino acids. The quantity of protein required to maintain a particular growth rate increased as the pattern became more unbalanced. When, as shown in Figure 4, growth rate was plotted against only the balanced portion of amino acids in the diet, the scatter was greatly reduced, indicating that the amino acids present in excess of the requirement in the diets that had unbalanced amino acid patterns were used only

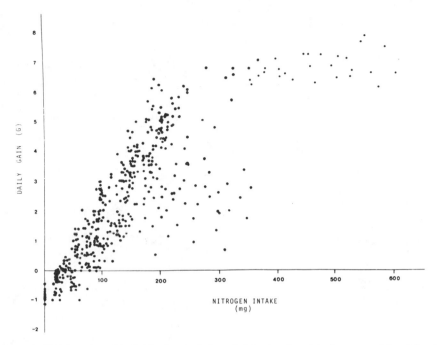

Figure 3. Weight gains of individuals rats fed graded levels of protein from a veriety of foods, food components and food mixtures (Uribe-Peralto, A. Ph.D. Thesis, University of Wisconsin, 1978).

for energy. The similar and maximum growth rates of rats to the right of the 200 mg intake of nitrogen point on this plot, indicates that, as intake of balanced protein increased above this value, efficiency of utilization for tissue protein synthesis declined sharply [15].

The question of efficiency of protein utilization has been a troubling one. Most measurements of efficiency are made using diets that contain an inadequate amount of protein. Evidence from both growth studies and nitrogen balance studies indicates that the proportion of nitrogen retained per increment of protein fed falls off as intake approaches the level at which maximum response is attained. Thus, the generally accepted standard measures of efficiency of protein utilization determined with less than adequate protein intakes, overestimate efficiency of utilization at the requirement level - the level of major interest in nutrition.

Thus, two of the major biological factors that influence amino acid utilization are total quantity of amino acid consumed and the proportion consumed in relation to the intakes of other amino acids. These factors, determine how much of the amount of an amino acid consumed will be used for protein synthesis and how much will be oxidized as a source of energy, provided there is no impairment of amino acid absorption and that the supply of other energy sources is adequate.

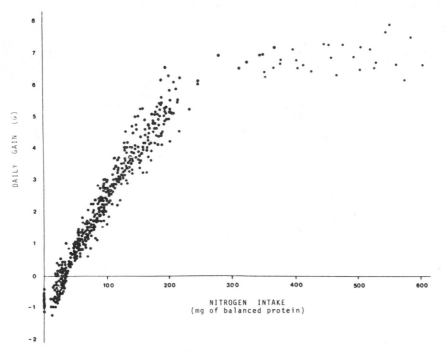

Figure 4. Weight gains of individual rats from Figure 3 plotted as a function of balanced protein intake, estimated using an amino acid scoring pattern based on the amino acid composition of rat's milk (Uribe-Peralto, A. Ph.D. Thesis, University of Wisconsin, 1978).

One other obvious factor that influences amino acid utilization is the extent to which the amino acid is absorbed. Amino acids may be biologically unavailable owing to either low digestibility of proteins [6, pp. 169-194] or chemical interactions that occur between amino acids and carbohydrates or among amino acids during heat processing or storage of foods [6, pp. 239-260]. Amino acids that are released during digestion are absorbed efficiently.

Also the energy supply of the organism can influence amino acid utilization. As energy supply falls below the amount needed for growth or maintenance the proportion of amino acids oxidized as a source of energy will increase. Efforts to quantify this effect are confounded by the difficulty in establishing accurately both energy and protein requirements and the contribution of energy from body stores. Nevertheless, results of a series of studies on human subjects indicate that when energy intake of adults was varied over the range of plus or minus 15% of the requirement, nitrogen retention decreased between 1 and 2 mg for each kcal of restriction. When energy intake was severely curtailed (less than 60% of the requirement) nitrogen retention fell by about 6 mg for each kcal of restriction. As caloric deficit becomes more severe, the proportion of protein or amino acids used for energy increases sharply [6, pp. 148-168]. As the subjects in these studies presumably were not depleted of fat, a substantial proportion of their energy needs must have been met from body reserves as even under the most severe caloric restriction reported, protein utilization could account for only a small proportion of the total energy requirement. It is well known that during starvation, protein is conserved while fat is depleted. As animal studies have shown, some amino acids are channelled into protein synthesis even when restriction of energy intake is severe [24].

Metabolic Aspects of Amino Acid Utilization

Survival of an organism under different nutritional and physiological conditions depends upon its ability to control the extent to which amino acids are used for tissue protein synthesis and as sources of energy.

When protein intake is not excessive, as with the breast-fed infant, but energy (kcal) intake is adequate, the primary need is to ensure that amino acids will be used preferentially for tissue protein synthesis, rather than being diverted into catabolic pathways and being degraded.

When protein or amino acids are consumed in amounts considerably in excess of those needed for tissue protein synthesis, channeling of the surplus amino acids rapidly into degradative pathways is necessary in order to provide energy and prevent their accumulation in body fluids.

Whenever protein intake is inadequate, conservation of amino acids and high efficiency in their use for tissue protein synthesis is essential for survival.

During starvation, or if the intake of energy sources is severely inadequate, the major need of the body is for energy and for an adequate supply of glucose to maintain normal functioning of the central nervous system. Survival under such conditions depends on the channeling of amino acids that are released during the breakdown of tissue proteins, or those from whatever limited amount of food may be consumed, into glucose-producing and energy-yielding pathways.

The high efficiency of utilization of amino acids for tissue formation when intake is low, the rapid rate of clearance of amino acids from blood when intake is high, the stability of plasma fasting amino acid concentrations, and the rarity of either ammonia toxicity or adverse effects from accumulations of amino acids in healthy individuals consuming large amounts of protein, all attest to the fact that amino acid utilization is influenced rapidly and effectively by the nutritional and physiological state of the organism.

Control of Amino Acid Utilization

The number of sites and mechanisms for control of amino acid utilization in the body is limited.

For minerals such as calcium and iron, absorption increases when intake is low, and decreases to prevent overloading when intake is high. Thus, control of the proportion of the ingested nutrient absorbed represents a major regulatory system.

Regulation of stomach emptying controls the rate of flow of amino acids to sites of absorption and thereby reduces the probability of overloading of the metabolic systems of the body. But there is no regulation of amino acid metabolism by the gastrointestinal tract of the type observed for many minerals. Most food proteins, unless they have been heat-damaged, are digested almost completely. The amino acids released during digestion are also absorbed almost completely. Even when the amino acid intake of experimental animals reaches a toxic level, absorption is essentially complete. The gastrointestinal tract is thus a unidirectional trapping system for amino acids [12, 13].

Control of excretion is a major mechanism for regulation of plasma concentrations of the electrolytes, sodium and potassium. Reabsorption of amino acids from the glomerular filtrate, however, is a highly efficient process. Amino acids are excreted in the urine in significant quantities only when the blood concentration is in the range that will cause adverse effects. Renal excretion, like intestinal absorption, is basically a unidirectional process for conservation of amino acids, not a regulatory system [12,13].

For energy sources (carbohydrates, fats) consumed in amounts in excess of immediate needs, storage as glycogen or fat is a major mechanism for removing surpluses from the circulation.

A high protein intake, however, does not lead to accumulation of either body proteins generally or unique storage proteins. In fact, if one amino acid is deleted from a meal and is provided a few hours later, growth and nitrogen retention are depressed. This provides evidence for the fact that there is little reserve of amino acids and that amino acids not used immediately for synthesis of proteins are removed rapidly from the circulation and degraded to provide energy.

Tissue proteins are, nevertheless, degraded when the body is subjected to a period of deprivation. Muscle in particular undergoes degradation during prolonged starvation; amino acids are released and are used to maintain critical organs in a functional state and for synthesis of glucose to support the metabolism of the central nervous system. This, however, represents loss of functional tissue not the utilization of a "protein reserve" [12,13].

With absorption of amino acids from the intestine into the portal blood serving only as an efficient trapping mechanism, with the excretion of amino acids in the urine occurring only after blood concentrations approach levels that cause adverse effects, and with no mechanism for storage of amino acids when intakes are high, control of protein synthesis and control of amino acid degradation are left as the major mechanism for controlling amino acid utilization.

If these major regulatory systems are defective or become overloaded, control of food intake is the one remaining mechanism for preventing inordinate accumulations of amino acids in body fluids.

Basic Mechanisms for Control of Metabolism

There are relatively few basic mechanisms for control of metabolic processes. Regulation of the concentrations of solutes in body fluids is primarily through control of enzymatic reactions and the transport of substrates to sites of metabolism.

The amount of enzyme or transport catalyst may be constitutive, i.e. fixed. The rate of the process depends then on the concentrations of substrates —or solutes— entering into the reaction.

The enzyme or transport catalyst may be adaptive; that is, the amount of the catalyst —enzyme or transport carrier— may increase or decrease in response to a change in the metabolic demand. The capacity of the system would thereby be altered.

Two characteristics of enzymatic or transport systems are important in relation to control of amino acid metabolism [40]. First, the rate of an enzymatic reaction increases as the concentration of the substrate for the reaction increases, up to the point at which the enzyme is saturated. The rate of the reaction at that point approaches the maximum.

The concentration of substrate required for half the maximum rate or velocity —the Michaelis constant or Km— differs for different enzymes. Comparison of the Km values for different enzymes of amino acid metabolism provides a guide to the relative rates that would be expected with a given concentration of amino acid. If the concentration of substrate is low, well below the Km value, the rate of the reaction will be low. If the concentration of substrate is high, well above the Km value, say by tenfold, then the rate of the reaction will approach the maximum.

Secondly, the rate of an enzymatic reaction also increases directly in proportion to the amount of enzyme present. Thus, if the amount of enzyme doubles, the time required for removal of a given amount of substrate should be halved.

Thus, factors that alter either amino acid concentrations or the quantities of amino acid degrading enzymes or transport proteins would be expected to influence amino acid utilization.

Role of Substrate Supply in Amino Acid Utilization

Comparison of the hepatic concentrations of two amino acids for rats fed a low protein diet is shown in Table I together with the concentrations required for half-maximum velocity of the amino acid activation reaction, the initial step for channeling amino acids into protein synthesis, and for the reaction representing the first step in the pathways for their degradation [30].

With normal liver amino acid concentrations, the rate of amino acid activation for protein synthesis should be close to the maximum. With the same con-

TABLE I *Comparison of Michaelis Constants for Amino Acyl*
Synthetases and Catabolic Enzymes With Hepatic
Amino Acid Concentrations

	Km of acyl synthetase	Hepatic concentration	Km of catabolic enzyme
	μM	μM	μM
Arginine	1.2 − 3.0	20 − 30	3000 [1]
Isoleucine	5	140	840 [2]

(Selected from Rogers, 1976) [10].

1. *Arginase*
2. *Branched-chain aminotransferase*

centrations of amino acids, however, the rates of the initial reactions in the degradative pathways would be only a fraction of their maxima. Catabolic reactions would not approach their maximum rates unless liver amino acid concentrations rose greatly above the "normal" values such as during absorption of amino acids from a high protein meal.

The properties of these two sets of enzymes —amino acid-activating enzymes with Michaelis constants 1/10 or less the normal concentration of free amino acids in liver and the initial enzymes in the degradative pathways having Michaelis constants several times the concentrations of free amino acids in liver— ensures that amino acids will be channeled preferentially into the initial step for synthesis of proteins even when protein intake is low.

Protein synthesis is influenced by diet in another way. The formation of polyribosomes —the protein-synthesizing systems of cells consisting of a chain of ribosomes attached to m-RNA— depends on a continuous supply of amino acids. During starvation the polysomes disaggregate to give small ribosomal units, free ribosomes and ribosomal subunits and the rate of protein synthesis is depressed. Feeding a complete amino acid mixture results in aggregation of the ribosomes and restores the rate of protein synthesis [26].

Jefferson and Korner [17] and more recently Flaim et al. [10] have examined this phenomenon in the perfused liver. They observed that the rate of protein synthesis was a function of the concentration of amino acids in the medium perfusing the liver. They also showed that there was a close association between the degree of aggregation of the ribosomes and the rate of protein synthesis. They [10] concluded from detailed studies of the components of the system that low concentrations of amino acids did not result in depletion of m-RNA needed for polysome formation but probably led to impairment of protein synthesis by affecting some component required for initiation of polypeptide chain formation.

In young growing organisms, channeling of amino acids into tissue proteins is an important mechanism for regulation of amino acid concentrations in body fluids. Preferential use of amino acids for synthesis of tissue proteins, rather than in reactions that shunt them into degradative pathways, depends on the amino acids that are ingested being channeled into the system for amino acid activation -the formation of aminoacyl-tRNAs. This occurs efficiently even at low amino acid concentrations [10], presumably because of the low Km's of the synthetases for these reactions (Table I). Peptide chain formation depends, then, upon an intact system for protein synthesis. When the quantities of amino acids consumed are somewhat below the amounts required for the maximum rate of growth, the available amino acids can be incorporated into proteins with an efficiency that approaches 90% of the amount consumed [5] with the proportion oxidized being low. An adequate amino acid supply ensures highly efficient utilization for this purpose [10] but the proportion of amino acids oxidized increases directly as the amount consumed increases above that required for maximum rate of growth.

Factors that affect insulin release also influence amino acid utilization. Ingestion of food, particularly high carbohydrate foods, stimulates insulin release. Insulin, in turn, stimulates uptake of amino acids, particularly by muscle, and also stimulates incorporation of amino acids into proteins [18]. Thus, the influence of insulin on transport of amino acids results in channeling of amino acids primarily into tissues that have only limited ability to degrade them. A variety of mechanisms thus ensures that ingested amino aicds will be used preferentially for synthesis of tissue proteins.

McCance [23] has pointed out that highly efficient utilization of amino acids for tissue synthesis can be considered a major mechanism for maintaining homcostasis of blood amino acid concentrations in infants. He emphasized that this is a particularly important protective mechanism that prevents the immature kidney of the young infant from being overloaded with solutes that would arise from extensive degradation of amino acids.

Utilization of Amino Acids for Energy

When amino acids are consumed in excess of the amounts needed for tissue-protein synthesis, efficient channeling of the extra amino acids into energy-yielding pathways and disposal of the nitrogenous end products is critical for preventing amino acids from accumulating in the body in amounts that might be injurious to health. Since amino acid-degrading enzymes function at their maximum rate only when amino acid concentrations are high, rate of amino acid degradation would be expected to increase substantially in response to increasing amino acid intake and the resulting elevations of tissue amino acid concentrations. This can be demonstrated *in vivo* in experimental animals.

When rats were fed increasing increments of histidine in an otherwise complete diet, growth rate increased directly with increasing dietary histidine content until the level in the diet exceeded 0.25% [19]. With higher dietary histidine levels, histidine consumption was in excess of the amount needed for protein synthesis and growth. Blood histidine concentration remained low until the dietary level of histidine exceeded 0.25% (Fig. 5). It then increased rather sharply but began to plateau as the dietary level approached 0.4%. Muscle histidine concentration behaved similarly and liver showed the same trend but the points of inflection were less sharp.

When histidine intake was low, growth rate was low, blood and tissue histidine concentrations were low, and very little of the histidine consumed was oxidized, less than 10% [9], as measured by the amount of radioactivity released from ^{14}C-histidine included in the diet (Fig. 6). When histidine intake exceeded the amount needed for protein synthesis, blood and tissue histidine concentrations began to rise, and the rate of histidine oxidation increased. It increased directly with increasing histidine intake of the animals, once the basic requirement had been met.

This occurred even in the presence of an adequate supply of energy from carbohydrate and fat. Similar results have been obtained with tryptophan [27], lysine [8], and threonine [20]. These observations indicate that amino acids are used efficiently as an energy source when intake is high and that they are used preferentially for energy in the presence of other energy sources. This is further evidence that surplus amino acids are not conserved.

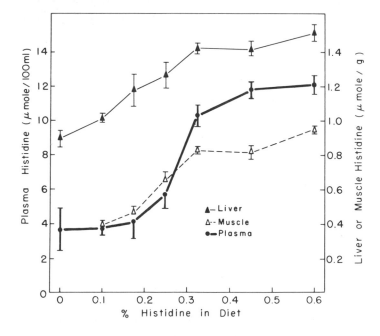

Figure 5. Plasma and tissue concentrations of histidine in rats fed a series of diets with increasing histidine content (After 19).

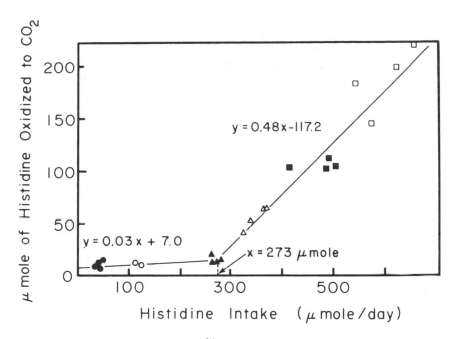

Figure 6. Changes in amount of ingested ^{14}C-histidine oxidized to CO_2 by rats fed increasing increments of histidine in the diet (After 19).

Substrate control of amino acid-degrading enzymes, i.e. a high rate of reaction when substrate supply is high and a low rate when substrate supply is low, contributes to conservation of amino acids for tissue protein synthesis when the supply is low and to rapid utilization of surpluses for energy when the supply is excessive [1,13,22]. The capacity of these enzyme systems is nevertheless finite; so, despite the responses to increased amino acid intake the capacity of the systems will be exceeded if intake is very high.

The rate of an enzymatic reaction is also directly proportional to the amount of enzyme that participates in the reaction. Hence, the capacity for amino acid degradation will increase if the amount of enzyme increases. Many of the enzymes of amino acid degradation in the liver are adaptive [11,22], i.e. the amount of enzyme changes in response to dietary or hormonal stimuli. The amounts of most amino acid-degrading enzymes in the liver change in response to changes in protein intake, increasing as protein intake rises and decreasing as protein intake falls.

Histidase, the enzyme that catalyzes the first step in histidine degradation, increases in the liver in response to an increase in protein intake (Fig. 7) and falls to low activity if protein intake is low [33]. The rate at which a load of histidine can be cleared from the body increases as histidase activity rises (Fig. 8). A given load of histidine, in this example 50 mg or about 1.3 times the daily requirement of the rat, was cleared from blood much more rapidly by rats that

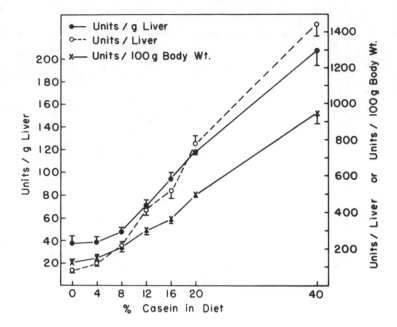

Figure 7. Change in histidase activity in liver in response to change in protein (casein) intake in the rat (After 22).

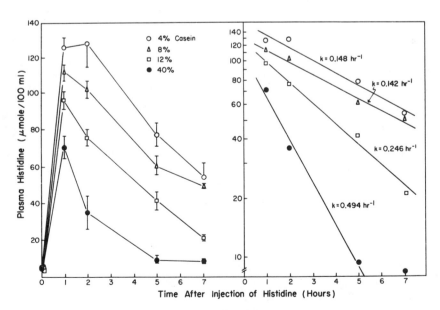

Figure 8. Changes in plasma histidine concentration over time after injection (i.p.) of 50 mg (322 μmoles) of histidine into rats allowed to adjust for 10 days to diets containing different amounts of protein (After 21). ○ 4% Casein △ 8% □ 12% • 40%.

had previously been fed a high protein diet than by those previously fed a low protein diet [21]. The rates of clearance for animals fed different levels of protein depended on the extent of induction of histidase.

This type of induction does not occur, as a rule, in response to an increased supply of substrate. It occurs, with very few exceptions, only in response to increased intake of protein or to treatment with glucagon or glucocorticoids [11]. Thus animals fed a low protein diet have low amino acid-degrading capacity and, as with children who have inborn errors of amino acid metabolism, degrade amino acids slowly [7]. A large load of histidine, one that exceeds the capacity for histidine degradation, causes a substantial rise in histidine concentration in body fluids (Fig. 9). Nevertheless, in animals in which amino acid-degrading enzymes have been induced either by feeding them a high protein diet or injecting them with cortisol and glucagon, the load of histidine is cleared from the body effectively over a six- to nine-hour period [25]. In those in which the enzyme has not been induced, tissue histidine concentrations remains greatly elevated even after 12 hours, a situation resembling that in patients with genetic defects of histidine catabolism. The difference in the ability of the two groups of animals to clear histidine from tissues is associated with a substancial difference nearly five-fold in their capacity for histidine oxidation.

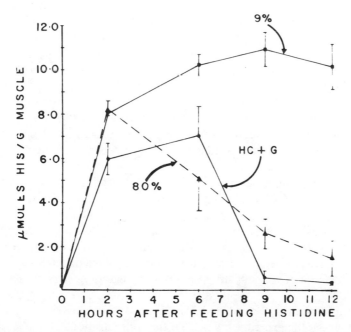

Figure 9. Changes in muscle histidine concentration of rats previously fed low protein (9% casein) or high protein (80% casein) diets or injected with hydrocortisone and glucagon (HC + G), with time after ingestion of a meal containing a load of 750 mg of histidine (After 25).

Control of Food Intake

Relationships among diet composition, amino acid utilization and food and protein intakes are complex. Both the protein content and the amino acid pattern of the diet can influence amino acid utilization, and depending upon the nutritional state of the organism, can affect food intake or protein selection.

Effects of Dietary Protein Content on Food Intake

Ingestion of a large amount of protein, even protein of high nutritional quality, increases blood amino acid concentrations, and if the quantity of protein consumed is great enough, amino acid concentrations will remain elevated for several hours. Plasma amino acid concentrations of rats that have previously been fed a low protein diet are greatly elevated [4] during the absorptive period, particularly on the first day after the casein content of their diet has been increased from 5% to 50%. The greatly elevated plasma amino acid concentrations are associated with severely depressed food intake.

For groups of rats fed experimental diets containing 25,50 or 75% casein, the degree of depression of food intake increased with the increasing casein content of the diet [4]. Yet, despite the severe depressions in food intake, the protein intake of each of the experimental groups was higher than before the diets were changed. Elevated protein intake stimulates transport of amino acids into the liver [35]. Values for uptake of the non-metabolizable amino acid, α-aminoisobutyric acid (AIB), by liver slices from rats fed a moderate or an exceedingly high protein diet are shown in Fig. 10. Hepatic uptake of AIB was elevated within one hour in those that had been fed a high protein meal. This response should facilitate amino acid catabolism and thereby utilization of amino acids for energy by increasing uptake of amino acids by liver. Glucagon exerts a similar effects. A high protein diet has been shown to stimulate glucagon production. In these studies the high protein diet was shown to increase the liver content of cyclic-AMP, a response that also occurs after glucagon injection.

Threonine dehydratase, a hepatic amino acid-degrading enzyme that is induced in animals consuming a high protein diet, was measured in the study of effects of changing protein intake on food intake [4]. The response of the enzyme in the various groups of animals was roughly proportional to their protein intakes. This type of induction, as was shown above for histidase, increases the capacity of the liver to degrade amino acids and clearance of amino acids from body fluids occurs more rapidly after amino acid-degrading enzymes have been induced (Fig. 9).

As the amino acid-degrading capacity of rats fed the high protein diet increased throughout the experimental period, the concentrations of amino acids in plasma rose less. Within a few days, food intake was restored nearly to that of control animals fed a low protein diet (Fig. 11). At this time, protein intake

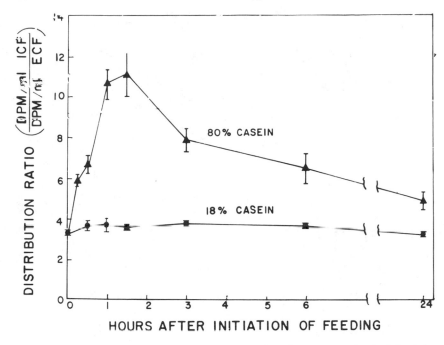

Figure 10. Uptake of α-aminoisobutyric acid by liver slices from rats previously fed an adequate (18% casein) or a high (80% casein) protein diet. Uptake is expressed as the ratio of intracellular to extracellular concentration (After 35).

had risen several-fold; despite this rise, plasma amino acid concentrations did not rise nearly as high on day five as they did on day one, when protein intake of the animals was much less. After the animals had adapted to the high protein intake, homeostasis of blood amino acid concentrations was restored with a greatly elevated rate of amino acid catabolism and an increased capacity to use amino acids as a source of energy.

Thus, control of food intake serves as the final mechanism for preventing severe overloading of the amino acid-degrading systems of the body. In healthy, well-nourished organisms it provides temporary protection from accumulation of amino acids while the body adjusts to a high protein intake. During this period of adaptation amino acid-degrading enzymes are induced; subsequently, the organism functions well and is able to clear an excessive amino acid load from body fluids without either ammonia or amino acids accumulating to harmful levels.

Observations of this type, showing that food intake depressions under a variety of dietary conditions are associated with changes in plasma amino acid concentrations [16], have stimulated interest in the effects of blood amino acid concentrations and patterns on food consumption and in the effects of diet on the functioning of the central nervous system generally.

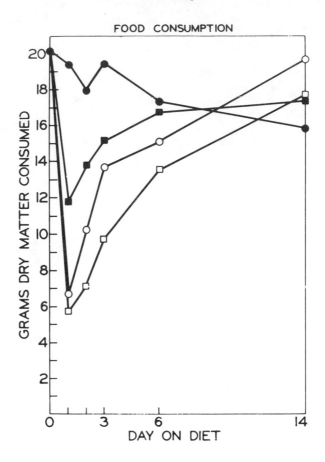

Figure 11. Food consumption of rats fed diets containing 25%, 50%, or 75% casein after being fed a low protein (5% casein) diet for 10 days previously (After 4). ● 5% casein diet ■ 25% casein diet ○ 50% casein diet □ 75% casein diet.

Effects of Amino Acid Pattern on Food Intake

Dietary surpluses of all but one of the indispensable amino acids cause an immediate and severe depression of food intake and growth associated with changes in blood and brain amino acid concentrations [28]. For example, addition of a mixture of amino acids devoid of histidine to a low protein diet depressed food intake and growth of rats (Fig. 12). A supplement of histidine restored growth and food intake.

The depressions in growth and food intake are associated with substancially elevated concentrations of amino acids other than histidine in blood. They are also associated with a marked drop in histidine concentration in the brain (Fig. 13). Concentrations of other amino acids in the brain changed very little. Ro-

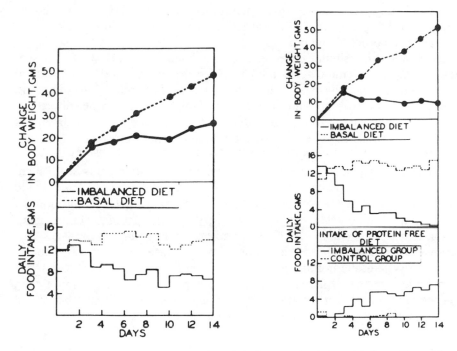

Figure 12. *Weight gain and food intake of rats fed a low protein (5% casein) diet, with or without addition of a mixture of amino acids devoid of histidine.*

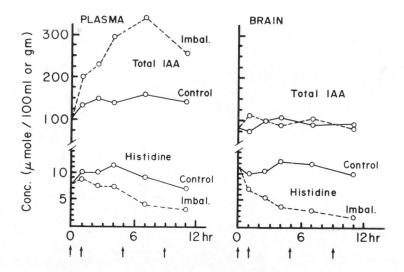

Figure 13. *Plasma and brain histidine and indispensable amino acid (IAA) concentrations of rats force-fed at intervals (indicated by arrows) small meals of a low protein diet with or without addition of a mixture of amino acids devoid of histidine (After 28).*

gers and Leung [31] observed that when rats fed diets of this type, food intake depression did not occur if bilateral lesions had been made previously in the prepyriform cortex of the brain.

These and other similar observations on animals fed a variety of diets suggested that certain amino acids in high concentrations in blood might be competing with another that was in low concentration for uptake into the brain, and that the altered brain amino acid pattern might initiate, either directly or indirectly, a signal for food intake depression [28]. Competition for uptake into the brain would be expected particularly among amino acids that were similar in structure and were transported into the brain by common transport system.

We [37] examined the effects of including various amino acids in the incubation medium on uptake of tryptophan into brain slices (Fig. 14). As would be anticipated from knowledge of amino acid transport systems, additions of large neutral amino acids, branched-chain (BCAA), or aromatic amino acids to the incubation medium suppressed uptake of tryptophan into the slices. Addition of lysine and arginine, basic amino acids that are transported by another transport system, did not affect tryptophan uptake by brain slices. A series of observations of this type reinforced our assumption that competition among plasma amino acids for uptake into the brain could account for the altered brain amino acid patterns observed in the animal studies.

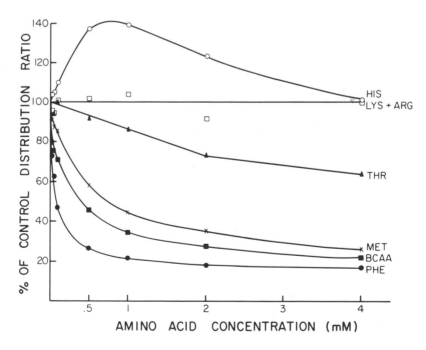

Figure 14. Effect of additions of amino acids to the incubation medium on uptake of tryptophan by rat brain slices. Uptake is expressed as distribution ratio which is the ratio of intracellular to extracellular tryptophan (After 37).

If this were the case, and the resulting alteration in brain amino acid pattern initiated a signal for food intake depression, food intake of animals fed a diet marginal in tryptophan, to which a mixture of the amino acids shown in the brain slice studies to inhibit tryptophan uptake had been added, should be depressed. The depression should be associated with low brain tryptophan concentration and should be alleviated by supplementation of the diet with tryptophan.

Food intake of rats consuming a diet that contained only a limited amount of tryptophan to which a mixture of large neutral amino acids had been added was depressed (Table II). The depression was associated with low brain tryptophan concentration and was alleviated by supplement of tryptophan, although not compeletly [14]. Dietary addition of lysine and arginine, which did not compete with tryptophan for uptake into brain slices, did not cause depression of food intake or growth or brain tryptophan concentration.

Similar studies, in which food intake responses have been predicted from studies of competition among amino acids for uptake into brain slices, have now been done with threonine [38,39] and lysine [36], which are transported by other transport systems, and also with histidine [39], which is transported by the same one.

Wurtman and Fernstrom and their associates at the Massachusetts Institute of Technology [9] were led by a different line of research to similar conclusions about the potential for dietary modifications influencing brain amino acid concentrations. In studies of tryptophan uptake into the brain, they noted that either an increase in plasma tryptophan concentration or a decrease in plasma BCAA concentrations was associated with increased tryptophan concentration in the brain. When they plotted brain tryptophan concentration against the

TABLE II Effect of Large Neutral Amino Acids on Food Intake and
Weight Gain of Rats Fed A Diet Limiting in Tryptophan

		Food Intake (gm)		Wt. Gain (gm)
		Day 1	Day 2	7 Days
I	Low trp diet *	14 ± 1	13 ± 1	28 ± 4
II	Diet I + 4.5 large neutral amino acids +	7 ± 2	6 ± 1	7 ± 1
III	Diet II + 0.05% L-trp	9 ± 1	10 ± 1	20 ± 1

* Basal diet contained 6% casein, 0.2% L-met, 0.2% L-thr, 0.1% L-his.
+ Large neutral amino acids = Leu, ile, val, phe, tyr, met in equal amounts.

ratio of the plasma concentrations of tryptophan to large neutral amino acids (LNAA), they found that there was a direct relationships between brain tryptophan concentration and the plasma ratio of tryptophan to large neutral (trp/LN) amino acids. They also observed that there was a direct relationship between brain serotonin concentration and this ratio. This provided evidence that the concentration of a neurotransmitter in the brain could be influenced by changes in the pattern of amino acids in plasma, which in turn could be influenced by changes in the pattern of amino acids in the diet.

They have suggested that this provides the potential for modifying central nervous systems function and, thereby, behavior by dietary manipulation. They noted research showing that animals treated in ways that lower brain serotonin concentration have a heightened response to pain and that this is suppressed by injecting them with sufficient tryptophan to elevate brain serotonin concentration [9].

Anderson and associates [3] and Fernstrom [9] have postulated that altered plasma trp/LN ratio, by influencing brain serotonin concentration, may provide a signal for altered food or protein intake by animals fed high protein diets. Although under some conditions such relationships have been observed [3], relationships between food intake or protein intake and brain tryptophan or serotonin concentration have not been consistent [29,32]. In a study of associations between brain serotonin concentration and protein intake in our laboratory [29] no significant correlation was observed. Overall, the evidence does not support the serotonin hypothesis for control of food and protein intake even though modifications in the protein content and amino acid pattern of the diet can influence both food and protein intake, blood and brain amino acid concentrations and brain serotonin concentration.

These effects of dietary protein content and amino acid pattern represent unique effects of nutritional factors on the utilization of amino acids for highly specific functions.

SUMMARY

Biological factors that influence the utilization of amino acids are of two types: one, dietary, e.g. the amounts of protein and sources of calories, the amino acid pattern and the bioavailability of the amino acids in the protein; two, metabolic, e.g. the nutritional and physiological state of the organism.

From a strictly nutritional viewpoint, effects of dietary factors on amino acid utilization are measured in terms of efficiency of nitrogen retention, i.e. the gross efficiency with which ingested amino acids are used for tissue protein synthesis. Efficiency, in this sense of the term, declines with 1) increasing protein intake above the requirement; 2) with increasing deviation of the dietary amino acid pattern from the pattern of amino acid requirements; 3) with decreasing energy intake; and, 4) with decreasing bioavailability of the amino acids in the diet.

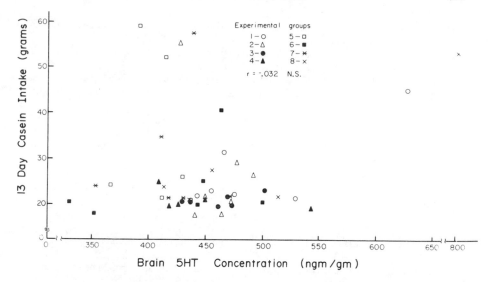

Figure 15. Relationship between brain serotonin concentration and protein (casein) intake of individual rats allowed to select between diets containing 15% or 55% casein with or without various amino acid supplements. Experimental groups 1−○, 2−△, 3−•, 4−▲, 5−□, 6−■, 7−, 8−×; r = .032 N.S. (After 29).*

From a metabolic viewpoint, major interest is in the regulatory responses that either protein synthesis or energy-yielding pathways when the nutritional or physiological state of the organism changes. The properties of enzymes of amino acid metabolism are such that oxidation is suppressed when amino acid intake is inadequate to barely adequate but is stimulated rapidly when intake exceeds the needs for protein synthesis. Adaptive responses that increase the quantity of amino acid-degrading enzymes and depress food intake occur if intake is so high that the capacity to degrade amino acids is exceeded. These adaptations enable the body to adjust to intakes of amino acids that would have adverse effects if adaptations did not occur.

Changes in body fluid amino acid concentrations, as the result of changes in either the quantity or quality of the mixture of amino acids provided in the diet or owing to impairment or limitations of amino acid-degrading enzymes can alter the amino acid supply to the brain and the utilization of amino acids for formation of neurotransmitters. This raises the possibility that dietary protein and amino acid modifications and certain pathologic states that impair amino acid metabolism can lead to behavioral changes.

REFERENCES

1. Aguilar, T.S., N.J. Benevenga and A.E. Harper. Effect of dietary methionine level on its metabolism in rats. *J. Nutrition 104:* 761-771, 1974.

2. American Academy of Pediatrics, Committee on Nutrition. Special diets for children with inborn errors of amino aicd metabolism. *Pediatrics 57:* 783-791, 1976.

3. Anderson, G.H. Regulation of protein intake by plasma amino acids. *In:* Advances in *Nutrition Research,* H.H. Draper, editor. *1:* 145-166, 1977.

4. Anderson, H.L., N.J. Benevenga and A.E. Harper. Associations among food and protein intake, serine dehydratase, and plasma amino acids. *Am. J. Physiol. 214:* 1008-1013, 1968.

5. Block, R.J. and H.H. Mitchell. The correlation of the amino acid composition of proteins with their nutritive value. *Nutrition Abstr. Rev. 16:* 249-278, 1946-47.

6. Bodwell, C.E., J.S. Adkins and D.T. Hopkins. Protein Quality in Humans. Westport, Conn.: Avi, 1981.

7. Brand, L.M. and A.E. Harper. DL-α-Hydrazinoimidazolylpropionic acid: An irreversible inhibitor of hepatic histidine ammonia-lyase *in vivo. Arch. Biochem. Biophys. 177:* 123-132, 1976.

8. Brookes, I.M., F.N. Owens and U.S. Garrigus. Influence of amino acid level in the diet upon amino acid oxidation by the rat. *J. Nutrition 102:* 27-36, 1972.

9. Fernstorm, J.D. Effects of the diet on brain neurotransmitters. *Metabolism 26:* 207-223, 1977.

10. Flaim, K.E., W.S. Liao, D.E. Peavy, J.M. Taylor and L.S. Jefferson. The role of amino acids in the regulation of protein synthesis in perfused rat liver. *J. Biol. Chem. 257:* 2932-2946, 1982.

11. Freedland, R.A. and B. Szepesi. Control of enzyme activity: Nutritional factors. *In:* Enzyme Synthesis and Degradation in Mammalian Systems, M. Rechcigl, Jr., editor. Baltimore: University Park Press, pp. 103-140, 1971.

12. Harper, A.E. Amino acid requirements and plasma amino acids. *In:* Protein Nutrition, H. Brown, editor. Springfield: C.C. Thomas, pp. 130-179, 1974.

13. Harper, A.E. Control mechanisms in amino acid metabolism. *In:* The Control of Metabolism, J.D. Sink, editor. University Park, PA: The Pensylvania State University Press, Chap. 4, pp. 49-71, 1974.

14. Harper, A.E. Influence of dietary and plasma amino acid patterns on brain amino acid concentrations. Proceedings, Conference on Commonalities in Substance Abuse and Habitual Behavior. Washington D.C.: NAS/NRC, pp. 39-59, 1977.

15. Harper, A.E. McCollum and directions in the evaluation of protein quality. *J. Agric. Food Chem. 29:* 429-435, 1981.

16. Harper, A.E., N.J. Benevenga and R.M. Wohlbueter. Effects of ingestion of disproportionate amounts of amino acids. *Physiol. Rev. 50:* 428-558, 1970.

17. Jefferson, L.S. and A. Korner. Influence of amino acid supply on ribosomes and protein synthesis of perfused rat liver. *Biochem. J. 111:* 703-712, 1969.

18. Jefferson, L.S., J.B. Li and S.R. Rannels. Regulation by insulin of amino acid release and protein turnover in the perfused rat hemicorpus *J. Biol. Chem. 252:* 1476-1483, 1977.

19. Kang-Lee, Y.A. and A.E. Harper. Effect of histidine intake and hepatic histidase activity on the metabolism of histidine *in vivo. J. Nutrition 107:* 1427-1443, 1977.

20. Kang-Lee, Y.A. and A.E. Harper. Threonine metabolism *in vivo:* Effect of threonine intake and prior induction of threonine dehydratase in rats. *J. Nutrition 108:* 163-175, 1978.

21. Kang-Lee, Y.A. and A.E. Harper. Effect of inductions of histidase on histidine metabolism *in vivo. J. Nutrition 109:* 291-299, 1979.

22. Krebs, H.A. Some aspects of the regulation of fuel supply in omnivorous animals. *In:* Advances in Enzyme Regulation, Vol. 10, G. Weber, editor Oxford: Pergamon Press, pp. 397-420, 1972.

23. McCance, R.A. Unconsidered mechanisms responsible for maintianing the stability of the internal environment. *Can. Med. Assoc. J.* 75: 791, 1956.

24. Miller, D.S. and P.R. Payne. Problems in the prediction of protein values of diets. Caloric restriction. *J. Nutr.* 75: 225-230, 1961.

25. Morris, M.L., S-C Lee and A.E. Harper. Influence of differential induction of histidine catabolic enzymes on hidsitidine degradation *in vivo*. *J. Biol. Chem.* 247: 5793-5804, 1972.

26. Munro, H.N. A general survey of mechanisms regulating protein metabolism in mammals. *In:* Mammalian Protein Metabolism, Vol. IV. New York: Academic Press, pp. 3-130, 1970.

27. Patterson, J.I. and A.E. Harper. Effect of tryptophan intake on oxidation of [$7a$-^{14}C] tryptophan and urinary excretion of N'-methylnicotinamide in the rat. *J. Nutr. 112:* 776-781, 1982.

28. Peng, Y., J.K. Tews and A.E. Harper. Amino acid imbalance, protein intake, and changes in rat brain and plasma amino acids. *Am. J. Physiol. 222:* 314-321, 1972.

29. Peters, J.C. and A.E. Harper. Protein and energy consumption, plasma amino acid rations, and brain neurotransmitter concentration. *Physiol. and Behavior 27:* 287-298, 1981.

30. Rogers, Q.R. The nutritional and metabolic effects of amino acid imbalances. *In:* Protein Metabolism and Nutrition, D.J.A. Colem K.N. Boorman, P.J. Buttery, D. Lewis, R.J. Neale and H. Swan, editors. London: Butterworths, 1976.

31. Rogers, Q.R. and P.M.B. Leung. The influence of amino acids on the neuroregulation of food intake. *Fed. Proc. 32:* 1709-1719, 1973.

32. Romsos, D.R., K.M. Chee and W.C. Bergen. Protein intake regulation in adult abese (ob/ob) and lean mice: effects of nonprotein energy source and of supplemental tryptophan. *J. Nutr. 112:* 505-513, 1982.

33. Schirmer, M.D. and A.E. Harper. Adaptive responses of mammalian histidine-degrading enzymes. *J. Biol. Chem. 245:* 1204-1211, 1970.

34. Stanbury, J.B., J.B. Wyngaarden and D.S. Frederickson. The Metabolic Basis of Inherited Disease, 3rd edition. New York: McGraw-Hill Book Co., 1972.

35. Tews, J.K. and A.E. Harper. α-Aminoisobutyric acid transport in liver slices from rats fed low protein meals. *J. Nutrition 106:* 1497-1506, 1976.

36. Tews, J.K:, A.M. Bradford and A.E. Harper. Induction of lysine imbalance in rats: Relationships between tissue amino acids and diet. *J. Nutrition 11:* 968-978, 1981.

37. Tews, J.K., S.S. Good and A.E. Harper. Transport of threonine and tryptophan by rat brain slices: relation to other amino acids and concentrations found in plasma. *J. Neurochem. 31:* 581-589, 1978.

38. Tews, J.K., Y-W. L. Kim and A.E. Harper. Induction of threonine imbalance by dispensable amino acids: Relationships between tissue amino acids and diet. *J. Nutrition, 110:* 394-408, 1980.

39. Tews, J.K., Y-W. L. Kim and A.E. Harper. Induction of threonine imbalance by dispensable amino acids: Relation to competition for amino acid transport into brain. *J. Nutrition 109:* 304-315, 1979.

40. White, A., P. Handler, E.L. Smith, R.L. Hill and J.R. Lehman. Principles of Biochemistry, 6th edition. New York: McGraw-Hill Book Co., 1978.

HUMAN AMINO ACID NUTRITION

Selma E. Snyderman*

Department of Pediatrics
New York University School of Medicine
Medical Center
New York, N.Y.

INTRODUCTION

The subject of "Human Amino Acid Nutrition" is much too large for the period of time allotted to me. Hence, I will confine my remarks to those facets which have the greatest relationship to the theme of this meeting.

Amino acids have an unique position in nutrition. They are necessary for the integrity of every body cell and also have a role in such special functions as the formation of enzymes, coenzymes, hormones and antibodies. However, there is virtually no storage of amino acids in the body. This poses certain problems. It makes it mandatory that any excess above the body's requirement be metabolized, thus setting in motion a complex metabolic chain that ends ultimately in the excretion of urea. The consequences of excess amino acid intake become apparent whenever there is some deficiency of enzyme activity, thus the premature infant whose enzyme systems are immature, will respond with the elevation of plasma amino acid levels [24] and the accumulation of ammonia [9]. The lack of stores allows for little reserve for periods of stress or inadequate intake. At such times, some type of readjustment which involves the rates of synthesis and degradation of tissue proteins must take place and prompt reduction in nitrogen balance also occurs. These considerations have led to extensive study of amino requirements and the factors that influence them. The factors include the balance of amino acids, the adequacy of caloric intake; the adequacy of all other nutritional factors including the total nitrogen intake; growth, the presence of illness, the route of alimentation, whether

Supported in part by Project 317, Maternal and Child Health Training Grant, United States Public Health Service.

food is supplied enterally or parenterally; and the age of the individual. Both the quantities of essential amino acids and the number which are essential are influenced by the age of the subject. When amino acid requirements are expressed per unit of body weight there is a sharp decline during the first stages of life, being very high in the premature infant, lower during the first months of life, with a further fall during the preadolescent years and young adulthood. Figure 1 illustrates the magnitude of these reductions in requirements, the figures for the premature and young infants are from the studies of our group at NYU Medical Center [14, 20-28], that for the 10 to 12 year olds from the data of the Japanese group, and those for the adults are a composite of the various young adults studies [8]. Figures for the elderly have not been included because of the large range of values that have been obtained. All of these studies followed similar protocols; the use of diets the protein moiety of which was a mixture of amino acids and the use of nitrogen balance as a criterion of adequacy.

The premature infant and some full term infants require two amino acids not usually considered to be essential. The complete removal from the diet of

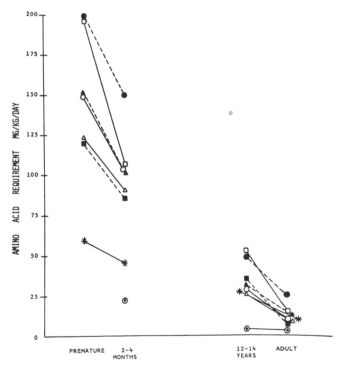

Figure 1. The relationship of essential amino acid requirements to age, when expressed in term of body weight. The greatest reduction in requirements takes place in the first months of life. ○—○ Isoleucine, ●—● Leucine, □—□ Lysine, ■—■ Threonine, △—△ Phenylalanine, ▲—▲ Valine, ⊙—⊙ Tryptophan, *—* Methionine.

either cystine or tyrosine results in the classical manifestations of amino acid deficiency; a reduction in the rate of weight gain, the retention of less nitrogen and a fall in the plasma level of either cystine or tyrosine [19]. Plasma level has not been uniformly accepted as a criterion of adequacy of intake of an amino acid, however, we have found it particularly useful in our studies of infants and children. It usually falls with inadequate intake and returns to the normal range at intakes slightly greater than those which are sufficient to permit a normal rate of weight gain and of nitrogen retention. There are fewer difficulties with metabolic balance studies in the infant subject than at other times of life. A formula feeding, divided into equal feedings is the normal mode of feeding, there is very little daily variation in activity and they are not subjected to the stress that the metabolic situation imposes at other ages. Figures 2 and 3 represent

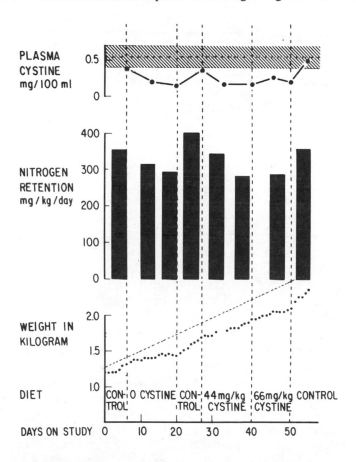

Figure 2. The protocol of a study demonstrating that cystine is essential for the premature infant. Removal of cystine from the diet results in a reduction in the rate of weight gain and the amount of nitrogen retained and a fall in the plasma cystine level. The hatched area represents 1 standard deviation above and below the average normal plasma level, designated by the dashed line.

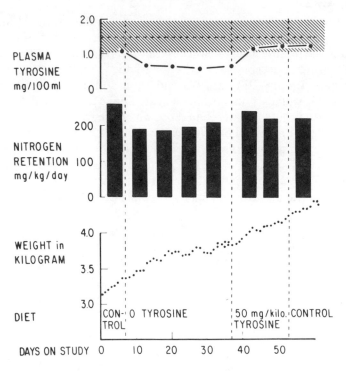

Figure 3. The protocol of a study demonstrating that tyrosine is essential for a full term newborn infant. A reduction in the rate of weight gain and the amount of nitrogen retained result from the removal of tyrosine from the diet. The plasma tyrosine level also falls, the hatched are represents 1 standard deviation above and below the normal average designated by the dashed line.

studies that demonstrated the essentiality of cystine and tyrosine. This does not apply to all newborn infants but is probably a reflection of the maturation of the enzyme systems necessary to synthesize these two amino acids.

The essentiality of histidine for the human has posed a particular problem ever since the studies of Rose [17] in adult men; he demonstrated the weight and nitrogen retention could be maintained on a diet devoid of histidine for relatively short periods of time. At a later date, Nasset and Gatewood [13] demonstrated that histidine deficiency resulted in anemia in adult rats and speculated that the subjects in Rose's studies maintained nitrogen balance by the breakdown of hemoglobin, a tissue rich in histidine. Growing animals do require histidine, and every species studied, chick [1], rat [16], salmon [7], mouse [29] and pig [15], has manifested the usual signs of an amino acid deficiency when it is removed from the diet. This is true also of the human infant who not only manifests the usual signs of an amino acid deficiency, but has a specific manifestation, the appearance of a rash which is very similar to that of ordinary infantile eczema [23]. Figures 4 and 5 illustrate protocols of studies illustrating the essential nature of histidine for the infant. We know that histidine remains essential for at least the first year of life, but do not know when if ever, it is no longer essential. The ease with which it is possible to control the plasma histidine level for the first years of life of histidinemic infants suggest that it is still essential for this period of time (Figure 6). The Japanese investigators concluded that it was unessential for 10 to 12 year old boys [12]. However, it has since been demonstrated by several groups of investigators that is is required by uremic adults [2, 4, 6]. Its essentiality in other disease states seems not to have been investigated, however plasma histidine levels are below normal in rheumatoid arthritis [15]. Whether it is essential for the normal adult has still not been finally resolved. In recent studies, removal of histidine from the diet has resulted in a negative nitrogen balance, a fall in plasma and muscle histidine, in body weight, in serum albumen and hematocrit [10]. Clinical symptoms were also observed, these included malaise, anorexia, memory loss and a skin

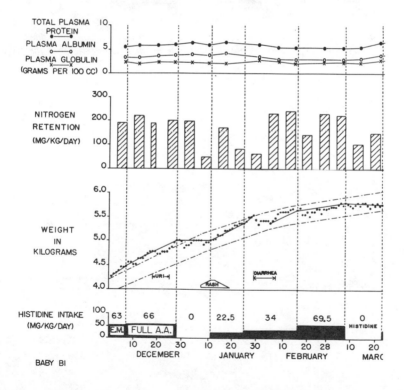

Figure 4. A study that demonstrated that histidine is essential for the infant. There was immediate cessation in weight gain and a reduction in the amount of nitrogen retained. The rash which appeared six days after histidine was removed from the diet improved with the re-introduction of histidine into the diet. This infant's requirement of histidine was 34 mg/kg/day. URI (upper respiratory infection) and diarrhea were intercurrent infections.

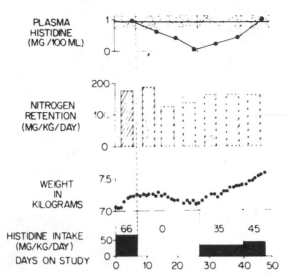

Figure 5. A histidine requirement study demonstrating the response of the plasma histidine level to adequate and inadequate amounts of histidine. This infant's histidine requirement was considered to be between 35 and 45 mg/kg/day.

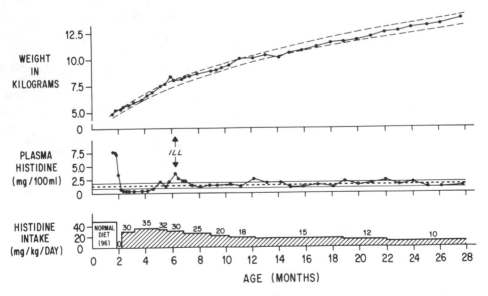

Figure 6. The treatment of an infant with histidinemia. The ease with which it was possible to maintain the plasma histidine level within normal limits suggests that it remains essential for this period of time. Average normal histidine level is represented by the dashed line; the solid lines represent one standard deviation above and below the average. The patient's weight fell between the 50th and 75th percentiles, represented by the dashed lines.

lesion. However, it took a relatively long time for these manifestations to appear, usually 15 to 20 days; this is in contrast to the prompt appearance of definite signs of deficiency when other essential amino acids are deleted from the diet. This slow appearance of the manifestations of histidine deficiency may be due to the use of other sources of histidine such as that obtained from the break down of hemoglobin and of the degradation of muscle carnitine. A decrease in muscle carnitine has been demonstrated in adult dogs depleted of histidine [3]. The situation is further complicated by the demonstration of incorporation of orally administered $^{15}NH_4Cl$ into imidazole ring of the histidine in globin, obtained from a parenterally fed (to eliminate gastrointestinal bacteria as a source of histidine) histidine depleted human subject [30, 18]. Thus it would seem that there is some synthesis of histidine in the normal adult, although possibly not sufficient to provide adequate amounts for a prolonged period of time. This apparent ability of the human adult to synthesize an amino acid which cannot be synthesized by any other animal species is of special interest since it has usually been considered that every animal species from unicellular protozoa to man required the same set of essential amino acids [11].

One of the strongest links between nutrition and genetics occurs in the understanding and treatment of the anomalies of amino acid metabolism. Elucidation of the site of the block has increased knowledge of the catabolic pathways of amino acids in the normal, and information about amino acid requirements has enhanced the treatment of these disorders. Experience with the therapy of the various disorders involving essential amino acid requirements of normal children. The aim of therapy of children with metabolic errors is to provide enough of the amino acid to take care of all body needs and allow normal growth but not to provide any excess wich may accumulated in the body as a result of the metabolic block. Thus, the minimal requirement is provided. This is true of the classical variety of the disorder when the enzyme activity is close to zero; for variants of the disease with measurable amounts of enzyme activity, the tolerance for the amino acid is greater and hence these intakes will be above requirement. Phenylketonuria results from deficient activity of phenylalanine hydroxylase, the enzyme which normally converts excess phenylalanine to tyrosine. As a result, phenylalanine accumulates in body fluids and in ways, still not completely understood, causes a number of clinical symptoms the most important of which is mental retardation. Control of the plasma level of phenylalanine can prevent the retardation. Our experience with 125 phenylketonuric infants treated from the first days of life demonstrated that their requirement is the same as the normal infant at a similar age and that there is a decrease in requirement in terms of body weight as the child grows older (Figure 7). It is surprising how little variation in requirement there is between these patients who are from very diverse ethnic backgrounds. The accumulation of this type of data should be able to fill in the gaps in our knowledge which were apparent in Figure 1. We have been collecting similar data for histidine from patients with histidinemia (Figure 8), for the branched chain amino acids

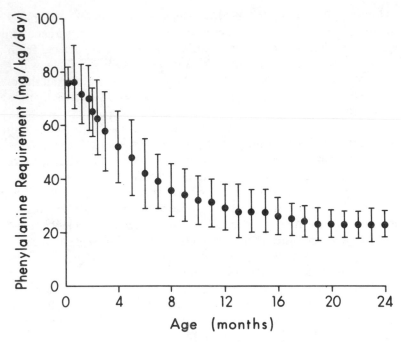

Figure 7. The phenylalanine requirements of 125 phenylketonuric infants treated from earliest in-
fancy, average. This illustrated the reduction in phenylalanine requirement that occurs during the
first months of life.

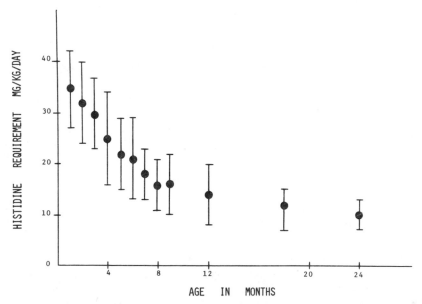

Figure 8. The histidine requirement of 15 histidinemic infants treated from early infancy. Average
and one standard deviation above and below average are illustrated.

in patients with branched chain ketoaciduria (Maple Syrup Urine Disease) and for methionine in those with hemocystinemia; there will be fewer figures for these dieseases which occur much more rarely but still more data than that obtained from the usual requirement study in the normal which involves 4 to 6 subjects.

In several disorders, amino acids usually considered to be unessential became essential as a result of the site of the metabolic block. This is true for tyrosine in phenylketonuria and cystine in homocystinuria. Nutritional information could be obtained by systematic study of requirements in these diseases. In a similar fashion, more information about minimal protein requirements can be obtained from the treatment of metabolic disorders amenable to protein restriction such as the defect in the urea cycle and the specific organic acidurias such as methylmalonic aciduria, and propionic aciduria.

Thus, therapy of these genetic disorders of amino acid mctabolism can extend our knowledge or requirements at different ages, can help differentiate unessential from partially essential amino acids, and can provide quantitative information about unessential amino acids. Knowledge of the nutritional needs of the less severe variant in the general population may be enhanced by these examples of extreme genetic variation in the tolerance for nutrients.

REFERENCES

1. Almoquist, H.J. Evaluation of amino acid requirements by observations in the chick. *J. Nutr.* 34:543, 1947.
2. Bergstrom, J., Furst, P., Josephson, B., Noree, L.O. Improvement of nitrogen balance in a uremic patient by the addition of histidine to essential amino acid solutions given intra venously. *Life Sciences* 9, Pt II:787, 1970.
3. Cianciaruso, B., Jones, M.R. and Kopple, J.D. Histidine, and essential amino acid for adult dogs. *J. Nutr.* III:1074, 1081.
4. Furst, P. ^{15}N-studies in severe renal failure II. Evidence for the essentiality of histidine. *Scand J. Clin. Lab. Invest.* 30:307, 1972.
5. Gerber, D.A. Low free serum histidine concentration in rheumatoid arthritis. A measure of disease activity. *J. Clin. Invest.* 55, 1164, 1975.
6. Giordano, C., DeSanto N.G., Rinaldi, S., DePascale, C., Pluvio, M. Histidine and glycine essential amino acids in uremia. *In* "Uremia" (R. Kluthe, G. Geryle and B. Burton, eds). p1 128. Thieme, Stuttgart, 1972.
7. Halver, J.E. and Shankds, W.E. Nutrition of salmonoid fishes: VIII Indispensable amino acids for sockeye salmon. *J. Nutr.* 72:340, 1960.
8. Irwin, M.I., and Hegsted, D.M. A conspectus of research on amino acid requirements of man. *J. Nutr.* 101:541, 1971.
9. Johnson, J.D., Albritton, W.L., and Sunshine, P. Hyperammonemia accompanying parenteral nutrition in newborn infants. *J. Pediat.* 81, 154, 1972.
10. Kopple, J.D. and Swenseid, M.E. Evidence that histidine is an essential amino acid in normal and chronically uremic man. *J. Clin. Invest.* 55:881, 1978.
11. Munro, H.N. An introduction to protein metabolism during the evolution and development of mammals. *In* "Mammalian Protein Metabolism" (H.N. Munro, ed.,), pp. 3-19. Academic Press, New York, 1969.

12. Nakagawa, I.T., Takahashi, T., Suzuki, T. and Kubayashi, K. Amino acid requirements of children: minimal needs of trytophan, arginine and histidine based on nitrogen balance method. *J. Nutr.* 80:305, 1963.

13. Nasset, E.S. and Gatewood, V.A. Nitrogen balance and hemoglobin of adult rats fed amino acid diets low in LD histidine. *J. Nutr.* 53:163, 1964.

14. Pratt, E.L., Snyderman, S.E., Cheung, M.W., Norton, P.M. and Holt, L.E. Jr. The threonine requirement of the normal infant. *J. Nutr.* 56:231, 1955.

15. Recheigl, M. Jr., Lossli, J.K., and Williams, H.H. Histidine requiremtns of baby pigs. *J. Nutr.* 60:619, 1956.

16. Rose, W.C. and Cox, G.J. The relation of arginine and histidine to growth. *J. Biol. Chem.* 59. 14, 1924.

17. Rose, W.C. Haines, W.J., Warner, D.T., and Johnson, J.E. The amino acid requirements of man. II. The role of threonine and histidine. *J. Biol. Chem.* 188:49, 1951.

18. Sheng, Y.B., Badger, T.M., Asplund, J.M., and Wixom, R.L. Incorporation of 15NH$_4$ Cl into histidine in adult man. *J. Nutr.* 107:621, 1977.

19. Snyderman, S.E. The protein and amino acid requirement of the premature infant. *In* "Metabolic Processes in the Foetus and Newborn Infant" (J.H.P. Janoxis, H.K.A. Visser and J.A. Troelstrar, eds), pp. 128-141. H.E. Stenfert Kroese, Leiden, 1971.

20. Snyderman, S.E., Boyer, A., Norton, P.M., Roitman, E. and Holt, L.E. Jr. The essential amino acid requirements of infants. X. Methionine. *J. Clin. Nutr.* 15:322, 1964.

21. Snyderman, S.E., Boyer, A., Norton, P.M., Roitman, E. and Holt, L.E. Jr. The essential amino acid requirements of infants. IX. Isoleucine. *J. Clin. Nutr.* 15:313, 1964.

22. Snyderman, S.E., Boyer, A., Phansalkar, S.V. and Holt, L.E. Jr. Essential amino acid requirements of infants: Trytophan. *Am. J. Dis. Child.* 102:163, 1961.

23. Snyderman, S.E., Boyer, A., Roitman, E., Holt, L.E. Jr., and Prose, P.H. The histidine requirement of the infant. *Pediatrics* 31:876, 1963.

24. Snyderman, S.E., Holt, L.E. Jr, Norton, P.M., and Phansalkar, S.V. Influences of the protein intake on the free amino acid content of the plasma and the red blood cells. *Am. J. Clin. Nutr.* 23:890, 1970.

25. Snyderman, S.E., Holt, L.E. Jr., Smellie, F., Boyer, A., and Westall, R.G. The essential amino acid requirements of infants: Valine. *AMA J. Dis. Child.* 97:186, 1959.

26. Snyderman, S.E., Norton, P.M., Fowler, D.I. and Holt, L.E. Jr. The essential amino acid requirements of Infants: Lysine. *AMA J. Dis. Child.* 97:175, 1959.

27. Snyderman, S.E., Pratt, E.L., Cheung, M.W., Norton, P.M., and Holt, L.E. Jr. The phenylalanine requirement of the normal infant. *J. Nutr.* 56:253, 1955.

28. Snyderman, S.E., Roitman, E., Boyer, A., and Holt, L.E. Jr. Essential amino acid requirement of infants: Leucine. *Am. J. Dis. Child.* 102:157, 1961.

29. Totter, J.R. and Berg, C. Influence of optical isomerism on utilization of tryptophan, histidine and lysine for mouse growth. *J. Biol. Chem.* 127:375, 1939.

30. Wixom, R.L., Anderson, H.G., Terry, B.E., and Sheng, Y.B. Total parenteral nutrition with selective histidine depletion in man. *Am. J. Clin. Nutr.* 30:887, 1977.

OBSERVATIONS ON PROTEIN TURNOVER

John C. Waterlow

Department of Human Nutrition
London School of Hygiene and Tropical Medicine
London, England

INTRODUCTION

The Purpose of Protein Turnover

My justification for introducing the word 'purpose' is the stament of Atkinson [2] with which I fully agree: *'In any field of biology, the concept of evolutionary teleology is the best guide available'.*

Protein turnover appears to be obligatory for the tissue proteins of eukaryote organisms, and I call it a mystery because it is not at all clcar what function it fulfils. In the liver a large part of the intracellular protein is stated to consist of enzymes, many if not most of which are inducible by diet or hormones (e.g. 45). This is considered to confer flexibility of responsc to dietary and other changes. Then there is the theory that protein breakdown is a scavenging mechanism for removing abnormal protein molecules produced by miscoding. However, as will be apparent later, the physiological changes in protein turnover which occur under various conditions show clearly that scavenging cannot be its only function or even its main one.

In other tissues the purpose, if there is one, of protein turnover is even more obscure. The proteins of the mature brain turn over, albeit on average rather slowly. Are we to infer from this that functions such as learning and memory cannot have a lasting structural basis, in terms of connections between one cell and another?

Muscle is an extremely interesting tissue. I find it difficult to reconcile conceptually the highly organized structure of the myofibril [21] with the fact that its proteins are constantly being broken down and renewed. The turnover rate is increased during growth [28, 32], which allows remodelling; it is also increased in muscles kept under stretch [19], but apparently not in active excercise. The proteins of heart muscle, which presumably does more mechanical work in a day than most muscles, turn over faster than those of skeletal muscle.

These relations between function and turnover rate are only just beginning to be explored, initially in terms of differences between different fibre types [56].

Plasma albumin is another example in which it is interesting to raise the question of purpose. Many books have been written about albumin turnover [55], and we know that its intravascular mass is maintained by a very sensitive mechanism of regulation. The rate of albumin synthesis is extremely sensitive to amino acid supply [22], but a fall in synthesis is quickly compensated by a reduction in the rate of breakdown. When one sees a homeostatic mechanism of this kind, it is natural to suppose, following Claude Bernard, that the function being regulated is important for the maintenance of 'la vie libre'. But what is this important function? Is it the maintenance of fluid exchange between tissues and blood, as originally proposed by Starling? Many clinical observations fit in with this idea, but many do not. Is the function to act as a reserve of amino acids, or as a carrier for vitamins, minerals, free fatty acids, etc? The fact that patients with congenital analbuminaemia show little or no disability [50] makes one wonder whether plasma albumin, although so closely regulated, really has any function.

Regulation of Protein Turnover

The second mystery about protein turnover is the way in which, in the normal steady state, rates of synthesis and breakdown are matched. This, of course, holds not only for the sum of body proteins but all individual proteins, and it is this matching which makes possible conventional nitrogen balance and the maintenance of constant body composition.

We have two cycles, as shown in Figure 1: the input-output cycle, which exchanges with the environment; and the synthesis breakdown cycle, which exchanges with body protein. The cycles overlap in the amino acid pool.

These cycles are *connected,* in the sense that a net change in the one must imply a corresponding imbalance in the other provided, of course, that the free amino acid pool size is regulated within fairly narrow limits.

However, the cycles are also *disconnected,* because we can show that the turnover cycle may speed up or slow down without any necessary relationship to the rate of flux through the input-output cycle. This is a very interesting situation.

When it comes to regulation, the balance in the input-output cycle depends upon mechanisms which have been well studied - the rates of amino acid degradation and urea formation, adaptive enzyme changes, etc. These are discussed by other speakers. Where the cycles overlap, it has been suggested that changes in the rate of protein synthesis may be controlled by changes in the rate of amino acid input, or in amino acid concentration. These ideas present some difficulties. Under usual dietary conditions the intake of any aminoacid is only about 25% of its flux, so that a change in intake will by itself make little diffe-

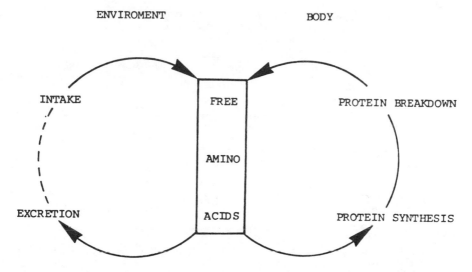

ENVIROMENT   BODY

Figura 1. Two cycles are shown. In the first, nitrogen exchanges with the environment. In the second, nitrogen exchanges with body proteins. The central area of overlap represents the free amino acid pool.

rence to the overall flux. It is also hard to understand how changes in amino acid concentration can have much effect on the rate of synthesis. The $k_M s$ of the first enzymes in the synthetic process, the aminoacyl-tRNA ligases, are so slow that the enzymes must presumably be saturated at all physiological amino acid concentrations.

I turn now to some variables which relate to, and in a sense determine, the overall rate of protein synthesis in a cell. This rate may usefully be related to the DNA content of the cell.

The concept of DNA unit, introduced by Cheek [7], makes it easier to express results in tissues with multinucleate cells, such as muscle, or in tissues with polyploidy, such as liver. The amount of synthesis controlled by a unit of DNA depends in the first place on the cell's content of ribosomal RNA, which Millward has called the 'capacity' for protein synthesis [31]. Under physiological conditions the amount of protein synthesized per unit RNA —the RNA 'activity'— seems to be relatively constant from one tissue to another [57], so that differences in the absolute rate of protein synthesis per unit DNA depend largely on the RNA/DNA ratio of the tissue. This is shown by the comparisons between liver, muscle and kidney in Table I. Synthesis per unit DNA (line E) is similar in kidney and muscle, and two to three times as great in liver. Although ribosomal RNA is itself rapidly turning over, it is not too difficult to visualize genetic mechanisms which determine the RNA/DNA ratio, and hence the *absolute* rate of protein synthesis per unit DNA in different tissues. However, the relationship of RNA to DNA tells us nothing about the

TABLE I Rates of protein synthesis in tissues of the adult
rat in relation to RNA and DNA concentrations

	Liver [a]	Muscle	Kidney
A Protein/DNA (mg/mg)	70	452	28
B RNA/protein (mg/g)	46	4.1	26
C RNA/DNA (mg/mg)	3.22	1.85	0.73
D Protein synthesis rate per unit RNA $(mg.d^{-1}/mg)$ (RNA 'activity')	17.5	10.9	19.9
E Protein synthesis rate per unit DNA $(mg.d^{-1}/mg)$ (DNA 'activity')	56.3	20.2	14.5
F protein synthesis rate per unit protein (mg/mg/) (fractional synthesis rate)	0.80	0.045	0.52

[a] No allowance has been made for the synthesis of export proteins, which probably amounts to about 30 per cent of total protein synthesis in the liver [53].

fractional synthesis rate (line F), which is inversely related to the amount of protein in the cell. The protein content per cell or DNA unit thus seems to be determined by two independent variables, the ratio of RNA to DNA and the fractional turnover rate (FTR). In this way we get a DNA unit in muscle which is 15 times the size of that in kidney, although the absolute rate of protein synthesis per unit DNA in the two tissues are not very different. Kidney has a small amount of protein per unit DNA, turning over fast, while muscle has a large amount per unit DNA, turning over slowly. One may perhaps ask: which is the regulated variable, FTR or cell size? This seems to me a fundamental question. One might speculate that the determining factor, both for the total and the individual proteins of the cell, is the rate of production and availability of messenger RNA. There is some evidence to suggest that this can be a rate-controlling factor, e.g. in the synthesis of serum albumin [40]. However, Pain and Clemens [39] regard variations in concentration of mRNA species as a mechanism of qualitative rather than quantitative regulation.

Turning to breakdown, we find a wide variety of proteinases [27], but the central role is probably played by the lysosome. Here again there is the problem of selectivity. It has been proposed that specific rates of breakdown are determined by properties of the protein molecule such as its size, larger molecules being degraded more rapidly [10]. This cannot, however, be a general rule, since it would not account for the slow degradation rate of some very large proteins such as myosin. Moreover, one and the same protein may be degraded at different rates in different tissues, as has been shown for the iso-enzyme lactic dehydrogenase 5 [13]. The position, therefore, is a very peculiar one: we have two machines, the ribosome and the lysosome, whose activities appear to be matched, but as far as present knowledge goes there is no connecting link between them.

Kinetics

The only connecting link that has been proposed is not a biochemical one but a model that depends on the supposed kinetics of the two processes. It is usual to regard protein synthesis as a zero order reaction and breakdown as a first order one. These assumptions lead to a self-regulatory system. In the steady state, when the amount of protein is constant,

$$S = kP,$$

where S is the absolute rate of protein synthesis (g/unit time), P is the amount of protein [g], and k is the first order rate constant, i.e. the fractional rate of breakdown, in units of t^{-1}. It is self-evident that if either S or k changes, P will change until a new steady state is reached, in which kP is again equal to S. It is therefore of some importance to examine whether the kinetic assumptions are correct.

In theory it seems very reasonable to suppose that synthesis is a zero order reaction in which the velocity depends on the activity of the enzyme system and is independent of the substrate concentration. The first enzymes of the synthetic pathway encountered by amino acids in the cell are the aminoacyl-rRNA-transferases, which have extremely low $k_M s$, much lower than the physiological concentrations of amino acids in cells so that one would not expect substrate to be limiting. In practice it is not so easy to demonstrate zero order kinetics for synthesis. For example, in the perfused liver preparation, in which substrate concentrations can be varied over a wide range, alterations in aminoacid concentration alter rates of protein breakdown [34], in addition to any effect they may or may not have on synthesis.

I find it much less easy to accept the concept of first order breakdown. This concept seems to be based on two propositions: first, the exponential decay of label in a protein which has been pre-labelled; secondly, the fact that a compartmental model in which the exchanges between pools follow first order kinetics is intellectually satisfying and can be analysed mathematically. In such a model all the rate constants and pool sizes can be derived from serial observations on a single pool, provided only that the arrangement of the pools is known or can be postulated [44]. In my view the evidence for first order degradation of proteins is rather thin. In the steady state, as Steele has pointed out [47], it is totally fallacious to suppose that exponential decay of label implies first order exchange of the labelled metabolite. This subject has been dealt with in more detail elsewhere [53]. It is enough to state here that only in the non-steady state is it possible to prove unequivocally that a reaction, whether it be degradation or transfer, is occuring at a constant fractional rate, i.e. is following first order kinetics. Experimentally it is very difficult to fulfil these conditions in biological systems. Most studies which claim to show exponential decay have been done in the steady state, or a steady state has been assumed. When a non-steady state is deliberately provoked, as, for example, by plasmaphoresis in studies of albumin kinetics, compensatory reactions come into play, such as shifts from the extra- to the intravascular pool and alterations in the rate of synthesis, which obscure the picture. However, I think the demonstration by Waldmann [50] that massive infusion of albumin in a congenitally hypoalbuminaemic patient produced absolutely no change in the decay curve of labelled albumin, is one of the few convincing pieces of evidence that degradation is a first order process. Another promising non-isotopic approach to this problem is by analysis of the rate of change in amount of an enzyme after applying or removing an inducing stimulus [9,12,49]. However, to my knowledge studies of this kind have not been conducted in a rigorous enough way for firm conclusions to be drawn about kinetics.

There is a different type of kinetic behaviour-life-span kinetics-exemplified by the red blood cell and the light sensitive pigment of the rods of the retina [20]. We suggested earlier the possibility of a pattern of degradation intermediate between first order and life-span, which we called 'multiple event kinetics', an idea due to Garlick [53]. Suppose that a protein molecule is only degraded after it has undergone a finite number, A, of consecutive stresses or injuries, in the way that a piece of wire only breaks after it has been bent a number of times. These 'injuries' are supposed to occur randomly at an average rate of N per unit time. The average time, T_d, needed for A events to occur, so that the molecule is destroyed, will be A/N. However, since the events are supposed to be occurring randomly, the actual number occuring in this time will be $A \pm \sqrt{A}$. The satistics are the same as those of radio-active counting. The 'half-life' of the process is determined by the ratio of A to N. The shape of the decay curve depends on the absolute value of A. If A is large, the decay curve resembles that of life-span kinetics. If it is unity, the decay is exponential. Which small values of $A > 1$, the curve is convex. I find it difficult to visualize any other process which will produce a convex decay curve (Figure 2).

A possible example of this idea in practice is provided by some experiments of Gershon and co-workers [24]. They found that in the livers of young mice the decay curve of proteins labelled with ^{14}C-carbonate was exponential, where-

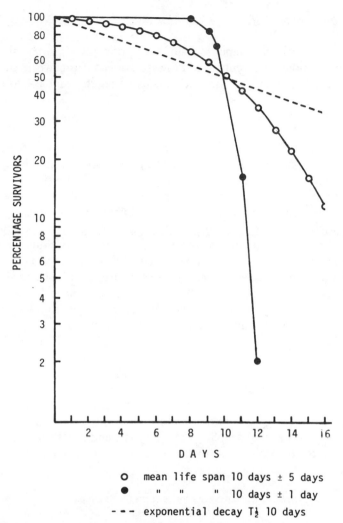

Figure 2. Kinetics of decay. ○ Mean life-span 10 + 5 days. ● Mean life-span 10 days ± 5 days.
- - - Exponential decay T ½ 10 days.

as in senescent mice it was convex. This observation, if confirmed, would suggest that in senescence more 'insults' are needed before a protein molecule is
degraded - an inference which may seem surprising.

I have devoted some time to the question of kinetics because I think it is far
from academic. By establishing the kinetics, which perhaps differ for different
proteins and different tissues, we may get some clues to the biochemical
mechanisms that enable rates of synthesis and breakdown to be co-ordinated
in a harmonious way.

Protein Turnover under Different Conditions

I turn now to a different theme. Measurements of rates of protein synthesis and breakdown under different conditions provide a framework of facts, within which any hypothesis about mechanisms of regulation have to fit.

Body size and protein turnover

Munro in 1969 [36] published a remarkable table with the title, 'The influence of body size on protein and energy metabolism, on the relative weights of individual organs and on the components of certain tissues'. In this table he states that whole body protein turnover varies as $Wt^{0.74}$- the same exponent as for basal energy metabolism and the usual way of expressing active cell mass. Munro's value was based on measuments on only two species, rat and man, made with ^{15}N-glicine by Sprinson and Rittenberg [46] thirtythree years ago. Since then results have been obtained on a wider range of species by methods which may be more accurate, involving infusion of ^{14}C-labelled amino acids. Comparisons have to be made with caution, because one cannot always be certain that the measurements in different species were made under standardized conditions and on animals in the same physiological state. Table II shows the best estimates that we have at present. Many variants of this table have been published as new species are included and methods improved. The results lead to an exponent of 0.73 on a log-log plot, with a correlation coefficient of 0.998. Thus, with scanty materials Munro built well.

The fact that whole body protein turnover and basal metabolic rate bear the same relationship to body weight implies that they must also be related to each other. This point has been made many times [51,54], and it has been concluded that the energy cost of protein turnover may account for some 20 per cent of

TABLE II Whole body protein turnover in animals
of different sizes

Species	Weight kg	Weight g/day	Whole body protein turnover g/kg/day
Mouse	0.04	1.74	43.5
Rat	0.35	7.7	22
Rabbit	3.6	33	9.2
Pig	32	268	8.4
Sheep	63	351	5.6
Man	70	325	4.6
Cow	575	1740	3.0

Data from ref. (43), except for mouse, ref. (14)

the BMR [54]. Perhaps the relationship between these two aspects of metabolism is a very general one. For example, the studies of Haschemeyer on temperature adaptation in the toadfish suggested that there is a relationship between protein turnover and overall metabolic rate in poikilotherms [25], as there seems to be in mammals.

The picture is different when protein turnover is related to body size in animals of the same species but of different weights at different stages of maturity. Results in rat and man are shown in Table III. For each species there are only three data points, and the methods of measuring turnover are different. It seems remarkable, therefore, that they should give the same exponent 0.53. This means that increasing maturity (exponent 0.53) causes a greater decrease in turnover than does increase in size resulting from species differences (exponent 0.73). The reason presumably is that as animals mature there is a change in body composition; the proportion of muscle, with a relatively low turnover rate, rises and the proportion of visceral tissues with a high turnover rate falls.

A further point is that with increasing maturity the fractional turnover rate (FTR) of muscle falls very rapidly [32], whereas, as shown in Table IV, there is

TABLE III *The effect of growth on whole body protein turnover in man and rat*

A. MAN

	Weight kg	Total protein turnover g/kg/day	Reference
Prematures	2.0	16.3 [a]	(41)
Infants	10	6.3	(18)
Adults	70	3.0	(59)

All measurements were made with ^{15}N-glycine
Protein turnover $(g/d) = 21.1W^{0.53}$

[a] Mean of all groups

B. RAT

	Weight g	Total protein turnover g/kg/day
	37	43.4
	115	23.3
	510	12.6

Protein turnover $(g/d) = 0.96W^{0.53}$
From ref. (28,29)

TABLE IV Muscle composition and protein turnover in
adult rat and adult man

	RAT	MAN
Fractional turnover rate		
% d^{-1}	4.5	3.55
RNA/protein		
mg/g	4.13	2.2
RNA activity		
mg protein synthesis	10.9	16.1
d^{-1}/mg RNA		
Protein/DNA		
mg/g	452	666
DNA activity		
mg protein synthesis	20.5	24.2
d^{-1}/mg DNA		

Rat: data from ref. (5)

Man: unpublished results of Rennie and Millward.
The synthesis rates are the means of rates in the fed and fasted state.

much less difference in FTR in mature animals of different sizes. This relative constancy between species of the FTR in a given tissue is reflected by the relative constancy of RNA concentration (RNA/protein) in animals of different sizes. Table IV shows that over a weight range of 2-3 orders of magnitude the RNA concentracion in muscle falls by only about 50 per cent.

Diet and food

We have to distinguish between the effects of the immediate food intake and the effects of the prevailing diet. Recent studies by several groups have shown very clearly that protein turnover is extremely sensitive to food intake. Our findings are illustrated in Table V. Both synthesis and oxidation are increased during the day, when food is being taken in, and fall in the night, when there is no food intake. The results of several studies are summarized in Table VI. In spite of differences in method and protocol, there is general agreement on the differences between the fed and post-absorptive states, although the extent to which protein breakdown changes is still rather controversial for reasons discussed by Garlick [15]. This sensitivity to inmediate food intake has important practical implications; it follows that for all measurements of protein turnover the dietary conditions must be rigidly controlled. Failure to realize this may be the reason that earlier studies on the effects of prevailing diet present some contradictions.

TABLE V *Effect of feeding and fasting on leucine turnover in normal adults*

mmol leucine per h	Fed	Fasted
	mean $\pm$ SD n = 5	
Intake	4.07 ± 0.19	0
Oxidation	2.19 ± 0.38	0.96 ± 0.18
Synthesis	5.70 ± 1.24	4.15 ± 0.77
Breakdown	3.82 ± 0.95	5.11 ± 0.78
Apparent balance	$+1.88$	-0.96

Measurements by constant infusion of $1\text{-}^{14}C$-leucine over 24 hours.
Subjects were fed during the first 12 hours and fasted during the second 12 hours.
Reproduced by permission of Human Nutrition/Clinical Nutrition

Data from ref. (8)

TABLE VI *Ratio of whole body protein synthesis rates in fed and fasted adults*

	Fed/fasted	Reference
Matthews et al. (1981)	1.67	(26)
Motil et al. (1981)		(35)
Intake 1.5 g protein/kg/d	1.00	
'' 0.6 g '' '' ''	1.15	
Clugston and Garlick (1982)		(8)
Normal adults	1.33	
Obese adults	1.36	

Some of the results on the effects of protein intake are shown in Table VII. The two earlier studies ((a) and (c)) seem to show that even at protein intakes which are less than adequate, synthesis rates are mantained, and that as the intake increases the breakdown rate falls. The other two studies show a somewhat different picture: with increasing intake there is a rise in synthesis rate, and a concomitant, but smaller, rise in breakdown. These discrepancies emphasize that more work still needs to be done on the development of reliable methods. On the balance of evidence, I think it is probable that when the protein intake falls below a certain level, in the region of the maintenance requirement, synthesis is reduced. In the extreme case, when we put obese patients on protein-free diet, the synthesis rate fell to about 50 per cent of that found

TABLE VII *Effect of protein intake on whole body protein*
turnover in man

	g protein per kg per day			
	intake	synthesis	breakdown	balance
CHILDREN				
(a)	0.6	6.4	6.4	0
	1.2	6.2	5.5	+0.7
	3.6	6.1	4.7	+1.4
	5.2	6.6	4.4	+2.2
(b)	0.7	4.2	4.75	−0.55
	1.7	5.8	5.0	+0.8
ADULTS				
(c)	0.38	3.48	3.49	−0.01
	1.5	3.01	2.74	+0.27
(d)	0.1	3.29	3.52	−0.23
	0.6	4.49	4.44	+0.05
	1.5	5.30	4.51	+0.81

[a] *From Golden et al. (18). ^{15}N-glycine, end product urea*
[b] *From Jackson and co-workers (unpublished).*
  ^{15}N-glycine, end products ammonia and urea (11)
[c] *From Steffe et al. (48). ^{15}N-glycine, end product urea.*
[d] *From Motil et al. (35). 1-^{14}C-leucine*

on an adequate protein intake at the same low level of energy [16]. We observed also that when protein was removed from the diet, the turnover rate fell within one to two days, as would be expected from the findings summarized above on the sensitivity to the immediate food intake.

The effects of changes in energy intake have been less studied. In the investigations in Table VII the energy intakes may be considered adequate. Although the obese patients mentioned above were receiving only 500 kcal per day, since they were losing weight they were presumably drawing on fat stores. The only studies I know of in which the energy intake has been systematically varied in normal subjects are some measurements in children by Jackson and co-workers in Jamaica (unpublished). On a fixed and adequate protein intake variations in energy intake from 80 to 100 kcal per kg per day on average had no effect on the rate of whole body protein turnover. The lower level is adequate for maintenance but not for growth. However, in normally growing children aged one to two years, the net protein synthesis needed for growth is relatively small (about 0.2 g protein per kg per day) compared with the basal rate of turnover (about 6 g protein per kg per day), and would therefore be difficult to detect.

Growth

Since growth requires net protein synthesis, and the synthesis rate is sensitive to the inflow of food, it seems to follow that growth should occur in spurts, in relation to food intake. This fact was suggested by us a long time ago to explain observations on increased post-prandial oxigen uptake of mal-nourished children during catch-up growth [6]. It follows also that in young animals one can make short-term observations on growth simply by compa-ring protein synthesis rates in the fed and fasted state. From experiments of this kind by Millward and co-workers in muscle [4], a remarkable finding emerges, as shown in Table VIII. In order to maintain constant composition of the tis-sue there have to be marked changes in the relative rates of synthesis of the dif-ferent muscle proteins. To keep up with the demands of growth the synthesis rate of the proteins which turn over more slowly in the steady state (e.g. actin) has to increase above the basal level much more than that of the proteins which turn over more rapidly.

Just as food intake must be taken into account in any study of growth, so the growth status of the animal must be taken into account in any study of the effects of food intake on protein turnover. It is now well recognized that rapid growth involves an increase in the rate of protein breakdown as well as of syn-thesis [28]. For example, in children in the rapid growth phase of catchup from malnutrition, for every gram of protein deposited, 1.4 g of protein have to be synthesized [18,52]. This means that 0.4 g protein are being broken down, over and above the basal rate of breakdown at nitrogen equilibrium. A very similar figure has been found in young rapidly growing pigs [43]. In this example, the 'efficiency' of protein synthesis is 1/1.4, or 71 per cent. In the young growing rat the highest efficiency found for net protein deposition was 40 per cent [4].

TABLE VIII Differential rates of synthesis of different muscle
proteins in the rat at different rates of growth

Growth rate %.d⁻¹	Total muscle protein synthesis rate %.d⁻¹	Relative rate of synthesis of myofibrillar: sarcoplasmic proteins
−12.8	2.58	0.43
0 (steady state)	4.5	0.50
0.3	4.9	0.57
0.7	5.2	0.65
2.3	14	0.72
6.3	29	0.73

Data from ref. (4)

The term 'efficiency' used in this way represents (net synthesis of protein)/(increase in turnover), and is therefore quite different from the classical concept of the efficiency of utilization of food protein. This anabolic increase in protein breakdown, as it has been aptly termed [28], which prevents net protein synthesis from being 100 per cent efficient, has been studied in most detail in muscle, and has been found both in normal growth [28]. and in hypertrophy induced by various stresses [23].

Any proposed mechanism for the regulation of rates of synthesis and breakdown—what I have called the central mystery in this subject—must take account of these two phenomena: differential changes during growth in the synthesis rates of different protein, and an increase in breakdown concomitant with that of synthesis.

Effects of hormones

Finally, it is quite clear that in the intact animal a number of hormones play an important part in the regulation of protein turnover, in many cases interacting with the nutritional state [17]. We understand little about the mode of action of hormones on protein synthesis and breakdown at the cellular level. The literature on their effects is very large [58], and I will illustrate the theme only by some observations on muscle. Table IX shows that insulin, growth hormone, thyroid hormones, adrenal hormones and glucagon all affect rates of protein synthesis and/or breakdown in muscle. The question then arises: who conducts this orchestra? We might perhaps modify Barcroft's aphorism, 'Every adaptation is an integration' [3] to 'Every regulation is an integration'. Could this perhaps be a safety device? If one part of the mechanism fails, another takes over.

The only purpose in asking these at present unanswerable questions is to show what a large and exciting field there is here for future research.

ACKNOWLEDGMENTS

In this paper I have drawn freely on the work and ideas of many colleagues, particularly Drs Garlick, Golden, Jackson and Millward, for whose generous collaboration I am most grateful. I whish also to acknowledge the support of grants from the Medical Research Council, the Welcome Trust and the Rank Prize Funds.

REFERENCES

1. Albertse, E.C., Garlick, P.J., and Pain, V.M. Whole body protein synthesis and oxidation rates in streptozotocin diabetic rats. *Proc. Nutr. Soc.* 38:125A, 1979.
2. Atkinson, D.E. Adaptations of enzymes for regulation of catalytic function. *In* "Biochemical Adaptation to Environmental Change" (R.M.S. Smellie and J.F. Pennock, eds.), pp. 205-223. *Biochemical Society Symposia* No. 41. London, 1976.
3. Barcroft, J. "Features in the Architecture of Physiological Function", 367 pp. Cambridge University Press, 1934.

4. Bates, P.C., and Millward, D.J. Changes in the relative rates of protein synthesis and breakdown during muscle growth and atrophy. *Biochem. Soc. Trans.* 6:612, 1978.

5. Bates, P.C., and Millward, D.J. Characteristics of skeletal muscle growth and protein turnover in a fast-growing rat strain. *Br. J. Nutr.* 46:7, 1981.

6. Brooke, O.G., and Ashworth, A. The influence of malnutrition on the post-prandial metabolic rate and respiratory quotient. *Br. J. Nutr.* 27:407, 1972.

7. Cheek, D.B., Holt, A.B., Hill, D.E., and Talbert, J.L. Skeletal muscle cell mass and growth: the concept of the deoxyribonucleic acid unit. *Pediat. Res.* 5:312, 1971.

8. Clugston, G.A., and Garlick, P.J. The response of protein and energy metabolism to food intake in lean and obese man. *Human Nutr.: Clin. Nutr.* 36C:57, 1982.

9. Das, T.K., and Waterlow, J.C. The rate of adaptation of urea cycle enzymes, aminotransferases and glutamic dehydrogenase to changes in dietary protein intake. *Br. J. Nutr.* 32:353, 1974.

10. Dice, J.F., Hess, E.J., and Goldberg, A.L. Studies on the relationship between the degradative rates of protein in vivo and their isoelectric points. *Biochem. J.* 178:305, 1979.

11. Fern, E.B., Garlick, P.J., McNurlan, M.A., and Watelow, J.C. The excretion of isotope in urea and ammonia for estimating protein turnover in man with (^{15}N)glycine. *Clin. Sci.* 61:217, 1981.

12. Freedland, R.A. Considerations in the estimation of enzyme half-lives in higher animals by rates of change in activities. *Life Sciences* 7:499, 1968.

13. Fritz, P.J., Vesell, E.S., White, E.L., and Pruitt, K.M. The roles of synthesis and degradation in determining tissue concentrations of lactate dehydrogenase. *Proc. Nat. Acad. Sci.* 62:558, 1969.

14. Garlick, P.J. Protein turnover in the whole animal and specific tissues. In "Comprehensive Biochemistry", Vol. 19B. Part. I. (M. Florkin, A. Neuberger, and L.L.M. van Deenen, eds.), pp. 77-152. Elsevier, Amsterdam, 1980.

15. Garlick, P.J., and Clugston, G.A. Measurement of whole body protein turnover by constant infusion of carboxyl-labelled leucine. *In* "Nitrogen Metabolism in Man" (J.C. Waterlow, and J.M.L. Stephen, eds.), pp. 303-322. Applied Science Publishers, London, 1981.

16. Garlick, P.J., Clugston, G.A., and Waterlow, J.C. Influence of low energy diets on whole body protein turnover in obese subjects. *Am. J. Physiol.* 238:E235, 1980.

17. Goldberg, A.I., Tischler, M., DeMartino, G., and Griffin, G. Hormonal regulation of protein synthesis and degradation in muscle. *Fed. Proc.* 39:31, 1980.

18. Golden, M., Waterlow, J.C., and Picou, D. The relationship between dietary intake, weight change, nitrogen balance and protein turnover in man. *Am. J. Clin. Nutr.* 30:1345, 1977.

19. Goldspink, D.F. The influence of immobilization and stretch on protein turnover of rat skeletal muscle. *J. Physiol.* 264:267, 1977.

20. Hall, M.O., Bok, D., and Bacharach, A.E. Biosynthesis and assembly of the rod outer segment membrane system. Formation and fate of visual pigment in the frog retina. *J. Mol. Biol.* 45:397, 1969.

21. Huxley, A.F. "Reflections on Muscle" 111 pp. Liverpool University Press, 1980.

22. James, W.P.T., and Hay, A.M. Albumin metabolism: effect of the nutritional state and the dietary protein intake. *J. Clin. Invest.* 47:1958, 1968.

23. Laurent, G.J., Sparrow, M.P., and Millward, D.J. Turnover of muscle protein in the fowl: changes in rates of protein synthesis and breakdown during hypertrophy of the anterior and posterior latissimus dorsi muscles. *Biochem. J.* 176:407, 1978.

24. Lavie, L. Reznick, A.Z., and Gershon, D. Decreased protein and puromycinyl-peptide degradation in livers of senescent mice. *Biochem. J.* 202:47, 1982.

25. Matthews, R.W., and Haschemeyer, A.E.V. Temperature dependency of protein synthesis in toadfish liver *in vivo.* Comp. Biochem. *Physiol.* 61B:479, 1978.

26. Matthews, D.E., Bier, D.M., Rennie, M.J., Edwards, R.H.T., Halliday, D., Millward, D.J., and Clugston, G.A. Regulation of leucine metabolism in man: a stable isotope study. *Science,* 214:1129, 1981.

27. Millward, D.J. Protein degradation in muscle and liver. *In* "Comprehensive Biochemistry", Vol. 19B, Part. I. (M. Florkin, A. Neuberger, and L.L.M. van Deenen, eds.), pp. 153-232. Elsevier, Amsterdam, 1980.

28. Millward, D.J., Bates, P.C., Brown, J.G., Cox, M., and Rennie, M.J. Protein turnover and the regulation of growth. *In* "Nitrogen Metabolism in Man" (J.C. Waterlow, and J.M.L. Stephen, eds.), pp. 409-418. Applied Science Publishers, London, 1981.

29. Millward, D.J., Bates, P.C., and Rosochaki, S. The extent and nature of protein degradation in the tissues during development. *Reprod. Nutr. Develop.* 21:265, 1981.

30. Millward, D.J., Brown, J.G., and Odedra, B. Protein turnover in individual tissues with special emphasis on muscle. *In* "Nitrogen Metabolism in Man" (J.C. Waterlow, and J.M.L. Stephen, eds.), pp. 475-494, Applied Science Publishers, London, 1981.

31. Millward, D.J., Garlick, P.J., James, W.P.T., Nnanyelugo, D.O., and Ryatt, J.S. Relationship between protein synthesis and RNA content in skeletal muscle. *Nature* (Lond.) 241:204, 1973.

32. Millward, D.J., Garlick, P.J., Stewart, R.J.C., Nnanyelugo, D.O., and Waterlow, J.C. Skeletal muscle growth and protein turnover.
Biochem. J. 150:235, 1975.

33. Millward, D.J., Holliday, M.A., Bates, P.C., Dalal, S., Cox, M., and Heard, C.R.C. The relationship between dietary state, thyroid hormones, oxygen consumption and muscle protein turnover. *Proc. Nutr. Soc.* 38:33A, 1979.

34. Mortimore, G.E., and Mondon, C.E. Inhibition by insulin of valine turnover in liver. Evidence for a general control of proteolysis. *J. Biol. Chem.* 245:2375, 1970.

35. Motil, K.L., Matthews, D.E., Bier, D.M., Burke, J.F., Munro, H.N., and Young, V.R. Whole body leucine and lysine metabolism: response to dietary protein intake in young men. *Am. J. Physiol.* 240:E712, 1981.

36. Munro, H.N. Evolution of protein metabolism in mammals. *In* "Mammalian Protein Metabolism" Vol. III (H.N. Munro, ed.), pp. 133-182. Academic Press, New York, 1969.

37. Odedra, B., Bates, P.C., Nathan, M., Rennie, M. and Millward, D.J. Glucocorticoid administration and muscle protein turnover. *Proc. Nutr. Soc.* 39:82A, 1980.

38. Odedra, B.R., Dalal, S.S., and Millward, D.J. Muscle protein synthesis in the streptozotocin-diabetic rat. *Biochem. J.* 202:363, 1982.

39. Pain, V.M., and Clemens, M.J. Protein synthesis in mammalian systems. *In* "Comprehensive Biochemistry" Vol. 19B, Part. I. (M. Florkin, A. Neuberger, L.L.M. van Deenen, eds.), pp. 1-76. Elsevier, Amsterdam, 1980.

40. Pain, V.M., Clemens, M.J., and Garlick, P.J. The effect of dietary protein deficiency on albumin synthesis and on the concentration of active messenger ribonucleic acid in rat. liver. *Biochem. J.* 172:129, 1978.

41. Pencharz, P.B., Masson, M., Desgranges, F., and Papageorgiou, A. Total body protein turnover in human premature neonates: effects of birth-weight, intra-uterine nutritional status and diet. *Clin. Sci.* 61:207, 1981.

42. Preedy, V.R., Pain, V.M., and Garlick, P.J. Sensitivities of rat gastrocnemius and soleus muscles to starvation, insulin and glucagon. *Proc. Nutr. Soc.* 39:83A, 1980.

43. Reeds, P.J., and Harris, C.I. Protein turnover in aminals: man in his context. *In* "Nitrogen Metabolism in Man" (J.C. Waterlow, and J.M.L. Stephen, eds.), pp. 391-408. Applied Science Publishers, London, 1981.

44. Shipley, R.A., and Clark, R.E.
"Tracer Methods for *in vivo* Kinetics", pp. 239.
Academic Press, New York and London, 1972.

45. Soberon, G. The physiological significance of tissue enzyme activities as affected by diet. *In* "Metabolic Adaptation and Nutrition", pp. 45-72. Scientific Publication No. 22, Pan American Health Organization, Washington DC, 1971.

46. Sprinson, D.B., and Rittenberg, D. The rate of interaction of the amino acids of the diet with the tissue proteins. *J. Biol. Chem.* 180:715, 1949.

47. Steele, R. "Tracer Probes in Steady State Systems", 236 pp. CC. Thomas, Springfield, 1971.
48. Steffee, W.P., Goldsmith, R.S., Pencharz, P.B., Scrimshaw, N.S., and Young, V.R. Dietary protein intake and dynamic aspects of whole body nitrogen metabolism in adult humans. *Metabolism* 25:281, 1976.
49. Szepesi, B., and Freedland, R.A. Time-course of enzyme adaptation: II. The rate of change in two urea cycle enzymes. *Life Sciences* 8:1067, 1969.
50. Waldmann, T.A., Gordon, R.S., and Rosse, W. Studies on the metabolism of the serum proteins and lipids in a patient with analbuminemia. *Am. J. Med. Sci.* 37:960, 1964.
51. Waterlow, J.C. Observations on the mechanism of adaptation to low protein intakes. *Lancet* ii:1091, 1968.
52. Waterlow, J.C., and Jackson, A.A. Nutrition and protein turnover in man. *Br. Med. Bull.* 37:5, 1981.
53. Waterlow, J.C., Garlick, P.J., and Millward, D.J. "Protein Turnover in Mammalian Tissues and in the Whole Body", pp. 197-207. North Holland Publishing Co., Amsterdam, 1978.
54. *Ibid* p. 451.
55. *Ibid* pp. 482-488.
56. *Ibid* p. 533.
57. *Ibid* pp. 540, 541.
58. *Ibid* chaps. 18, 19.
59. Young, V.R., Steffee, W.P., Pencharz, P.B., Winterer, J.C., and Scrimshaw, N.S. Total human body protein synthesis in relation to protein requirements at various ages. *Nature* (Lond.) 253:192, 1975.

DISCUSSION[1]

In the discussion, Cohen commented on the selectivity with which intracellular protein degradation occurred. Velázquez wondered if there might be mutants as regards selective protein degradation. Such individuals might, for example, be especially susceptible to kwashiokor; Waterlow agreed but expressed doubt they could yet be identified with the necessary accuracy. Harper and Cederbaum stressed the need for many control sites for protein and amino acid breakdown and synthesis, including in particular an initiation factor for polypeptide chain formation, with which Waterlow agreed.

[1]*Summary of the discussion prepared by J. Neel.*

THE USE OF STABLE ISOTOPES TO STUDY NITROGEN METABOLISM IN HOMOZYGOUS SICKLE CELL DISEASE

Alan A. Jackson

Tropical Metabolism Research Unit
University of the West Indies
Mona, Kingston
Jamaica

INTRODUCTION

Stable Isotopes

The discovery of stable isotopes in the early 1930's and their application to biomedical research over the subsequent two decades marks one of most notable advances in sciences [29]. Their use made possible the delineation of specific metabolic pathways which led to major conceptual developments. Isotopes of hydrogen, carbon and nitrogen were used to trace the movement of compounds within the body leading to an appreciation that the material from which the organism was formed was in a constant state of flux, with a continuing exchange between the dietary components and the substance of the tissues themselve [47]. As a logical consequence the processes whereby the dynamic state of the body constituents was maintained and controlled became a fitting subject for study. Many metabolic pathways were discovered, both synthetic and degradative, and an appreciation of intermediary metabolism was born.

The methods themselves were laborious and required painstaking attention to detail in the processing of specimens suitable for analysis. Nevertheless, the value of the approach was reflected in its gradual advance, so that by 1950 a number of schools around the world were using this tool to address a variety of problems.

However, the advent of radioactive isotopes rapidly superseded the use of stable isotopes. Radioactive isotopes appeared to be able to address all the problems for which stable isotopes had been used for far less effort. They were considerably cheaper and easier to manufacture. Their detection was technically simpler, so that the doses were correspondingly smaller. The obvious advantage overall was that for the same expenditure of effort it was possible to make rapid progress in a wide range of fields of enquiry. Radioactive isotopes were not without their limitations. Frequently, scientists ask questions which they are reasonably confident they have the ability to answer. Radioactive isotopes of carbon and hydrogen are available. But not of oxygen and nitrogen. Thus attention was directed to the activity of carbon compounds, which could be investigated using[14]C. In terms of protein metabolism this represented a shift of interest from the study of the activity of the amino or nitrogen grouping to that of the carbon skeleton. A further problem of practical concern in human or clinical studies is the potential hazard to health in the use of radioactive tracers for *in vivo* studies. This limits the types of subjects that can be studied using radioactive tracers and excludes most normal groups, in particular children and adults in the reproductive years. Our Unit was created to investigate the metabolic problem faced by children with severe malnutrition. One of the most striking features of that condition is the marked, extensive depletion of body protein. Perforce we have taken an active interest in the use of stable isotopes for *in vivo* metabolic studies, with particular emphasis on nitrogen: an interest that started around 1960.

Stable isotopes are simply investigative tools and so the uses to which they can be put are many and varied. In principle they can be used to follow virtually any metabolic pathway and the constraints imposed are of a technical nature. The major limitation is the ability to isolate, in a pure form, sufficient quantities of the material under investigation to allow for an accurate measurement of enrichment. A number of methods are available for the quantification of stable isotopes in biological samples [6], although in practice the measurement of enrichment has been most frequently carried out either by emission spectrometric analysis [46] or mass spectrometric analysis [15]. We only have experience with the latter, using an isotope ratio mass spectrometer. With this instrument sample size may be a limitation, although we have been able to get reliable readings with a sample size as small as 2.5 μml [21]. The more recent introduction of gas chromatograph mass spectrometers has put a very powerful tool in the hands of research workers giving them the capacity to carry out analyses on a much wider spectrum of compunds than previously. One particular advantage of this technique is that it only requires a relatively small quantity of sample, enabling analyses to be carried out on biological specimens which had been beyond the reach of our investigations. These technical developments along with the conceptual progress in the field have led to an increased interest and expanding literature on the use of stable isotopes in biomedical science [28,54].

The technical support required to run and maintain a mass spectrometer is not easy to come by in the developing world. Our experience has been that considerable attention and financial support is required to ensure continuing satisfactory performance. Our studies have tended to focus on measurements in the whole body and we have used a variety of approaches in trying to elucidate the metabolic problems of severe malnutrition, for example whole body protein turnover [41], urea kinetics [17,19], total muscle mass [40] glucose turnover [25] and bile salt deconjugation (Tarauvinga, Golden & Jackson, unpublished). Each approach has generated data that could not have been acquired in any other way, and contributed practically to the improved management of malnourished children. In the last seven years our attention has been directed increasingly to a study of aspects of intermediary nitrogen metabolism [13,14,18, 22]: a field that we feel holds considerable promise in the future for deepening our understanding of metabolic processes in health and disease. In this paper I would like to concentrate on the most common genetic condition of clinical importance that we come across in our region, that is homozygous sickle cell haemoglobinopathy (HbSS).

Sickle Cell Disease

HbSS is a prime example of a molecular disease, the result of a single substitution in the haemoglobin molecule. Glutamic acid is replaced by valine at the 6th position from the N terminal of the β chain [16]. This changes the properties of the protein in such a way that under appropiate conditions the haemoglobin polymerises, a process known as sickling because of the characteristic morphological appearance of the red blood [48]. The polymerisation in potentially reversible, but with each cycle of sickling there is damage to the red cell, which leads ultimately to the formation of irreversibly sickled cells. These cells are removed from the circulation and destroyed. The clinical and pathological features of the disease are protean. Our consideration centers on the effect that an increased breakdown, and hence turnover of red cells has on metabolism generally. More particularly we are interested in the turnover of a single protein, haemoglobin, in relation to the nitrogen status of the whole body.

The reduction in the life span of the red cell in HbSS was first demonstrated by London et al [31] using the tracer ^{15}N-glycine. The actual kinetics of the situation are variable depending upon the status of individual patients, although the determinants of this variability are unknown. Serjeant [48] gives the mean life span of the red cell as being of the order of 10 days, as compared to 120 days in the normal. From this he calculates an increase in effective haemoglobin synthesis rate from the normal 6.25 g/d (15 mg N/kg/d) to 40 g/d (116 mg/N/kg/d) in HbSS. There is a difficulty in making comparisons with normal values brought about by the uncertainty as to what would be an appropriate choice of references measurement. In HbSS there are important alterations in body habitus and composition [4]. Body weight has been chosen as a reference base in full appreciation of the potential limitations that this imposes.

There are very few data available on the effect of a significant increase in the turnover of the single protein, haemoglobin, on metabolism generally. Sometime ago we studied a young male with HbSS who was suffering from chronic renal disease and was receiving a low protein diet as part of his therapeutic management. We noted that his nitrogen balance was worse than two other patients with severe renal disease [16]. In particular, there was a marked increase in the faecal nitrogen losses in HbSS, so that the apparent absorption of dietary protein was only 33%, as compared to 74% in the other patients (Table I). A similar pattern of increased faecal nitrogen losses has been observed in West Africa, [37]. Adolescents, normal and HbSS, were given three levels of protein intake. At each level the faecal nitrogen was increased in HbSS compared to normal and thus the apparent absorption of the dietary protein was reduced. We have tried to account for this difference in faecal nitrogen based upon the known metabolism of haemoglobin. The Haemoglobin molecule is catabolised to the globin chains and haem ring. The haem ring is degraded to bilirubin, which is effectively and end product of metabolism, being excreted in the bile and lost from the body in the stool [22]. A bilirubin production rate of 300 mg/d in the normal would be increased to 1920 mg/d in HbSS, giving rise to a faecal nitrogen loss of 0.46 and 3.49 mg/kg/d respectively. In HbSS the increased bilirubin production is insufficient to account for more than 10 to 15% of the differences. Therefore in HbSS there is an apparent malabsorption of dietary protein, according to standard nutritional concepts.

Protein Turnover in HbSS

In 1967, Waterlow [50] reported the used of a continuous infusion of ^{14}C-lysine to measure whole body protein turnover in the young adult male sicklers in Jamaica. He obtained a value of 505 mg N/kg/d, far greater than in a normal adult of 250 mg N/kg/d, and more than could be accounted for solely on the basis of a theoretical increase in haemoglobin turnover of 100 mg N/kg/d, *vide supra*. A number of variables, such as age, race and life style could have accounted for the differences, apart from the contribution of HbSS itself.

TABLE I *Apparent absorption of dietary protein in HbSS compared to normals at varying protein intakes, in chronic renal disease [16] and adolescents [37].*

| State | Intake mg N/kg/d | Faecal Nitrogen mg N/kg/d | | Aparent Absoption % | |
		Normal	HbSS	Normal	HbSS
Renal	45	12		73	
	59		40		33
Adolescent	90	10	30	89	67
	135	21	37	84	73
	180	30	40	83	78

We have recently measured whole body protein turnover in a group of normal young men and repeated the study on the same two sicklers reported by Waterlow in 1967, some 15 years later (Badaloo, Jahoor & Jackson, unpublished observations).

The technique used was a modification of that introduced by Picou & Taylor Roberts [41]. A prime/intermittent infusion of a tracer dose of ^{15}N-glycine was given and the enrichment measured in urinary ammonia used to calculate turnover [53]. Using this method plateau enrichments are achieved by 12 hours in both urinary ammonia and urinary urea, Fig. 1, and results can be obtained within 12 to 18 hours. For the duration of the study all subjects were given regular intermittent feeds at 3 hourly intervals, at the same time as the dose of ^{15}N-glycine. The whole body turnover in HbSS was 633 mg N/kg/d, a value similar to that derived by Waterlow previously. This was 135 mg N/kg/d greater than that found in six normal subjects, 498 mg N/kg/d, the increase being within the range expected from the theoretical contribution coming from increased haemoglobin turnover. This difference is more marked if it is related to the dietary protein intake. Fig. 2 shows that in the normals there was significant positive linear relationship between turnover and dietary nitrogen intake.

Nitrogen turnover = 1.22x Nitrogen intake + 251   r = 0.94, p < 0.01.

With this method it is possible to calculate the rate of protein breakdown in the whole body. In the normals protein breakdown is almost constant over the

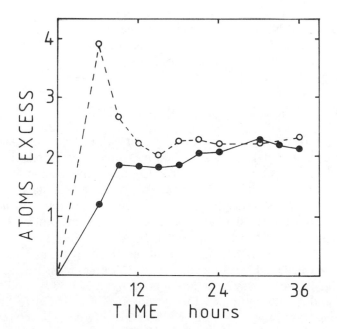

Figure 1. Rise to plateau enrichment in urinary ammonia (○) and urinary urea (●), following a prime/intermittent infusion of ^{15}N-glycine, over 36 hours.

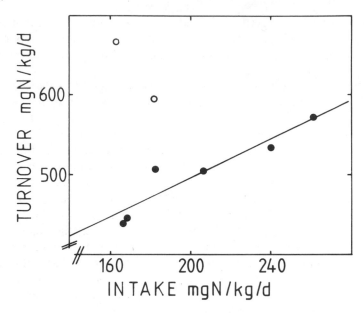

Figure 2. The rate of whole body protein turnover in relation to the dietary protein intake in HbSS (○) and normals (●) derived from the plateau enrichment in urinary ammonia, using ^{15}N-glycine.

range of protein intakes, Fig. 3, and is on average 308 mg N/kg/d, much less than is HbSS, 461 mg N/kg/d. In a steady state breakdown is equal to synthesis. Thus protein synthesis, whereas in HbSS this is increased to 25% of the total. Hence the increase in haemoglobin synthesis in HbSS represents a considerable metabolic demand.

Urea Kinetics in HbSS

In the study referred to above on a young man with HbSS, taking a low protein diet for chronic renal disease, we had measured urea kinetics. We were surprised to find that the rate of urea production was higher than in normals on their habitual protein intake [17]. Therefore we have been measuring urea kinetics in HbSS, at different protein intakes (Jackson, Landman & Stevens, unpublished observations). The method used was that introduced by Picou and Phillips [39] as modified by ourselves [17]. A prime/intermittent infusion of ^{30}N-Urea was given over 36 hours. The rate at which urea is produced in the liver, P, can be calculated from the dilution of ^{30}N-urea, measured in the urinary urea, Fig. 4. The urinary excretion of urea over a 24 hour period was measured, Eu, and a value obtained for the proportion of the urea produced which approximates to the urea which has been hydrolysed in the colon to ammonia, T, and thus made metabolically available as a source of non-essential nitrogen [8,26]. It is possible to measure the extent to which ammonia libera-

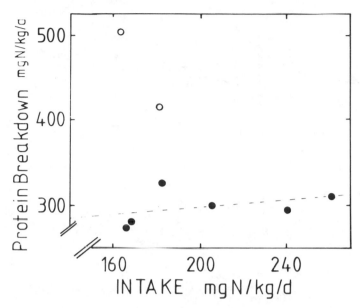

Figure 3. The rate of whole body protein breakdown in relation to the dietary protein intake in HbSS (○) normals (●).

ted from urea hydrolysis in the colon is resynthesised to urea, P_R, by measuring the enrichment of ^{29}N-urea in urinary urea.

We have data on four patients with HbSS, studied on nitrogen intakes ranging from 60 to 400 mg N/kg/d. Urea production rate showed a linear relationship to dietary intake, Fig. 5.

HbSS Urea production = 0.33 x N intake + 134   r = 0.96, p < 0.01.

In the normal, urea production was also related to intake, but at each level of intake was lower than in HbSS.

Normal Urea production = 0.59 x N intake + 2   r = 0.99, p ≤ 0.01.

In the normals the rate at which hydrolyzed urea was being recycled to urea synthesis, P_R, was low. A completely different pattern was seen in HbSS, where P_R was high (60 mg N/kg/d) and varied little with dietary intake. If PR is subtracted from the total production rate then the expression (P-P_R) may be taken to represent the rate at which dietary and endogenous nitrogen compounds are being catabolized to urea, Fig. 6. In HbSS, P-P_R is still greater than in the normal, although the differences is less dramatic than that for total production. Again there is a close linear relationship to dietary intake for both states.

HbSS 32 P-P_R = 0.29 x N intake + 86   r = 0.98, p < 0.01

Normal   P-P_R = 0.43 x N intake + 37   r = 0.99, p ≤ 0.01

A compilation of the four relationships total productions and P-P_R, in HbSS and normal, is shown in Fig. 7. The pattern is clearly different in HbSS compared to normal.

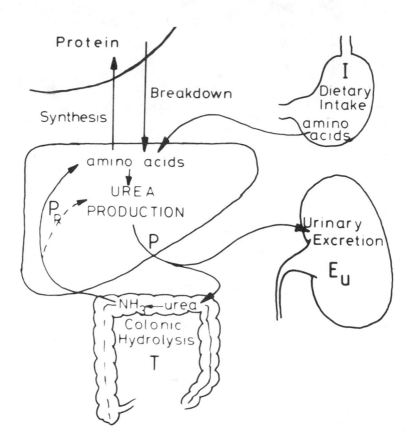

Figure 4. Schematic diagram representing the kinetics of urea metabolism in the body.

The rate at which urea is hydrolyzed in the colon, T, in normal subjects is inversely related to the nitrogen intake. On a normal intake about 70% of production is excreted in the urine and 30% hydrolyzed. As the intake of nitrogen is reduced below about 70 mg N/kg/d, and increasing proportion of the urea produced is hydrolyzed in the colon rather than being lost to the body in the urine [17]. This was not the situation in HbSS, where there was found to be an almost constant rate at which urea was hydrolyzed in the colon, 135 mg N/kg/d, over a fivefold range of dietary intake.

In a steady state the rate of urea production is thought to relate directly to the dietary intake of nitrogen, based upon the urinary excretion of urea [1]. The finding that in HbSS both total urea production and $(P-P_R)$ are greater than normal at the levels of dietary intake studied, lead to the conclusion that the absorption of dietary nitrogen in HbSS must be at least as efficient as in the normal and possibly more efficient. This suggestion is supported by the

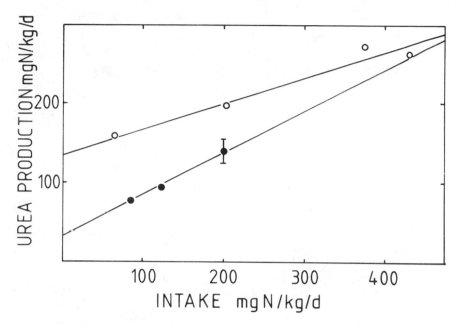

Figure 5. The rate of total urea production in relation to the dietary intake of protein in HbSS (○) and normals (●), as measured with a prime/intermittent infusion of ^{30}N-urea.

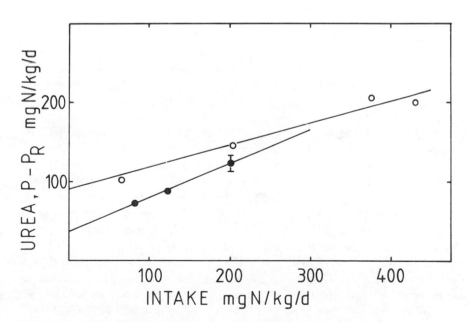

Figure 6. The rate of urea production from dietary and endogenous amino acids (P-P$_R$) in relation to the dietary intake of protein in HbSS (○) and normals (●).

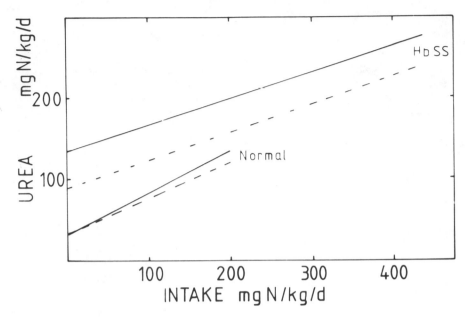

Figure 7. The relationship between total urea production(———————) and P-P_R (--------) in HbSS and normals.

derived value for flux of nitrogen through the urea precursor pool which was increased nearly two times in HbSS. Thus the finding of a relatively low apparent absorption of dietary protein in HbSS, based upon nitrogen balance data is not supported by consideration of the urea kinetics data. Rather, we would suggest that the increased faecal losses of nitrogen in HbSS represent endogenous losses of nitrogen, rather than protein malabsorption.

There is little direct evidence available on the factors that control the rate at which urea is hydrolyzed in the colon. We have suggested that the main determinants of this activity may be the availability of energy and nitrogen substrates being offered to the colonic flora through the ileo-caecal value [17]. The fixed high rate of hydrolysis seen in the colon in HbSS, even at relatively high dietary levels of nitrogen intake, and the extent to which this nitrogen is reincorporated into urea, is unusual. There is only one clinical condition in which a similar situation has been described. In patients with a blind loop syndrome, where there is intense bacterial activity at a high level of the small intestine, there is a very high rate of urea production, hydrolysis and reincorporation of the nitrogen into urea synthesis [24]. When the condition is corrected by appropriate antibiotic treatment the urea kinetics revert to a more normal pattern. We have no evidence to suggest that patients with HbSS are not suffering from a functional small bowel over-growth. However, clinically they do not present a picture that suggests this condition. Furthermore, the finding that

P-P$_R$ is, if anything, higher than normal would indicate the dietary protein itself is being digested and absorbed very efficiently, and of itself maintains an unusually high rate of urea production. A more likely explanation for the increase in colonic hydrolysis of urea would be that it is a manifestation of the intensity of protein metabolism brought about by the demands for haemoglobin synthesis.

The ultimate fate of the ammonia generated by urea hydrolysis is uncertain, and itself depends upon the overall metabolic state of the organism. An oral load of ammonia may be fixed as urea on an adequate protein diet or, if the dietary protein intake is reduced, the ammonia is made available as a source of non-essential nitrogen, fixed in amino acids and thence used for protein synthesis [50]. Hydrolyzed urea nitrogen enjoys a similar fate, dependent upon the dietary intake [8]. The finding of a high value P$_R$ in HbSS at all levels of protein intake appears contradictory. It could be explained if P$_R$ actually represented nitrogen that had been fixed in amino acids and protein, and was returning to urea, through, for example, the catabolism of rapidly turning over proteins. One possible source of marked increased in rapidly turning over proteins might be in ineffective erythropoiesis. In situations where so called "stress reticulocytes" are produced ineffective erythropoiesis can increase by as much as twenty times normal [44,55]. It is generally stated that ineffective erythropoiesis is not a feature of HbSS [48], but this is in comparison to other haemolytic states [32]. Malamos et al [32] give the efficiency of erythropoiesis in HbSS as being about 82%. If P$_R$ does represent a measure of ineffective erythropoiesis then our data would suggest a value of at least 70% for effective erythropoiesis.

Amino Acid Balance

Consideration has to be given to the pattern of amino acids required for haemoglobin synthesis. In this sense haemoglobin is a particularly unbalanced protein with respect to branched chain aminoacids [48]. Valine and Leucine together comprise one fifth of the total amino acid residues, whereas both the α and β chain are completely devoid of isoleucine.

One of the more important features of the molecule is the specific requirement for the synthesis of the haem ring. Each of the four nitrogen atoms in the rings is derived from a glycine molecule, which also contributes one carbon atom [34].

Four further carbon atoms are each derived from glycine [35]. Hence the synthesis of one haem ring requires eight molecules of glycine. As this is ultimately lost to the body as bilirubin it represents a persistent drain on the glycine pool of the body. In the normal this would amount to 5 mg glycine/kg/d, but increase in HbSS to 38 mg glycine of 2 to 4 g/d, and about twice that for the total intake of glycine plus serine. Therefore the need for glycine to satisfy the irrecoverable demands for haemoglobin synthesis may represent a considerable proportion of the dietary intake. This is unlikely to present a problem if glycine and/or serine can be readily synthesized as non-essential amino acids in the body. Very few diets are likely to present a balanced pattern of amino acids to satisfy the specific requirements for branched-chain amino acids and glycine of patients with HbSS.

Glycine Synthesis

The metabolic pathways that lead to the net synthesis of glycine and serine are far form clear [2]. There is evidence to suggest that in situations where the metabolic demand for these amino acids is increased there may be difficulty in increasing synthesis sufficiently to satisfy the need, if adequate quantities are not available from the diet. Glycine is an essential amino acid for optimum growth in chicks [36]. It is thought that this reflects the demands for uric acid synthesis, an excretory end product of metabolism. Rats may require dietary glycine for optimal growth and recovery from injury [7,48]. There appears to be a narrow margin between the amount of glycine synthesized and the demand [3] and the availability of folic acid may be critically important in this respect [2,3]. When the protein content of most diets is reduced, the availability of non-essential nitrogen may become the first limiting factor. A dietary source of non-essential nitrogen in the form of ammonium salts improves growth and nitrogen balance, but even greater improvement is seen if glycine is given as an additional source of non-essential nitrogen [26]. The anaemia associated with chronic renal disease has been found to improve in response to a dietary supplement of glycine [12]. It has been suggested that glycine may be acting as the first limiting nutrient for the growth of preterm infants taking donor human breast milk [9].

The major pathway for glycine synthesis is the glycine cleavage system, which utilizes folic acid as a cofactor [27]. Folic acid deficiency is not an unusual finding in HbSS, although megaloblastic changes in the peripheral film, appear with varying frequency [48].

The activity of the glycine cleavage system *in vitro* is profundly affected by the metabolites produced in the catabolism of branched-chain amino acids [30,37]. On most diets there would be a relative excess of isoleucine, relative to the demands for haemoglobin synthesis. The potential exists for the metabolites produced in the catabolism of excess isoleucine to interfase with the glycine cleavage system and limit the endogenous production of glycine. It is not known whether this happens to an extent that is functionally important.

Glutathione in Red Cells

We reasoned that if glycine were limiting in the diet of patients with HbSS, and if the capacity to make glycine endogenously were insufficient to satisfy the demands, then there should be evidence of inadequate synthesis of compounds rich in glycine. One of the amino acid residues of the tripeptide glutathione is glycine. Glutathione is found in all cells where it plays an important role in maintaining the oxido-reductive potential and hence protecting the cell in the face of oxidant stress [33]. Virtually all of the glutathione in red cells is usually in the reduced state [51].

We used the method described by Beutler [5] to measure the glutathione content of red cells taken from adult patients with HbSS, at a time when they were in a steady clonical and haemotological state (Jackson, Foster & Serjeant, unpublished observations). The results are given in Table II. In HbSS the glutathione content of whole blood was greatly reduced, but this was due to anaemia. When expressed per unit red cell or unit haemoglobin there was no difference between HbSS and normal. However, Powers and Thurnham [42] have shown that if red cells are separated by age on a density gradient that the glutathione content of the oldest cells is only about 50% that of the youngest cells. As the red cells in the samples from HbSS are on average considerably younger than those from normals, 6 to 12 days compared with 60 days, one would expect the glutathione content in HbSS to be higher than normal. If a correction is made for the relative age of the cells then the red cells from HbSS contain significantly less glutathione than the normal; only about 77% of that expected for their age. Patients with congenital defects leading to severe reductions in the glutathione content of red cells suffer from a haemolytic anaemia and metabolic acidosis [33]. The low level of glutathione in HbSS is not decreased sufficiently to produce problems on its own. However, the integrity of the red cell is related to its capacity to withstand oxidative stress. Each cycle of sickling and unsickling damages the membrane further, and there is evidence that Heinz body formation, and the progressive membrane changes brought about by a reduced capacity to protect against lipid peroxidation are related to the production of irreversibly sickled cell [9]. The glutathione content of the red cell may be another factor of importance in this situation, as has been suggested in haemoglobin H disease [43] and for unstable haemoglobins associated with hereditary Heinz body anaemias [20]. Maybe it is too much to suggest that the

TABLE II *The glutathione (GSH) content of red cells in adults with HbSS compared to normal adults. Values are means + S.D.*

	GSH mg/l	GSH/Red Cell mg/10^{12}	GSH/Haemoglobin mg/g
Normal	377 ± 36	85 ± 11	2.0 ± 0.3
n	11	10	11
HbSS	219 ± 29	84 ± 14	2.8 ± 0.6
n	16	10	16

increased haemolysis which increases the demands for glycine is itself produced in part by the limited availability of glycine, thus making a relative glycine deficiency both the cause and the result of the same process.

CONCLUSIONS

The patients with HbSS that we have studied probably suffer from relatively mild disease. They compensate well for their disease state, in that they have all enjoyed comparatively good health and lived through to adulthood. They are a self selected population. Even so, they have at one time or another experienced complications of a greater or lesser degree. If there is any basis to the hypotheses advanced above, it may be expected that the changes would be manifest in a much more dramatic form in those whose disease had followed a much more malignant course and had succumbed at a relatively early age. Even with expert experienced care the mortality from HbSS is high at all ages. This is particularly marked in childhood when at least 10% die in the first year of life, and a further 5 and 3% in the second and third years respectively [45]. Growth is poor, maturation delayed and body composition abnormal. Of those who survive to adulthood many develop progressive chronic renal failute at an early age. On the basis of the data that we have so far, a number of conclusions may be drawn that have a direct bearing on the progress of the disease.

1. Nitrogen balance, and the interpretation of data derived from nitrogen balance studies in HbSS are affected by the demands for the synthesis of an excessive amount of a single protein, haemoglobin. Altogether haemoglobin synthesis may account for no less than 25% of the total protein synthetic activity in the body. The situation is aggravated by the fact that haemoglobin is an unbalanced protein, being totally deficient in isoleucine, and exerting and excessive demands for glycine. The demand for glycine is accentuated by the irreversible loss of the end product of haem metabolism, bilirubin in the stool.

2. Increased faecal losses of nitrogen contribute significantly to the poor nitrogen balance. Although there is a low apparent absorption of dietary protein this is not in fact due to poor digestibility *per se,* and the concept is not helpful in this situation. Rather, the increased faecal losses represent losses of endogenous nitrogen in the stool. Only a small part of this can be attributed to the increased losses as bilirubin, and it is necessary to invoke other mechanisms to explain the major component of faecal nitrogen.

3. Ingested protein is digested and absorbed as efficiently as in the normal, but is used with less efficiency for metabolic processes, as shown by the increased urea production rate. The main reason for this is likely to be that the balance of amino acids in the ingested protein does not match

the balance needed for the synthesis of all the proteins in the body. A further contribution to urea synthesis may be coming from a group of proteins that are turning over rapidly, in particular proteins associated with ineffective erythropoiesis.

4. The adaptive processes that are active in HbSS to conserve body nitrogen at normal levels of proteins intake, are similar to those usually seen in normals when ingesting a low protein intake, e.g. increased recycling of urea through the colon. In practice the effectiveness of this mechanism may be offset either by the demands of ineffective erythropoiesis or because the nitrogen coming from hydrolyzed urea can not be utilized efficiently and is directed back to urea synthesis. In either case the patient with HbSS may be perceived as existing in a state where the diet is chronically short of protein, relative to the metabolic demands.

There might be at least two important clinical implications of this relative chronic dietary deficiency of protein. Firstly many adult patients with HbSS go on to develop chronic renal failure. Part of the standard therapeutic regime for this condition a low protein diet. However, a patient with HbSS may not be able to tolerate this approach and standard treatment may be particularly pernicious. This consideration requires careful evaluation. Secondly, the classical explanation for the persistence of the HbSS genotype is that it offers a selective advantage in terms of resistence to malaria [48]. The mechanism whereby this apparent protection is brought about is far from clear although a number of possible suggestions have been made [48]. In rats given rodent malaria under controlled conditions the severity of the parasitaemia, mortality and superinfection are all reduced in animals fed a protein deficient diet [10,11]. It is not known how this protection is afforded, and a concept is introduced which seems to fly in the face of conventional wisdom. However, it raises another possibility for the relatively low prevalence of malaria in HbSS; the possibility that in HbSS the relative dietary protein deficiency affords protection in a manner similar to that observed in rats.

5. The extent to which the demands for haemoglobin synthesis are satisfied in HbSS must have implications for the body's ability to carry out its other functions at a satisfactory level. Should glycine indeed prove to be semi-essential in this situation, then one could anticipate a secondary effect on a wide number of tissues and systems. These considerations may have importance in the pathophysiology of the disease process itself, unrelated to the vascular effects of the sickling per se.

Our understanding of genetics and molecular biology has been advanced considerably by the study of haemoglobinopathies. As yet these developments seem to have made very little impact on the quality of life enjoyed by the individuals suffering from the diseases. Hopefully an appreciation of the adaptations in metabolism that are compatible with survival may lead to approaches for nutritional therapeutic intervention of benefit.

ACKNOWLEDGEMENTS

I am appreciative of many fruitful discussions held with colleagues, especially M. Golden, J. Landman, F. Jahoor, G. Serjeant and S. Terry. The generous assitance of the Wellcome Trust is gratefully acknowledged. The mass spectrometer was a gift from the Medical Research Council.

REFERENCES

1. Allison, J.B., & Bird, J.W.C.: Elimination of nitrogen from the body, *In* "Mammalian Protein Metabolism I" (edits. H.N. Munro & J.B. Allison). Academic Press, New York, 1964, pp. 483-512.

2. Arnstein, H.R.V.: The metabolism of glycine. *Advances in Protein Chemistry,* 9.1, 1952.

3. Arnstein, H.R.V. & Stankovic, V.: The effect of certain vitamin deficiencies on glycine deficiency. *Biochem. J.,* 62, 190, 1956.

4. Ashoroft, M.T. & Serjeant, G.R.: Body habitus of Jamaican adults with sickle cell anaemia. *Southern Medical Journal,* 65, 579, 1972.

5. Beutler, E., Duron, O. & Kelly, B.M.: Improved method for the determination of blood glutathione. *J. Lab. & Clin. Med.* 61, 882, 1963.

6. Bier, D.M.: Stable isotope methods for nutritional diagnosis and research. *Nutr. Rev.,* 40, 129, 1982.

7. Breuer, L.M., Pond, W.G., Warner, R.G. & Loosli, J.K.: The role of dispensable amino acids in the nutrition of the rat. *J. Nutr.* 82, 499, 1964.

8. Close, J.H.: The use of amino acid precursors in nitrogen accumulation disease. *New Eng. J. Med.,* 290, 663, 1974.

9. Das, S.K. & Nair, R.C.: Superoxide dismutase, glutathione peroxidase, catalase and lipid peroxidation of normal and sickled erythrocytes. *Br. J. Haematol.,* 44, 87, 1980.

10. Ediringhe, J.S., Fern, E.B. & Targett, G.A.T.: Dietary suppression of rodent malaria. *Transac. Roy. Soc. Trop. Med. & Hyg.,* 75, 591, 1981.

11. Edirisinghe, H.S., Fern, E.B., & Targett, G.A.T.: Resistance to superinfection with Plasmodiubergheir in rats fed a protein-free diet. *Transac. Roy. Soc. Trop. Med. & Hyg.,* 75, 591, 1982.

12. Giordano, C., De Santo, N.G., Rinaldi, S., De Pascale, C. & Pluvio, M. Histidine and glycine essential amino acids in uraemia. *In* "Uremia" (edit r. Kluthe, G. Berlybe & B. Burton) Georg Thieme Verlag K.G., Stuttgart, 1972, pp. 138-143.

13. Golden, M.H.N. & Jackson, A.A.: Tissue enrichments and protein turnover measured with ^{15}N-glycine, *Nature,* 265, 563, 1977.

14. Golden, M.H.N., Jahoor, P. & Jackson, A.A.: Glutamine production rate and its contribution to urinary ammonia in normal man. *Clin. Sci.,* 62, 299, 1982.

15. Halliday, D. & Read, W.W.C.: Mass spectrometric assay of stable isotope enrichment for the estimation of protein turnover in man. *Proc. Nutr. Soc.,* 40, 321, 1981.

16. Ingram, V.M.: Gene mutations in human haemoglobin: The chemical differences between normal and sickle cell haemoglobin. *Nature,* 180, 326, 1957.

17. Jackson, A.A.: The measurement of urea kinetics using ^{15}N-urea in patients with chronic renal disease. M.D. disertation, University of Cambridge, 1982.

18. Jackson, A.A. & Golden, M.H.N.: ^{15}N-glycine metabolism in normal man: the metabolic α-amino nitrogen pool. *Clin. Sci.,* 58, 517, 1980.

19. Jackson, A.A., Shaw, J.C.L., Barber, A. & Golden, M.H.N.: Nitrogen metabolism in preterm infants fed human donor breast milk: the possible essentiality of glycine. *Pediat, Re.,* 15, 1454, 1981.

20. Jacob, H.S., Brain, M.C., Dacie, J.U., Carell, R.W. & Lehmann, H.: Abnormal haem binding and globin SH gropu blockade in unstable haemoglobins. *Nature* 218, 1214, 1968.

21. Jahoor, F., Jackson, A.A. & Golden, M.H.N.: A method for the isolation of the amide nitrogen of glutamine from biological samples for mass spectrometry. *Analyt. Biochem,* 121, 349, 1982.

22. Jahoor, F.: Ammonia metabolism *in vivo* in the rat. *In* "Nitrogen metabolism in man" (eds. J.C. Waterlow & J.M.L. Stephen). Applied Science Publishers, London, 1981. pp. 173-196.

23. James III, G.W.: Stercobilin and hematopoiesis. *Amer. J. Clin. Nutr.* 3, 64, 1955.

24. Jones, E.A., Smallwood, R.A., Craigie, A. & Rosenoer, V.M.: The enterohepatic circulation of urea nitrogen. *Clin. Sci.,* 37, 825, 1969.

25. Kerr, D.S., Stevens, M.C.G. & Picou, D.I.M.: Fasting metabolism in infants: II. The effect of severe undernutrition and infusion of alanine on glucose production estimated with $U-^{13}C$-glucose. *Metabolism* 27, 831, 1978.

26. Kies, C.: Nonspecific nitrogen in the nutrition of human beings. *Fed. Proc.,* 31, 1172, 1972.

27. Kikuchi, G.: The glycine cleavage system: composition reaction mechanism and physiological significance. *Molecular and Cellular biochemistry,* 1, 169, 1973.

28. Klein, E.R. & Klein, P.D.: A selected bibliography of biomedical an environmental applications of stable isotopes, 1977-1978. *Biochemical Mass Spectrometry,* 6, 515, 1979.

29. Klein, P.D., Hachey, D.L., Kreek, M.J. & Schoeller, D.A.; stable isotopes: essential tools in biological and medical research. *In* "Stable Isotopes": Applications in Pharmacology, Toxicology and Clinical Research" ed. T.A. Baillie) Macmillan, London, 1978, pp. 3-14.

30. Kilvraa, S.: Inhibition of the glycine cleavage system by branched-chain amino acid metabolites. *Pediat. Res,* 13, 889, 1979.

31. London, J.M., Shemin, D., West, R. & Rittenberg, D.: Heme synthesis and red blood cell dynamics in normal humans and in subjects with polycythaemia vera, sickle-cell anaemia, and pernicious anaemia. *J. Biol. Chem.,* 179, 463, 1949.

32. Malamos, B., Belcher, E.H., Gyftake, E. & Binopoulos, D.: Simultaneous radioactive tracer studies of erythropoiesis and red-cell destruction in sickle-cell disease ans sickle-cell haemoglobin/thalassaemia. *Brit. J. Haematol.* 9, 487, 1963.

33. Meister, A. & Tate, S..: Glutathione and related glutamyl compounds: biosynthesis and utilization. *Ann. Rev. Biochem.* 45, 559, 1976.

34. Muir, H.M. & Neuberger, A.: The biogenesis of porphyrins: The distribution of ^{15}N in the ring system. *Biochem. J.,* 45, 163, 1949.

35. Muir, H.M., & Neuberger, A.: The biogenesis of porphyrins 2. The origins of the methyne carton atoms. *Bioch. J.,* 47, 87, 1950.

36. Ngo, A., Coon, C.N., & Beecher, G.R.: Dietary glycine requirement for chicks and cellular development in chicks. *J. Nutr.* 107, 1800, 1977.

37. O' Brien, W.E.: Inhibition of glycine synthase by branched-chain α-Keto acids. *Arch. Biochem. Biophys,* 189, 291, 1978.

38. Odonkor, P.Q. & Addase, S.K.: Nitrogen balance in adolescent sockle cell patients. *Proc. Nutr. Soc.,* 1982.

39. Picou, D. & Phillips, M.: Urea metabolism in malnuurished and recovered children receiving a high or low protein diet. *Amer. J. Clin. Nutr.,* 25, 1261, 1972.

40. Picou, D., Reeds, P.J., Jackson, A.A. & Poutler, N.: The measurement of muscle mass in children using ^{15}N-creatine. *Pediat. Res.* 10, 184, 1976.

41. Picou, D. & Taylor-Roberts, T.: The measurement of total protein synthesis and catabolism and nitrogen turnover in infants in different nutritional states and receiving different amounts of dietary protein. *Clin. Sci.,* 36, 283, 1969.

42. Powers, H.J. & Thurnham, D.I.: Riboflavin deficiency in man: effects on haemoglobin and reduced glutathione in erythrocytes of different ages. *Br. J. Nutr.,* 46, 257, 1981.

43. Rigas, D.A. & R.D.: Erythocyte enzymes and reduced glutathione (GSH) in hemoglobin H disease: relation to cell age and denaturation of hemoglobin *H.J. Lab. & Clin. Med.,* 58, 417, 1961.

44. Robinson, S.J. & Tsong, M.: Hemolysis of "stress" reticulocytes a source of erythropoietic bilirubin formation. *J. Clin. Invest.,* 49, 1025, 1970.

45. Rogers, D.W., Clarke, J.M., Cupidore, L., Ramlal, A.M., Sparker, B.R. & Serjeant, G.R.: Early deaths in Jamaican children with sickle cell disease. *Br. Med. J.,* 1, 1515, 1978.
46. Salter, D.N.: Emission spectrometric analysis of [15]N. *Proc. Nutr. Soc.,* 40, 335, 1981.
47. Schoenheimer, R.: The dynamic state of body constituents. Harvard University Press, Massachusetts, 1942.
48. Serjeant, G.R.: The clinical features of sickle cell disease. *In* "Clinical Studies, 4, "(A.G. Bearn, D.A.K. Black & H.H. Hiatt, eds.) North Holland Publishing Company, Amsterdan, 1974.
49. Sitren, H.S. & Fisher, H.: Nitrogen retention in rats fed on diets enriched with arginine and glycine. Improved N retention after trauma. *Br. J. Nutr.* 37, 195, 1977.
50. Sprinson, D.B. & Rittenberg, D.: The rate of utilisation of ammonia for protein synthesis. *J. Biol. Chem.* 180, 707, 1949.
51. Srivastava, S.K. & Beutler, E.: Accurate measurement of oxidized glutathione content of human, rabbit and rat red blood cells and tissues. *Analyt. Biochem.* 25, 70, 1968.
52. Waterlow, J.C., Lysine turnover in man measured by intravenous infusion of L-/U-[14]C T lysine. *Clin. Sci.,* 33, 507, 1967.
53. Waterlow, J.C., Golden, M.H.N. & Garlick, P.J.: Protein turnover in man measured with [15]N: Comparison of end products and dose regimes. *Amer. J. Physiol,* 235, E165, 1978.
54. Waterlow, J.C. & Stephen, J.M.L.: Nitrogen Metabolism in Man. Applied Science Publishers, London, 1981.
55. Yannoni, C.Z. & Robinson, S.H.: Early labelled haem in erythroid and hepatic cells *Nature* 258, 330, 1975.

DISCUSSION[1]

Motulsky questioned the suggestion that the maintenance of sickle cell trait might be due to nutritional factors in people with sickle cell anemia. He pointed out that this was maintained in asymptomatic carriers with no protein calorie malnutrition. Jackson responded that no studies existed for nitrogen metabolism in sickle cell trait, but thought to assume it to be normal, as Motulsky had done was dangerous. Cohen raised a methodological question concerning the recycling of labelled ammonia produced by urease in the intestine and the influence that it might have on the results of these types of studies. Jackson stated that other data they have suggest that this is not a problem, but had too little time to elaborate. Nesheim pointed out that para-aminobenzoate influences parasitemia in mouse malaria and questioned how this might affect the results of nutritional manipulation in human malaria. Neither Jackson nor Solomons could recall studies of this issue. Garby asked what happens if the patients are supplemented with glycine. Jackson said that was not done because they were not sure that glycine was deficient in the patients and because there was a narrow margin of safety for the use of glycine. Both Snyderman and Cederbaum questioned the latter statement. Jackson responded that glycine might be risky in patients predisposed to hyperammonia, a situation that

[1]*Summary of the discussion prepared by S. Cederbaum.*

might exist in sickle cell disease. Cohen inquired about the benzoate content of the indigenous diet eaten by some of Jackson's patients, pointing out that benzoate could exaggerate incipient hypoglycinemia. Cederbaum inquired if new or simplifed techniques to study protein metabolism were on the horizon so that larger number of individuals, including "outliers", could be studied at an acceptable cost and convenience. Waterlow felt that [^{15}N]-glycine was cheap enough and the methods simple enough so that tests of 100 individuals posed no undue hardship, and the ascertainment of the degree of variability in protein turnover was at hand. Hillman agreed, stating that simpler sachines measuring ^{13}C as well as ^{15}N are becoming available and breath tests measuring release of labelled gases can be readily performed. He emphasized also that the impetus for these technological developments arose because of the existence of outliers or homozygotes with inborn errors of metabolism and methods developed for these patients can be applied more broadly to nutritional problems. Scrimshaw agreed, pointing out that simpler and cheaper methods will also be available to study ^{18}O and ^{2}H. Torún stated that recently they were prevented from doing just such studies measuring energy expenditure, for financial reasons. Cohen offered a perspective. He was wary of the efforts to identify a single technology to define and reflect a dynamic steady state when we recognize that the steady state is comprised of the interaction of many complex and regulated processes.

PART IV

ENERGY BALANCE

ENERGY BALANCE AND OBESITY

Lars Garby

Department of Physiology
University of Odense
Denmark

INTRODUCTION

The importance of hereditary factors in the development of obesity in human beings has been the subject of several studies. The more direct approach of twin and adoptee studies has not resulted in any clear-cut answers. Recognition of shortcomings of such studies and insistence that there ought to be clear-cut answers, have broadened the area of research and it now includes the whole field of energy exchange and energy metabolism in general, as well as a great many other aspects of obesity research.

The aim of the present paper is two-fold: I will try to summarize the present state of the art and I will also try to contribute to the discussion of the problems in this area of research; they are difficult and many.

Health Consequences of Overweight and Obesity

This subject is extremely difficult and, although there is fair agreement among investigators that overweight and obesity is associated with an increased risk of developing coronary heart disease, hypertension, diabetes and gallbladder disease, there is little evidence with respect to causality. Intervention studies which, at least in principle could solve the problem of causality, are extremely difficult to carry out and it would seem to me that twin studies could be used in this context. A recent critical review by the Royal College of Physicians Working Party on Obesity [36] deals extensively with the associations mentioned above, but is practically silent on the problem of causality.

Measuring Obesity

Obesity can be defined on the basis of a number of different measurements. The most common measurement includes body weight (W) and height (H), and division of the former with some function of the latter. The rationale behind this kind of operation is to obtain a measure which is highly correlated with weight but minimally correlated with height. Several such indices have been suggested over the years: W/H, W/H^2, W/Hp^3 and W/Hp, where p is the linear regression coeficcient of weight (dependent variable) or height (independent variable). The latter index was suggested by Benn [1] on the basis of the mathematical demonstration that this index is independent on height, provides that height and weight are linearly related. The relative merits of the different indices have recently been investigated by Lee, Kolonel and Hinds [28] in a study comprising several large population groups of various ethnic origin in the State of Hawaii. The authors found that Benn's index showed the lowest correlation with height and that its correlation with weight was not much smaller than that of W/H and W/H^2. They recommend that Benn's index be used as a routine. Dugdale and Lovell [9] have recently calculated the linear regression coefficient of logW on logH for the 50th percentile values of five major published sets of growth data of children. The average value was found to be 2.4 and the index W/H$^{2.4}$ was found to be independent of age and sex of the children, aged between 5 and 12 years.

Obesity can also be defined on the basis of more direct estimates of body fat (BF), *e.g.* through measurements of body weight and volume (V) or of total body potassium (TBK) and total body water (TBW), *i.e.*

$$BF = f' \ (W, V) \tag{1 a}$$
or $$BF = f'' \ (W, TBK, TBW) \tag{1 b}$$

Obesity can furthermore be defined in terms of measurements of the thickness of the layer of subcutaneous fat by skinfold measurements or soft tissue radiography or of other anthropometric parameters such as diameters and girths. The numbers obtained at various sites can be used directly or they can be combined in different ways.

It is clear that all these measurements show a relatively high degree of correlation. In fact, the statistical methods used to combine the measurements of skinfold, diameters and girths are based on the idea that the combination should predict, and thus correlate well with, other more direct estimates of body fat.

On the other hand, it is also clear that the different measurements cannot *a priori* be expected to express the same biological property. The standard error of estimate of the predicted body fat on the basis of measurements of body weight, height and age is a high as 15 - 20% in subjects from a nearly random sample and it is not much less when other anthropometric measures are included [32,6]. Part of the error must be due to random errors of the actual measurements, in particular V, TBK and TBW. Another part must be due to non-constancy of the parameters in the functions f' and f' in eqs. [1]. The remaining part is due to failure of the independent variables to estimate body fat, *i.e* to a variable body composition. Unfortunately, the partition of the errors is not known. Since obesity in human beings cannot *a priori* be considered to be a unique condition but, rather, several, one must entertain the possibility that the different measurements may correlate differently with the different conditions. This possibility has important implications because it means that the results of epidemiological studies on genetic factors and on relation to morbidity may well depend on the particular measurement chosen.

Heritability of Obesity in Humans

There is quite a high degree of familial aggregation in obesity, *i.e.* obesity runs in families. Foster infants of obese mothers are heavier than foster infants of normal weight mothers [35] and Griffiths and Payne [20] have made the interesting observation that non-obese 3-4 year old children of obese parents had an energy expenditure of some 22% less than that of matched children of non-obese parents.

Heritability studies of obesity aim at quantifying the relative importance of heredity and environment. The methodology consists in comparing the similarity in obesity of subjects with given genetic relationships.

There are several studies on twins in which the intra-pair variance of obesity indices in monozygotic pairs has been compared to the variance in dizygotic pairs, all pairs raised together. Obviously, if the monozygotic intra-pair variance is smaller than that of the dizygotic intra-pair variance, a certain degree of heritability may be inferred. The results of such studies [3.33] show that there is some evidence for a genetic influence on some of the induces of obesity but not for others and that the difference in intra-pair variance varies with sex and age.

There are also several studies on the correlation of obesity indices between parents and biological children and between parents and adopted children. Withers [41] and Biron, Mongeau and Berthrand [2] found the correlation to be higher for the biological pairs, but Garn, Bailes and Higgins [18] found no consistent differences. Hartz, Giefer and Rimm [21] carried out a very large study including 546 children not related to other children in the same family and 25554 children biologically related to all children in the same family. The measure of obesity was percentage overweight for given height, sex and age. The data were interpreted in terms of a simple model assuming that the total phenotypic variation, var (P), of the quantity is the sum of the variance due to heredity, var (H), the environment, var (E), and a component, var (E), unexplained by the other two. The heritability index, h^2, calculated in this model as the ratio of var (H)/var (P) was found to be quite small, 0.12, and not significant at the 0.05 level.

Estimation of heritability from the kinds of studies referred to above is very difficult. One major problem is that there are usually several different plausible models for partioning of the variance and it is extremely difficult to arbitrate on the merits of the different models which, applied to the same raw data, may give widely different results. The problems have recently been discussed in several papers by the Birmingham group [10, 11, 12, 17, 24, 29].

Another, and possibly more serious, problem relates to the fact that the models used for data reduction and inference assume, as they must that the variable that is investigated is an expression of one and the same biological entity. This is a rather bold assumption when it comes to the phenomenon of obesity in humans. When the problem is one of investigating the biochemical and physiological background for developing and mantaining obesity, an assumption of uniformity in cause may well be productive, but his is not the situation when it comes to investigating heritability. In fact, as long as our knowledge of obesity in humans is as superficial as it is, I would be hesitant to advise anyone to embark upon heritability studies.

Inherited Obesity in Laboratory Animals

Obesity can be inherited in many laboratory animals, particularly in rodents. Reviews on the subject are found in the papers by Bray and York [4, 5] and in a recent volume edited by Festing [13].

Obesity in laboratory animals has been classified in different ways. Festing [14] has suggested that the primary, and most important, distinction between different types should be between obesity inherited as a simple Mendelian gene and obesity inherited as a polygenic character.

Obesity is inherited in a single Mendelian manner in a number of mutants of mice and rats, e.g. the diabetes (db), the fat (fat) and the obese (ob) mouse and the fatty (fa) rat. In these cases, the obesity arises as a result of a point mutation. So far it has not been possible to detect the primary lesion in any of the mutants. The mentioned examples are those which have been most extensively studied with respect to the mechanisms of the disturbed energy balance.

Obesity may also be inherited as a polygenic character. In such cases, obesity arises as a result of having an extreme array of genes that determines factors such as growth rate, appetite, metabolic rate, physical activity and social reactivity. There is probably no single genetic lesion. The mode of inheritance is difficult to disentangle and environmental influences are generally strong. A number of inbred strains and F_1 hybrids of the mouse belong to this category and obesity with polygenic characteristics, has also been found on other rodents. This type of obesity has not been studied extensively with respect to energy balance.

There is a plethora of data on morphological, biochemical and physiological characteristics of obese rodents. The relevance of much of the data to the question of the mechanism responsible for the development and maintenance of obesity is, however, not clear; obesity as such, must be assumed to induce secondary changes in many systems of the body.

Characteristics of the Energy Balance in the obese (ob/ob) mouse

There has been a considerable increase, over the past 5 years, in the knowledge of how some rodents regulate their energy stores. It is now known that brown adipose tissue in many rodents has quantitatively a very significant capacity to dissipate chemical energy directly to heat [15, 16, 37], and that the mechanism of dissipation is an activation of a "shortcircuit" proton-conductance pathway in the mitochondria of this tissue [30, 31]. It has furthermore been established that cold [8, 15] and increased food intake [34] activates the dissipation and that a single meal increases the *in vitro* oxygen consumption of brown fat by almost three times [19].

Application of this new knowledge to the problems of the *ob/ob* mouse has established the following fact: the *ob/ob* mouse has a lower body temperature, about 2°C, over a wide range of environmental temperature [39]. Excess energy begins to accumulate from about 12 days of age [38] but food intake up to 4 weeks of age does not seem to be larger than in the lean siblings [7]. Hyperphagia is, however, a consistent feature in the later development. Indirect measurements of the activity of the proton-conductuance pathway in brown fat have shown that it is reduced [4] and that it does not show the normal increase on exposure to cold [22] or to increased food intake [40]. The noradrenaline turnover of brown adipose tissue is smaller than in lean siblings [27], an observation that may be taken as evidence for a lower sympathetic activity in the organ.

A Model for the Development and Maintenance of Obesity on the ob/ob mouse

The observations referred to above have naturally generated speculations about the primary defect in the *ob/ob* mouse. So far, however, no working hypothesis involving only a single defect has been suggested. I will propose one here, mainly because I want to illustrate a method of approach that appears to be helpful.

Figure 1 is a schematic diagram to illustrate the energy flows in a energy transforming system whose function it is to maintain a non-equilibrium situation with respect to differences in generalized potentials, $\triangle \pi_i$ (chemical potentials, electrical potentials, pressures, etc.), and with respect to the temperature in the system, T, the latter being assumed to be higher than that of the environment. The system receives a flux of chemical energy, $J^I {}_{ch.en.}$, but, for simplicity, it performs no external work. A fraction of the chemical energy flux, $f_2 . J^I {}_{ch.en.}$, is transformed directly into heat, $J^I{}_q$, by the element with the transfer function f_2, *e.g.* brown adipose tissue. THe remaining fraction, $f_1 J^I {}_{ch.en.} = J^{II} {}_{ch.en}$, is used in transporting (per unit time) extensive quantities, $\triangle \pi_i$, (moles of chemical species, charge, volume, etc.) against the conjugated potential differences $\triangle \pi_i$. To simplify the analysis, without violating principles, we assume that the coupling between chemical energy fluxes and generalized transport takes place without losses so that $J^{II} {}_{ch. en} = \Sigma \triangle k_i \triangle \pi_i$. Relaxation of the transport work

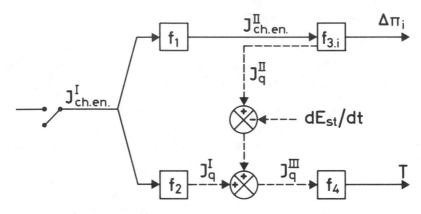

Figure 1. Illustration of an energy tranforming system whose function it is to maintain generalized potential differences $\triangle \pi_i = 0$ and a temperature T which is larger than the environment temperature. A fraction f_2 of the chemical energy flux J^I ch. en. is tranformed directly into heat J^I q. The remaining fraction J^{II} ch. en. performs work of different kinds to produce generalized potentials differences $\triangle \pi_i$. Relaxation of the work produces heat J^{II} q. The sum of the heat fluxes generates the temperature T, whose mgnitude depends on the heat conductance of the system boundaries. For details, see text.

takes place by the transport fluxes K_i'' in the opposite ("downward") direction with a dissipation of energy as heat, $J^{II}_q = \Sigma \triangle k_i'' \triangle \pi_i$. The relation between the input of chemical energy and the resulting potential differences is described by the transfer functions $f_{3,\ i}$, *i.e.* They are essentially flux resistances to relaxation of potential differences. The energy stored (or lost), dE st/dt, is equal to the difference in energy between the two transport fluxes and, in the steady state where $\triangle K_i' = \triangle K''_i$ (and d$\triangle \pi_i$/dt = 0), the total heat production, J^{III}_q, is equal to J^I ch, en,. The temperature of the system is obtained as the product of the heat production and the transfer function f_4; the latter is essentially a resistance to the heat flow across the system boundaries.

The system in Figure I will produce and maintain states with non-zero potential differences $\triangle \pi_i$ and a body temperature higher than the environment. However, in order to minimize effects of variations in the influx of energy and in the environmental temperature, there is a need for feed-back. Figure 2 illustrates the system with feed-back from the regulated quantities, $\triangle \pi_i$ and T. The temperature is sensed and feeds back (loop 1) to the transfer function f_4, for example by sympathetic nerve impulses to cutaneous blood vessels. The temperature also feeds back to the transfer function f_2 (loop 2) *i.e.* to brown adipose tissue, and finally to the influx of chemical energy (loop 3). One or several of the potential differences $\triangle \pi_i$ feed back to the transfer functions $F_{3,i}$ by loop 4, to influence the rate of the "downward" fluxes *e.g.* cation fluxes or peptide bond cleavage. Feed-back to brown adipose tissue takes place through loop 5 and to the intake of chemical energy through loop 6.

There are good reasons to believe that the generation and transmission of information to brown adipose tissue and to cutaneous blood vessels have com-

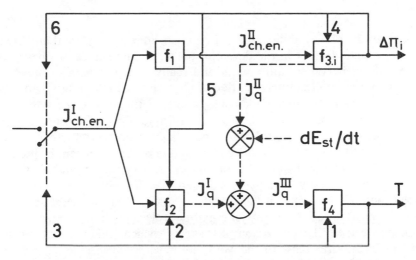

Figure 2. Illustration of the system in figure 1 with added feedback loops.

mon elements, *i.e.* those of noradrenergic nerve transmission. The observations on the *ob/ob* mouse can then be explained by assuming that one of these elements in defective such that loops 1, 2 and 5 are ineffective. A defect in the capacity of the cutaneous blood vessels to constrict will lead to a higher than normal heat loss and to subnormal body temperature. This will lead to a higher food intake since loop 3 is supposed to work normally. The increased food intake, which can normally be dissipated as heat through loops 4 an 5, can now only be dissipated throgh loop 4 and the capacity of the dissipating elements $f_{3,i}$ is overloaded. This leads to accumulation of energy, *e.g.* fat (which may be the least dangerous way to accumulate energy), and, in the struggle to maintain both a normal body temperature and a normal body weight, there is a compromise such that both become abnormal.

Observations in Man

The observations on the role of brown adipose tissue in rodents and the defect functioning of this tissue in the *ob/ob* mouse have led to several interesting observations in humans. Rothwell and Stock [34, see also 23] have observed, by thermography, an increase in the temperature over the back after stimulation with a sympathomimetric drug. Infusion of noradrenaline leads to an increase in oxygen consumption in normal subjects but this increase is much less in obese women [25, 26]. The postprandial increase in the heat output appears to be smaller in obese subjects [see 23]. All these observations show that there are heat dissipation mechanisms in humans which are different in obese subjects. Whether or not they are of quantitative importance for the development and maintenance of obesity in man remains to be studied.

Future Work

The results of heritability studies in human subjects indicate that there may well be genetic factors in the development and maintenance of obesity. This statement is, if course, quite weak and really does not help us very much.

Perhaps the simplest interpretation of the results is that obesity is an expression of several different genetic backgrounds, with some of the states having no heritability at all. Dr. Phillip James in Cambridge has recently suggested that the assumption of several states of obesity is counterproductive. Although I agree with this point of view in general, and in particular when the problem is to formulate working hypotheses with respect to biochemical and physiological mechanisms of obesity, it must be admitted that the assumption does give one explanation for the results of the heritability studies. In any case, it appears that work on mechanisms must play an important role in the future. Such work will hopefully lead to characterization of "defects" which, although not necessarily primary in the strict sense of the word, are much more specific than just overweight and sking fold thickness. The stage will then be open for new studies on heritability.

ACKNOWLEDGEMENTS

I am indebted to Mr. E. Steen Hansen, M. Sc., for hepful discussions of the proposed model.

REFERENCES

1. Benn, R.T. Some mathematical properties of weight-for-height indices used as a measure of adiposity. *Br. J. Prev. Soc. Med.* 25: 42, 1971.
2. Biron, P., Mongeau, J. G., and Bertrand, D. Familial resemblance of body weight/height in 374 homes with adopted children. *J. Ped.* 91: 555, 1977.
3. Borjesson, M. The aetiology of obesity in children. *Acta Ped. Scand.* 65: 279, 1976.
4. Bray, G.A. an York, D.A. Genetically transmitted obesity in rodents. *Physiol. Rev.* 51: 598, 1971.
5. Bray, G.A. and York, D.A. Hypothalamic and genetic obesity in experimental animals: An autonomic and endocrine hypothesis. *Physiol. Rev.* 59: 719, 1979.
6. Bruce, A., Anderson, M., Arvidsson, B. and Isaksson, B. Body composition. Prediction of normal potassium, body water and body fat in adults on the basis of body height body weight and age. *Scand. J. Clin. Lab. Invest.* 40: 461, 1980.
7. Contaldo, F., Gerber, H., Coward, W.A. and Trayhurn, P. in Obesity: Pathogenesis and Treatment (Enzi, G., Crepaldi, G., Pozza, G. and Renold, A.E., eds.) pp. 319-322. Academic, London, 1981.
8. Desautels, M., Zaror-Behrens, G. and Himmis-Hagen, J. Increased nucleotide binding, altered polypeptide composition, and thermogenesis in brown adipose tissue mitochondria of cold-acclimated rats. *Can. J. Biochem.* 56: 378, 1978.
9. Dugdale, A.E. and Lovell, S. Measuring childhood obesity. *The Lancet* II: 1224, 1981.
10. Eaves, L.J., Last, K.A., Martin, N.G. and Jinks, J.L. A progressive approach to nonadditivity and genotype-environmental covariance in the analysis of human differences. *Br. J. Math. Stat. Psychol.* 30: 1, 1977.

11. Eaves, L.J., Last, K.A., Young, P.A. and Martin, N.G. Model fitting approaches to analysis of human behaviour. *Heredity* 41: 149, 1978.

12. Eaves, L.J. Twins as a basis for the causal analysis of human personality. *In* "Twin Research" (W.E. Nance, G. Allen and P. Parisi, eds.), pp. 151-174. A.R. Liss, New York, 1978.

13. Festing, M.F.W. "Animal Models of Obesity" (M.F.W. Festing, ed.), MacMillan Press Ltd., London and Basingstoke, 1979.

14. Festing, M.F.W. The inheritance of obesity in animal models of obesity. *In* "Animal Models of Obesity" (M.F.W. Festing, ed.), pp. 15-37. MacMillan Press Ltd., London and Basingstoke, 1979.

15. Foster, D.O. and Frydman, M.L. Nonshivering thermogenesis in the rat. II: Measurements of blood flow with microspheres point to brown adipose tissue as the dominant site of the calorigenesis induced by noradrenaline. *Can. J. Physiol. Pharmacol.* 56: 110, 1978.

16. Foster, D.O. and Frydman, M.L. Tissue distribution of cold-induced thermogenesis in conscious warm abd cold-acclimated rats re-evaluated from changes in tissue blood flow: the dominant role of brown adipose tissue in the replacement of shivering by nonshivering thermogenesis. *Can. J. Physiol Pharmacol.* 57: 257, 1979.

17. Fulker, D.W. Multivariate extensions of a biometrical model of twin data. *In* "Twin Research" (W.E. Nance, G. Allen and P. Parisi, eds.), pp. 217-236. A.R. Liss, New York, 1978.

18. Garn, S.M., Bailes, S.M. and Higgins, J.T.T. Fatness similarities in adopted pairs. *Am. J. Clin. Nutr.* 29: 1067, 1976.

19. Glick, Z., Teague, R.J and Bray, G.A. Brown adipose tissue: Thermic response increased by a single low protein, high carbohydrate meal. *Science* 213: 1125, 1981.

20. Griffiths, M. and Payne, P.R. Energy expenditurre in small children of obese and nonobese parents. *Nature* 260: 698, 1976.

21. Hartz, A., Giefer, E. and Rimm, A.A. Relative importance of the effect of family environment and heredity on obesity. *Ann. Hum. Genet., Lond.* 41: 185, 1977.

22. Himms-Hagen, J. and Desautels, M. A Mitochondrial defect in brown adipose tissue of the obese *(ob/ob)* mouse: reduced binding of purine nucleotides and failure to respond to cold by an increased binding. *Biochem. Biophys. Res. Common.* 83: 628, 1978.

23. James, W.P.T. and Trayhurn, P. Obesity in Mice and Men. *In* "Nutritional Factors: Modulating Effects on Metabolic Processes" (R.F. Beers and E.G. Bassett, eds.), pp. 123-138, Raven Press, New York, 1981.

24. Jinks, J.L. and Fulker, D.W. Comparison of the biometrical, genetical, MAVA, and classical approaches to the analysis of human behaviour. *Psycol. Bull.* 73: 311, 1970.

25. Jung, R.T., Shetty, P.S., James, W.P.T., Barrand, M. and Callingham, B.A. Reduced thermogenesis in obesity. *Nature* 279: 322, 1979.

26. Jung, R.T., Shetty, P.S. and James, W.P.T. Heparin, free fatty acids and an increased metabolic demand for oxygen. *Postgrad. Med. J.* 56: 330, 1980.

27. Knehaus, A.W. and Romsos, D.R. Reduced norepinephrine turnover in brown adipose. tissue of *ob/ob* mice. *Am. J. Physiol.* 242: E253, 1982.

28. Lee, J., Kolonel, L.N. and Hinds, M.W. Relative merits of the weight-correscted-for-height indices. *Am. J. Clin. Nutr.* 34: 2521, 1981.

29. Martin, N.G., Eaves, L.J., Kearsay, M.J. and Davies, P. The power of the classical twin method. *Heredity* 40: 97, 1978.

30. Nicholls, D.G. Hamster brown-adipose-tissue mitochondria: purine nucleotide control of the ion conductance of the inner membrane, the nature of the nucleotide binding site. *Eur. J. Biochem.* 62: 223, 1976.

31. Nicholls, D.G. Brown adipose tissue mitochondria. *Biochem. Biophys. Acta.* 549: 1, 1979.

32. Noppa, H., Andersson, M., Bengtsson, C., Bruce, A. and Isaksson, B. Body composition in middle-aged women with special reference to the correlation between body fat mass on autheopometric data. *Am.J. Chin. Nutr.* 32: 1388, 1979.

33. Osborne, R.H. and DeGeorge, F.V. Stature, weight and ponderal index. *In* "Genetic Basis of morphological Variation", pp. 60-75. Harvard University Press, Cambridge, Mass., 1959.

34. Rothwell, N.J. and Stock, M.J. A role for brown adipose tissue in diet-induced thermogenesis. *Nature* 281: 31, 1979.
35. Shenker, J.R., Fisichelli, V. and Lange, J. Weight differences between foster infants and overweight and nonoverweight foster mothers, brief clinical and laboratory observation. *J. Pediat.* 84: 715, 1974.
36. The Royal College of Physicians Working Party on Obesity.
37. Thurlby, P.L. and Trayhurn, P. Regional blood flow in genetically obese *(ob/ob)* mice: The importance of brown adipose tissue ot the reduced energy expenditure of nonshivering thermogenesis. *Pflügers Arch.* 385: 193, 1980.
38. Thurlby, P.Ll and Trayhurn, P. The development of obesity in preweanling ob/on mice. *Br. J. Nutr.* 39: 397, 1978.
39. Trayhurn, P. and James, W.P.T. Thermoregulation and nonshivering thermogenesis in the genetically obese *(ob/ob)* mouse. *Pflügers Arch.* 373: 189, 1978.
40. Trayhuurn, P., Jones, P.M., McGuckin, M.M. and Goodboody, A.E. Effect of overfeeding on energy balance and brown fat thermogenesis in obese *ob/ob* mice. *Nature* 295: 323, 1982.
41. Withers, R.F.J. Problems in the genetics of human obesity. *Eugen. Rev.* 56: 81, 1964.

METABOLIC EFFICIENCY IN MUTANT MICE

Douglas L. Coleman*

The Jackson Laboratory
Bar Harbor, Maine

INTRODUCTION

Several different single gene mutations are known to cause similar diabetes and obesity syndromes in mice [8, 9]. Our studies with two mutations, obese (*ob*) and diabetes (*db*), have shown that the severity of the diabetes depends not only on the mutant gene itself but also on the interaction of the mutant gene with modifying genes in the host inbred background [5, 12, 19]. Thus on the C57BL/6J (BL/6) inbred background, both mutations produce a massive obesity with few diabetes symptoms, whereas on the C57BL/KsJ (BL/Ks) background, both mutations produce a severe and life-shortening diabetes as well as obesity. The development of severe obesity, rather than severe diabetes, appears to be related to the ability of the host to expand insulin supply sufficiently rapidly to maintain normal blood sugar concentrations [5, 8, 9].

The early events that occur in each mutant as the syndrome develops are similar. These include hyperphagia, hyperinsulinemia, and attempts to increase insulin supply by beta cell hypertrophy and hyperplasia. Hyperglycemia, obesity, and severe diabetes are secondary features that result from insulin resistance and the ability, or inability, of the host to sustain increased insulin secretion. Severe obesity, hyperinsulinemia, islet hypertrophy and hyperplasia characterize both the obese (*ob*) and diabetes (*db*) mutations maintained on the BL/6 background, whereas, on the BL/Ks background, islet hyperplasia and insulin supply cannot be sustained. Instead, beta cell necrosis occurs culminating in relative insulinopenia, and severe diabetes. Our studies suggest that different

This research was supported in part by research grants AM 14461 and AM 20725 from the National Institute of Arthritis, Diabetes, Digestive and Kidney Diseases. The Jackson Laboratory is fully accredited by the American Association for the Accreditation of Laboratory Animal Care.

genetic defects in both mutants lead to a hyperactive hypothalamus which triggers an excessive release of pancreatic insulin in response to normal stimuli [5, 11, 13]. Thus, hyperinsulinemia occurs even when mutants are restricted to the amount of food eaten by normal mice and or feeding, *ad libitum,* hiperphagia leads to still greater secretion of insulin, insulin resistance, more overeating, and further stimulation of insulin secretion. This vicious cycle is typical of the early stages of disease development in both mutants maintained on either background. Ultimately, either severe diabetes, or severe obesity with well-compensated diabetes occurs, depending upon the genetic background of the host. Establishing the nature of these obese gene-host interactions that control susceptibility or resistance to severe diabetes in mice should aid in our understanding of similar interactions that may occur in human diabetes.

The obese (*ob*) and diabetes (*db*) mutations in the mouse have been used extensively in studies involving perturbations in energy balance associated with obesity. Both mutants have the ability to become obese even when calories are severely restricted [1, 5, 8, 14, 25, 28]. Hyperphagia is not a prerequisite to obesity in these models, since mutants gain normal amounts of weight while depositing abnormal amounts of fat even when restricted to 50% of the amount of food eaten by normal mice [5, 20]. Several mechanisms have been proposed to explain this remarkable increase in metabolic efficiency exhibited by the mutants. A major saving of energy associated with the metabolism of both the obese and diabetes mutants could result from a defect in thermoregulatory thermogenesis [25 to 29]. At ambient environmental temperatures, the body temperature of the mutants remains lower than normal, and when exposed to the cold (4°), the obese mutants rapidly become hypothermic and die within a few hours [15, 22, 29]. An observed increased metabolic rate in obese mice adapted to 10° [27] and our observation [10] that such adapted mice will survive maintenance at 4° suggests that the defect in thermoregulatory thermogenesis is only partial. Even so, any defect in cold-induced nonshivering thermogenesis could contribute to increased metabolic efficiency by diverting those calories normally used to produce heat.

Efficiency studies

Feeding of either the obese or diabetes mutants exactly that amount of food normally eaten by a lean (+ / +) mouse still permitted an additional weight gain of 1-2 g in the mutant. Most of this additional weight gain was reflected in increased depot stores of adipose tissue [1, 14]. In attempts to quantify this increased metabolic efficiency associated with obesity mutants, we fed mutants the identical amounts of food on the same time schedule as normal mice [5, 8, 10]. This procedure effectively eliminated the stuff-starve regimen which, in itself, can lead to obesity. This schedule was accomplished by training a normal mouse to press a bar to obtain a single 20 mg pellet of food and yoking this system to food dispensers in cages in which the mutants were housed. Under these conditions, all mutants obtained their food in the amount and the schedule determined by the normal mouse. Even with this degree of control over the food intake, the mutants over a 4 week period still gained 1-2 g of weight than did normal mice (Table I, and see also ref. 5, 8 10). Carcass analysis demonstrated that most of this weight increment in the food restricted mutant consisted of lipid (Table I). When restricted further, to 2/3 or even 1/2 of the amount eaten by a normal mouse, weight gain remained either normal or only slightly below normal (lines 4 and 5, Table I) and the obese body composition was still retained. In order to assess the role of restricted feeding on the development of diabetes, pairfeeding at the 50% of normal was continued for periods up to 5 months using the mutants maintained on the BL/Ks background that typically become severely diabetic [10, 20]. Most mutants survived this prolonged period of severe food restriction and maintained average body weight only slightly lower than the normal controls (Fig. 1a.) Blood sugar concentrations of mutants rose gradually from 180 to over 300 mg/dl by 2 months (Fig. 1b). Other diabetes symptoms, glycosuria, polyuria and polydipsia occurred in the usual time sequence. On termination of the experiment, carcass analysis established that mutants defended the obese body composition in spite of the prolonged periods of extreme food restriction. Histological examination of the pancreas revealed islet atrophy similar to that observed in BL/Ks mutants fed *ad libitum*. These studies established that hyperphagia, although a major contributory factor to the rapid rate and amount of fat accretion, is not essential for the development of either obesity or diabetes. Other studies [20] indicate that it is the amount and type of carbohydrates fed rather than the total food intake that leads to the rapid development of the diabetes. Even severe underfeeding did not prevent this abnormal diversion of energy (food) into lipid deposition. This marked increase in efficiency in the utilization of energy

TABLE I. *Body weight and body fat on various feeding schedules*

| | Starting | Weight after 4 weeks | | Percent fat | |
Genotype	weight	Fed ab lib	Pair-fed	Ad lib	Pair-fed
1. BL/Ks - + / +	14.9g	26.1g (11.5)[1]	21.4g (6.8)	19.1	14.9
2. BL/Ks-ob/ob	17.0g	38.6g (21.6)	25.6g (8.6)	42.3	43.7
3. BL/Ks-db/db	16.8g	38.2g (21.4)	24.3g (7.5)	36.8	43.7
4. BL/Ks-db/db[2]	15.3g	—	26.2g (10.9)	—	47.4
5. BL/Ks-db/dab[3]	25.5g	—	24.3g (-1.2)	—	37.0

[1]Figures represent average obtained from 4 mice in each group. Weight gain per 4 week period is in parenthesis.
[2]Fed 2/3 the amount of food eaten by normal on same schedule.
[3]Fed 1/2 the amount of food on same schedule.
Reprinted from table 3, Coleman 1981 with permission of the author and Alan R. Liss Publisher.

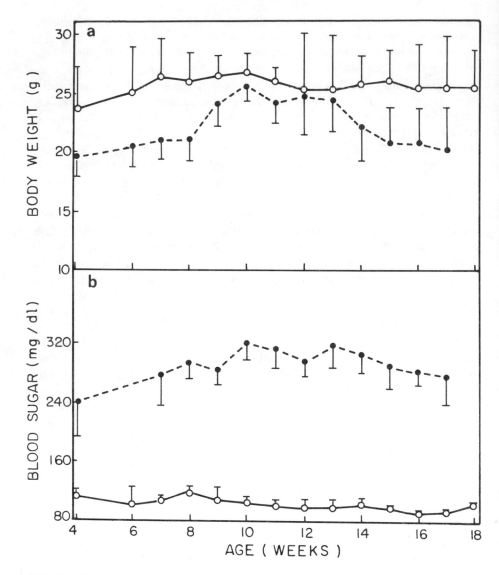

FIG. 1. Effect of long term diet restriction (50% of calories) on body weight and blood glucose. Values represent mean ± SEM. Operant males (+ / +) 0—0, restricted mutants (db/db), •—•. Body weight differences between genotypes are not significant, blood glucose differences are significant (P < 0.01). Fig. 1 from Leiter et al., 1981, with permission of the author and Metabolism.

occurring as a result of a spontaneous mutation becomes a liability under laboratory conditions where food is available *ad libitum*, but a similar change (in the wild) could be advantageous by increasing potential survival time during periods of prolonged food deprivation [4, 23].

Thermoregulation

If mutants were unable to thermoregulate, the calories normally used for thermoregulation could be diverted to fat synthesis and would be seen as an increase in metabolic efficiency. In attempts to quantify the contribution made by any defect in thermoregulation to the increased metabolic efficiency, we undertook pair-feeding studies at a thermoneutral temperature [10]. When maintained at thermoneutrality (33°), the normal (operant) mouse would consume sufficient energy only for maintenance, and none for thermoregulation. This mouse when yoked to our operant feeding device would then provide mutants only that amount of food required for maintenance and the mutants should maintain a rate of weight gain similar, if not identical, to the control mice. Daily food intake of the normal operant mouse decreased to 175 pellets at 33° (67% of normal consumption) from an average of 280 pellets at 23°. This established that 33% of the food intake of the normal mouse was required for thermogenesis [10]. Thus, pair-feeding at thermoneutrality effectively restricted the food intake of the mutant mice to 67% of the normal food intake of a mouse maintained at 23°. The additional weight gain attained in mutants pair-fed at thermoneutrality was similar, if not identical, to that seen in mutants restricted conventionally to 67% of the normal food intake. Both studies suggest that with either restriction regimen, 67% of normal food intake is sufficient to allow excess weight gain in mutants. These data strongly suggest that the energy required by the normal for thermoregulation (33%) was not sufficient to account for the increased metabolic efficiency in obese mutants [10].

Obese and diabetic mutants maintained in a thermoneutral environment (33°) decreased food consumption in amounts (33%) similar to normal mice. This demonstrated that mutants, as well as normal mice, decrease food consumption proportionately, and in a normal fashion, in response to temperature increases. Further, when placed in a colder environment (10°) both normal and mutant mice made consistent and similar increases in food consumption, again suggesting that mutants were increasing their food consumption in response to decreases in ambient temperature to meet the additional requirements for thermoregulation [10].

Mutants pair-fed to normal mice maintained at 33°, would only be provided sufficient food for maintenance, exclusive of any energy normally used for thermoregulation. Under these conditions mutants still gained more weight in 2 weeks than normal mice [10]. This observation demonstrates that even when deprived of the specific amount of food required by a normal mouse for thermogenesis, the food is not sufficient to correct the abnormal weight gain typical of mutants. This increased weight gain relative to normal mice, even when pair-fed at thermoneutrality suggests that any defect in thermogenesis in mutants makes only a minor contribution to increased metabolic efficiency.

In our studies, mutant mice maintained at ambient temperature had core temperatures (deep rectal) slightly, but not significantly, less than normal mice [10]. Upon cold exposure (4°) the temperature of normal mice decreased to a nadir of 32° and then returned to normal by 24 to 36 hr. In contrast, rectal temperatures of mutants maintained at 4° continued to fall and the mutants failed to survive 24 hr of exposure. However, if mutant mice were cold adapted for 2 days at 10° before exposure to 4°, all mutants survived and maintained near normal body temperatures. Maintenance of the body temperature at less than one degree below normal even in these extreme circumstances would not spare much energy. The failure to survive when abruptly exposed to temperatures of 4° supports the observation that both obese mutants are defective with respect to some acute response required to maintain body temperature [17, 18]. However, when cold adapted in a gradual fashion, secondary adaptive mechanisms must occur that increase heat production sufficiently to permit survival.

DISCUSSION

The data on food consumption by normal mice and both mutants raised at different environmental temperatures are consistent with the suggestion that both obesity mutants have a near normal energy requirement for thermoregulation. All mice (both mutants and normal) decreased food intake by about 33% when ambient temperatures were increased from 23° to thermoneutrality (33°C). When ambient temperatures were decreased, all mice increased their food consumption proportionately, again suggesting that equivalent amounts of energy were being used for heat production in mice of all genotypes. Apparently, mutants are capable of modifying food intake in a normal fashion to compensate for changing energy requirements.

Our data demonstrate that although both obesity mutants may have minor deficits in some specific aspects of thermogenesis, both mutants can increase thermogenesis sufficient to maintain body temperatures near normal even when maintained at 4° and the failure to thermoregulate is only partial. This defect (very minor under most laboratory conditions) would not contribute greatly to the large increase in metabolic efficiency observed in both mutants. Other possible energy saving mechanisms must be considered.

Under some environmental conditions obese and diabetes mutants were found to have a lower basal activity of the enzyme Na^+, K^+-ATPase and the basal activity was not induced in response to thyroid hormone as it is in normal mice [2, 21]. Na^+, K^+-ATPase is a component of the cell membrane that controls ion flux and, if operating rapidly could utilize considerable energy.

Any energy saved by decreased activity of this ATPase could be diverted to energy storage and would be seen as an increased metabolic efficiency. The continuous cycling of this ATPase in muscle has been suggested as a possible source of heat for the maintenance of body temperature [2]. A reduced activity of this ATPase could explain a lower metabolic rate and a lesser contribution to maintaining body temperature. Recent evidence suggests that the operation of this ATPase in muscle probably does not contribute significantly to body heat production. Present studies indicate that brown adipose tissue (BAT) in rodents is the primary tissue involved in nonshivering thermogenesis [16, 26]. It has been shown that mitochondria from the BAT of obese mice on acute exposure to the cold fail to increase the binding of purine nucleotides as do normal mice. Other than this defect, obese mutants can make all other appropriate secondary responses required for survival in the cold [17, 18]. My data suggest that the necessity for this acute adaptive response can be circumvented if cold exposure at 10° for as little as 24 hr precedes the exposure to 4°. Under extreme environmental conditions, mutant mice were able to compensate normally by increasing or decreasing the amount of energy required for body temperature maintenance.

All of the obesity mutants are grossly hyperinsulinemic. Severe hyperinsulinemia should favor anabolic processes and promote the synthesis of body constituents while inhibiting degradation. Normal metabolism involves the continuous breakdown and synthesis of body constituents. Much energy is consumed in both synthesis and degradation. In the hyperinsulinemic mutant the normal synthesis-degradation cycles could be shifted toward increased synthesis and reduced degradation. The saving of energy that would occur by the elimination of these normal metabolic cycles could be reflected in food restricted mutants as an increase in metabolic efficiency. Further, it may be that the hyperinsulinemia of mutants is antagonistic to the actions of a variety of catabolic hormones, especially glucagon and catecholamines. Such an antagonistic action could be indirectly responsible for the lack of norepinephrine initiated response in turning on both cold and diet-induced thermogenesis [3, 18, 24]. More critical studies, in vivo, are needed on the relative rates of all types of normal cycling in both mutant and normal mice before the individual contributions of each mechanism to the energy efficiency can be established.

Although the nature of each potential energy saving metabolic change has yet to be established, it is apparent that the spontaneously obese laboratory mutants may have similar, if not identical, metabolic changes brought about by mutation, as do a variety of desert rodents that have evolved by natural selection. Hyperphagia associated with more efficient ways of storing and utilizing energy would be beneficial when food is scarce. These same attributes become liabilities when food is in abundance. Hyperphagia exacerbates the excess systemic demand for insulin and increased carbohydrate intake taxes the ability of the beta cells to sustain insulin supply. Either obesity or diabetes develops depending on the ability of the host to respond adequately. Primitive man, living in austere environments where periods of famine were interspersed with periods of plenty could have envolved multiple efficiency mechanisms by natural selection similar to those seen in desert rodents and to those that occurred in laboratory rodents by spontaneous mutation.

The association of increased metabolic efficiency in obesity-diabetes syndromes lends credence to the thrifty gene hypothesis regarding the maintenance of deleterious diabetes genes in human populations [23]. The demonstration that mice heterozygous for a diabetes producing gene have a survival advantage over homozygous normal mice provides a mechanism whereby the deleterious diabetes genes can persist and even increase in human populations [6, 7]. An understanding of the biochemical pathways that are modified in both heterozygotes and homozygotes would have far-reaching consequences in understanding the human disease. Studies on these modifying factors are simpler using mutants maintained on standard well-defined inbred backgrounds than in human populations where many genes are interacting to contribute, either positively or negatively, to metabolic efficiency.

REFERENCES

1. Alonso, L. C., Maren, T. H. Effect of food restriction on body composition of hereditary obese mice. *Am. J. Physiol.* 183:284, 1955.
2. Bray, G. A., York, D. A., and Yukimura, Y. Activity of Na^+, K^+,-ATPase in the liver of animals with experimental obesity. *Life Sci.* 22:1637, 1978.
3. Brooks, S. L., Rothwel, N. J., Stock, M. J., Goodbody, A. E., and Trayhurn, P. Decreased protein conductance pathway in brown adipose tissue mitochondria of rats exhibiting dietary-induced thermogenesis. *Nature* 286:274, 1980.
4. Coleman, D. L. Diabetes and obesity: thrifty mutants? *Nutrition Rev.* 36:129, 1978.
5. Coleman, D. L. Obese and diabetes: two mutant genes causing diabetes-obesity syndromes in mice. *Diabetologia* 14:141, 1978.
6. Coleman, D. L. Obesity genes: beneficial effects in heterozygous mice. *Science* 203:663, 1979.
7. Coleman, D. L. Acetone metabolism in mice: increased activity in mice heterozygous for obesity genes. *Proc. Natl. Acad. Sci.* 77:290, 1980.
8. Coleman, D. L. Inherited diabetes syndromes in the mouse. *In* "Progress in Clinical and Biological Research" vol 45. (E. S. Russell, ed.), pp 145-158. The Jackson Laboratory 50th Aniversary Symposium. Alan R. Liss. Inc., New York, 1981.
9. Coleman, D. L. Diabetes-obesity syndromes in mice. *Diabetes* 31:(suppl 1), 1, 1982.
10. Coleman, D. L. Thermogenesis in diabetes-obesity syndromes. *Diabetologia* 22:205, 1982.
11. Coleman, D. L. and Hummel, K. P. Effects of parabiosis of normal with genetically diabetic mice. *Am. J. Physiol.* 217:1298, 1969.
12. Coleman, D. L. and Hummel, K. P. The influence of genetic background on the expression of the obese (ob) gene in the mouse. *Diabetologia* 9:287, 1973.
13. Coleman, D. L. and Hummel, K. P. Effects of parabiosis of obese with diabetes and normal mice. *Diabetologia* 9:294, 1973.
14. Cox, J. E. and Powley, T. L. Development of obesity in mice pair-fed with lean siblings. *J. Comp. Physiol. Psychol.* 91:347, 1977.
15. Davis, T. R. A. and Mayer, J. Imperfect homeothermy in the hereditary obese hyperglycemia syndrome of mice. *Am. J. Physiol.* 228:276, 1954.

16. Foster, D. O. and Friedman, M. L. Nonshivering thermogenesis in the rat. II. Measurement of blood flow with microspheres point to brown adipose tissue as the dominant site of the calorigenesis induced by noradrenalin. *Can. J. Physiol. Pharmacol.* 56:110, 1978.

17. Himms-Hagen, J. and Desautels, M. A. mitochondrial defect in brown adipose tissue of the obese mouse: reduced binding of purine nucleotides and a failure to respond to cold by and increase in binding. *Biochem. Biophys. Res. Comm.* 83:628, 1978.

18. Hogan, S. and Himms-Hagen, J. Abnormal brown adipose tissue in obese *ob/ob* mice: response to cold. *Am. J. Physiol.* 239:E301, 1980.

19. Hummel, K. P., Coleman, D. L., and Lane P. W. The influence of genetic background on expression of mutations at the diabetes locus in the mouse. I. C57BL/KsJ and C57BL/6J strains. *Biochem. Genet.* 7:1, 1972.

20. Leiter, E. H., Coleman, D. L., Eisenstein, A. B., and Strack, I. Dietary control of pathogenesis in C57BL/KsJ diabetes (*db*) mice. *Metabolism* 30:554, 1981.

21: Lin, P. Y., Romsos, D. R., Akera, T., and Leveille, G. A. Na⁺, K⁺-ATPase enzyme units in skeletal muscle from lean and obese mice. *Biochem. Biophys. Res. Comm.* 80:398, 1978.

22. Lin, P. -Y., Romsos, D. R., Vander Tuig, J. C., and Leveille, G. A. Maintenance energy requirements, energy retention and heat production in young obese (*ob/ob*) and lean mice fed a high fat or high-carbohydrate diet. *J. Nutr.* 109:1143, 1979.

23. Neel, J. V. Diabetes mellitus, a thrifty genotype rendered detrimental by progress. *Am. J. Human. Genet.* 14:353, 1962.

24. Rothwell, N. J., Stock, M. J. A role for brown adipose tissue in diet-induced thermogenesis. *Nature* 281:31, 1979.

25. Thurlby, P. L. and Trayhurn, P. The role of thermoregulatory thermogenesis in the development of obesity in genetically obese (*ob/ob*) mice pair-fed with lean siblings. *Br. J. Nutr.* 42:377, 1979.

26. Thurlby, P. L. and Trayhurn, P. Regional blood flow in genetically obese (*ob/ob*) mice. The importance of brown adipose tissue to the reduced energy expenditure on non-shivering thermogenesis. *Pflügers Archiv.* 385:201, 1980.

27. Trayhurn, P. Thermoregulation in the diabetic-obese mouse (*db/db*) mouse: the role of nonsshivering thermogenesis in energy balance. *Pflügers Arch.* 380:227, 1978.

28. Trayhurn, P. and Fuller, L. The development of obesity in genetically diabetes-obese (*db/db*) mice pair-fed with lean siblings. The importance of thermoregulatory thermogenesis. *Diabetologia* 19:148, 1980.

29. Trayhurn, P. and James, W. P. T. Thermoregulation and nonshivering thermogenesis in the genetically obese (*ob/ob*) mouse. *Pflügers Arch.* 373:189, 1978.

DISCUSSION[1]

Bray asked Coleman whether in his experience, hyperphagia (defined as increased food intake relative to appropiate lean controls) is ever a necessary component in the development of obesity in animal models. Coleman stated that all the animal models he has studied will become obese without extra calories; a normal intake is sufficient. He thinks this also holds for the Pima indians who are more efficient on a lower intake of food.

[1]*Summary of the discussion prepared by H. Bourges*

Bray commented that he knows of no animal model —rats, mice, pigs,— in which, with proper controls, hyperphagia is required for development of obesity; however, for humans there is no data of value in this regard. Coleman expressed his opinion that once the "thrifty" mechanisms involved in obesity are understood and means to uncouple them are deviced, obese people will be able to live a normal life and eat normally instead of starving themselves continuously and unsuccessfully.

Rosenberg agreed that the obesity phenotype could not be included within the conditions with a major exogenous component.

OBESITY — LESSONS FROM EXPERIMENTAL MEDICINE

George A. Bray
and
Janis S. Fisler

Division of Diabetes and Clinical Nutrition
U.S.C. School of Medicine
Los Angeles, California

INTRODUCTION

The different types of obesity illustrate as clearly as anything the influence of environment and genetics. I have selected three different types of obesity to discuss in detail. However, before doing that, let me put the entire problem into perspective. Table I shows the types of obesity which can be classified primarily as environmental in origin, those which have a mixed basis and those which are primarily genetic. The clearest example of environmental influences is hypothalamic obesity [11]. Experimentally this can be produced by damaging the ventromedial hypothalamus in almost any species. Genetic factors have not yet been shown to be significant in this form of obesity. At the other extreme are the types of obesity which are transmitted as dominant or recessive traits. Dietary obesity, on the other hand, clearly displays the influence of both envi-

TABLE I. Obesity classified on an environmental-genetic continuum

Environmental	Mixed	Genetic
Hypothalamic	Dietary	Recessive
Endocrine	Sucrose	Dominant
Drug-induced	High Fat	Polygenic
Viral-induced	Cafeteria	Polygenic
	Physical Inactivity	

ronmental factors such as the type of diet or degree of physical activity which is available, and the fact that only genetic subtypes of rodents, and probably man are susceptible to dietary obesity. In the discussion which follows, I will begin with the hypothalamic obesity, then discuss the dietary obesities and end with a discussion of genetic obesity.

Hypothalamic Obesity

Historical Perspective. The history of hypothalamic obesity began with the publication of two classic clinical cases one described by Frolich [32] in 1901 and the other by Babinski [3] in 1900. The association of hypothalamic disease and the development of hyperphagia has been studied periodically and has been reviewed a number of times during the past eighty years. A detailed clinical and physiological review of the findings in human begins with this syndrome was published in 1975 (II).

In spite of important clinical observations, the major impetus to study of hypothalamic obesity arose from experimental animals. In 1927, Smith noted that removal of the pituitary as compared to injury of the lower hypothalamus produced different syndromes. When obesity was produced by injecting chronic acid into the hypothalamus, symptoms of hypopituitarism were not seen. However, hypophysectomy without injury to the hypothalamus produced a picture of hypopituitarism with end-organ atrophy [101].

The next major advance in the study of hypothalamic obesity occurred with the demonstration that stereotaxic ventromedial hypothalamic lesions produced electrolytically were associated with obesity [42]. Several years following this discovery, Anand and Brobeck reported that injury to the lateral hypothalamus produced aphagia [1]. On the basis of these observations, Stellar proposed a "dual center hipothesis" to explain the functional relationship of these two areas [108]. This hypothesis served as the intellectual framework for 20 years of studies on the syndrome of hypothalamic obesity. The dual center hypothesis suggested that the ventromedial hypothalamus was a satiety area and that the lateral hypothalamus was a primary feeding center. Several observations made this simple hypothesis inadequate [5, 15]. First the demonstration that hyperphagia was not needed to produce obesity after hypothalamic injury was shown with both weanling rats [108] and in tube fed animals [39]. In addition, neuroanatomic studies revealed that the "dual centers" were involved with fibers running in the rostro-caudal direction, with little suggestion that important fibers ran between the ventromedial and lateral hypothalamic areas [119]. Finally, the demonstration that function of the automatic nervous system changed significantly after ventromedial or lateral hypothalamic injury, led to two new hypotheses, 1) the autonomic hypothesis by Bray and York [15] and by Inoue and Bray [47] and 2) the cephalic phase hypothesis proposed by Powley [87].

Vagus Nerve. One of the key experiments leading to the concept that neural control of the pancreatic beta-cells plays a primary role in the development of this syndrome, were the experiments with islet transplants reported by Inoue, Bray and Mullen [49, 50]. In these studies rats were made diabetic by injecting streptozocin. After diabetes was fully developed, the animals received transplants of fetal pancreatic tissue placed beneath the renal capsule. After recovery from the diabetes, the rats with transplanted islet tissue were divided into two groups, one of which received ventromedial hypothalamic lesions and the other sham lesions. Nontransplanted control groups were given similar electrolytic hypothalamic lesions or appropiate sham operations. In the animals with hypothalamic lesions and islet transplants the increase in food intake and the obesity were not observed or were markedly attenuated. The concentrations of insulin likewise did not rise as it did in the animals with VMH lesions wich became obese. This experiment strongly supports the importance of neural outputs from the hypothalamus to the beta cell as a primary determinant of food intake. Powley and Opsahl [89] reported earlier that subdiaphragmatic vagotomy would reverse hypothalamic obesity. Inoue and Bray [46] confirmed this effect of vagotomy and showed a correlation between acid secretion and insulin. In subsequent studies vagotomy performed prior to hypothalamic injury was found to attenuate but not block hyperphagia and obesity [123, 56]. Similary scopolamine, and atropine-like drug has also been found to attenuate the development of hypothalamic obesity [17]. On the other hand, vagotomy performed 30-60 minutes after acute electrolytic VMH lesions reverses the glucoseinduced hyperinsulinemia [7]. The most critical studies involve tube-feeding identical amounts of food to animals with or without hypothalamic lesions and with or without vagotomy [21]. The WMH-lesioned animal with a transected vagus does not become obese whereas the one with the intact vagus does become obese. These studies implicate the vagus nerve as a pivitol link in the pathogenesis of the hyperinsulinemia which follows hypothalamic lesions, but indicate that other factors may also be involved.

Sympathetic Nervous System. In animals with hypothalamic obesity the function of the sympathetic nervous system is also impaired. Evidence of diminished fuction of this component of the autonomic nervous system, comes from studies performed in several laboratories over the past few years [13, 51, 80, 15, 48]. Hypothalamic obese animals respond less well to stress than intact controls. Hypothalamic obese animals which are forced to swim, or are injected with 2-deoxy-d-glucose, or are exposed to the cold, showed a smaller rise in glycerol and free fatty acids than sham-operated animals receiving similar treatment [80]. In earlier studies Inoue, Campfied and Bray [51] had observed that the VMH lesioned animals had lower concentrations of circulating glucagon and smaller salivary glands, two findings which suggested the abnormalities in the sympathetic nervous system. The levels of dopamine beta hydroxilase have been reported to be an index of sympathetic activity. The concentrations of this enzyme showed a smaller rise after stress in animals with VMH lesions than in control animals [48]. Vander Tuig and Romsos [121] found a lower rate of norepinephrine turnover in heart, liver brown fat and pancrease of hypothalamic obese rats than in control rats. On the other hand, Young and Landsberg [129] have also measured the turnover of catecholamines in sympathetic nerve endings and reported that mice with hypothalamic lesions following gold-thioglucose had normal turnover rates for catecholamines. These findings cannot presently be reconciled with the earlier ones. Young and Landsberg [128] have also observed that in overfed animals given access to sucrose, the turnover of catecholamines is increased. It is obvious that additional studies of catecholamine concentrations and turnover and its relation to VMH hypothalamic obesity, will shed light on the development of obesity and control the autonomic nervous system.

Dietary Obesity

Experimental studies on dietary obesity have provided fewer clear insights than those on genetic obesity. Dietary obesity has been produced in experimental animals by high fat feeding, sucrose supplementation or by feeding a varied and palatable diet (supermarket or cafeteria diet).

High Fat Diets. When animals are fed a standard, low fat, laboratory chow diet they grow and accumulate fat at a steady rate. However, when laboratory animals are given a diet with fat content of 40% to 60%, most animals increase their food intake, are more efficient in energy utilization, and become markedly obese [94, 95]. In careful studies on the genetics of this phenomenon Fenton and Chase [31] showed that high fat diets promoted weight gain in genetically susceptible mice, but not in all strains of mice. Schemmel and her colleagues [95] have shown that feeding rats a diet containing 60% of its calories as fat, produces the greatest increase in body fat in Osborne-Mendel rats, an intermediate level of increase in body fat in animals of most other strains and only a very small weight gain in animals of the S 5B/P1 strain.

The effect of a high fat diet is related to the age at which the diet is offered. In young rats at or just after weaning, the effect of a high fat diet is much less than when fed to older animals. In early studies, it was suggested that when the high fat diet was withdrawn and replaced with a standard laboratory chow diet, animals lost weight. However, if the high fat diet is continued sufficiently long the number of adipocytes increase. When the animals are returned to the standard chow diet, food intake returns to normal. Weight loss occurs to the level at which the adipocytes reach the same size as those of the chow fed group [29]. Since the number of fat cell in the animals fed a high fat diet has increased, the total body fat is increased and this difference is maintained even though food intake remain normal.

Since most dietary fats are composed primarily of long-chain triglycerides, studies of fat feeding have dealt mainly with the effect of triglycerides of long-chain fatty acids on obesity. When a diet with an equivalent amount of lipid but composed of medium-chain triglycerides (8-10 carbon fatty acids) is substituted, little or no obesity is induced [94, 59, 12]. Food intake is lower for rats fed a medium-chain triglyceride diet than for rats fed corn oil or lard [12, 94, 124]. However, reduced food intake cannot account totally for the lack of weight gain. Food eficiency was also reduced in rats fed medium-chain trygly-cerides [94].

Dietary obesity induced by fat feeding has significant metabolic differences from other models of obesity. The hyperinsulinemia seen in hypothalamic and genetic obesity, is absent or much reduced in dietary fat induced obesity [8, 69]. Animals fed high fat diets show elevated serum glucose as well as an impaired glucose make in reponse to insulin [81]. The impaired glucose uptake is associated with decrease levels of hexokinase [6]. The oxidation of glucose to CO_2 is spared, with evidence of a compensatory decrease in the activity in other pathways [57, 133, 102].

Associated with the changes in carbohydrate metabolism are several abnormalities in lipid metabolism. Studies with ^{14}C-labeled substrates, suggest that there is a decrease in fatty acid synthesis from glucose associated with decreased insulin stimulated lipogenesis. The activity of enzymes which generate NADPH for fatty acid synthesis, specifically glucose-6-phosphate dehydrogenase and malic enzyme are [58]. In addition, acetyl CoA carboxylase, the rate limiting enzyme in lipogenesis, is inhibited by fat feeding. In spite of decreased lipolysis in response to norepinephrine [6] there is an increase in plasma free fatty acids, which is associated with increased hepatic triglyceride as well as an increase in ketones. The obesity associated with feeding diets high in long chain fatty acids occurs in association with a number of significant metabolic changes [58, 102, 124]. Decreased insulin levels and reduced sensitivity to insulin [59] along with enzyme changes described above produce a glucose sparing effect.

High Sucrose Diets. Increasing the percent of sucrose in a standard diet has little effect on body weight. However, when sucrose is available as a drinking solution and animals are given a choice between the solution of sucrose or tap water along with chow, there is a gradual increase in body weight and body fat in the animals allowed access to sucrose. In experimental studies by Kanarek and her collaborators [55] the percentage of protein above 18% in the diet did not influence the effects of feeding a solution of sucrose. Neither did changing the quantity of fat from 14.5% to 36.4%.

Supermarket or Cafeteria Diet. Sclafani and associates [33, 97] have noted, that when rats are allowed a variety of palatable snack foods in addition to standard laboratory chow, they will readily gain weight. A variety of foods have been used for this purpose including cookies, salami, cheese, bananas, marshmallows, candy, peanut butter and sweetened condensed milk. Rats fed this diet overeat and gain up to $2\frac{1}{2}$ times as much weight in the two month period as control animals fed only laboratory chow. Allowing rats access to a running wheel resulted in a 27% smaller weight gain than observed in the rats eating snack food diet with no access to a running wheel [97]. The effectiveness of the snack food diet was enhanced in older rats compared to younger animals. As with the high fat diet, access to a snack food diet increased both mean body weight and the variability of the body weight. Like the animals fed a high fat diet, the snack food weight gain could be reversed when laboratory chow became the only available form of calories. Whether reversal is complete is open to question since Rowe and Rolls [93] have reported that adult rats which became fat on a snack food diet maintained their elevated weights when given laboratory chow to eat.

The degree of obesity obtained with the cafeteria diet varies even though severe hyperphagia is induced in all animals. This suggests that differences in weight gain may be due to differences in energy utilization. Rothwell and Stock [91, 92] have used the cafeteria diet to examine dietary thermogenesis. They have found significant differences between the strains of rodents, in the ease with which these animals fatten on a cafeteria diet. Examining animals which gain weight only slowly under these conditions, these authors have documented the presence of dietary thermogenesis (luxus consumption) and have proposed that this may involve activity of the brown adipose tissue [92].

Genetic Obesity

Evidence from twin studies, as well as studies on adopted children and families with obesity, all support a role for genetics in obesity. Extreme examples of human obesity probably have a strong genetic component. One set of identical twins weighing 340 kg each have been circus performers in the United States for a number of years and have been depicted in newspapers riding bicycles and trying on clothes. Less extreme forms of obesity probably also have a genetic component, but it is clear that environment also plays a role.

The most clear-cut forms of genetic obesity have been developed with experimental animals. The first description of recessively inhereted obesity called the obese mouse (gene symbol = ob), was published by Ingalls, Dickie and Snell in 1950 [45]. The obese mouse (ob/ob) is now available throughout the world on a variety of different inbred backgrounds. In the United States, the most widely studied genetic background carrying the obese (ob) gene is the C57/B16J strain. In the United Kingdom and Europe, there are at least two other genetic backgrounds upon which this gene is carried. These genetic backgrounds may provide one explanation for some of the reported differences between these animals (Table II). This table lists the genetic types of obesity along with the presence and severity of some of the traits.

TABLE II. Summary of characteristics in syndrome of obesity

Features	VMH No genetic Basis	ob/ob Recessive Chromosome$_6$	db/db recessive Chromosome$_4$	fa/fa Recessive ?	A^y_a Dominant Chromosome$_2$	NZO Polygenic	KK Polygenic
Obesity	++	+++	++	+++	+	++	+
Hyperphagia	++	++	++	++	+	+	+
Finickiness	++	−	−	−	?	?	?
Hyperglycemia	−	+++	+++	−	±	±	+
Hyperinsulinemia	+	++	+	++	+	++	++
Insulin resistance	±	+++	+++	++	±	+	+
Hypercellular adipose tissue	--	++	±	+	--	--	--
Hypothermia	±	++	++	+	+	?	?
Impaired fertility	±	++++	++++	+++	±	--	--

++++Very severe. +++Severe. ++Moderate. +Mild. ±Variable. --Absent. ?No data.

Based on current concepts of molecular biology, the recessively inherited forms of obesity represent a single base change in the DNA sequence that codes for a single peptide, which may be either an enzyme or a structural protein (one gene-one peptide hypothesis). If this peptide is an enzyme, its presence might be manifested by either an increase or a decrease in the concentration of one or more intermediary metabolites.

Since the original discovery of the obese mouse, a number of hypotheses have been generated to provide a framework for identifying the basic biochemical abnormality in these animals [14, 15]. Some of these hypotheses include: 1) impaired oxidation of acetate, 2) abnormal response to growth hormone, 3) increased concentrations of glycerol kinase in adipose tissue, 4) increased cellularity of the adipose tissue, 5) triglyceride (fat) storage disease due to a decrease in lipolysis or to enhanced lipogenesis or esterification, 6) impaired response to insulin (*i.e.* insulin resistance), 7) increased insulin secretion, 8) decreased insulin receptors, 9) reduced sodium pump activity [deficiency in thyroid-induced ($Na^+ + K^+$) ATPase], 10) decreased response to thyroid hormone, 11) reduced levels of brain catecholamines, 12) decreased concentration of cholecystokinin in the brain, and 13) increased concentrations of endorphin in the pituitary and circulation. Many of these hypotheses have now been eliminated, while others are still under active investigation. Recent developments will be reviewed under the following headings: 1) Thermogenesis, 2) The Endocrine System, 3) The Brain, 4) Circulating Factors.

Thermogenesis. Diminished body temperature and rapid fall in core temperature in the cold were demonstrated during the early studies on the obese mouse [25]. Although this observation was made in 1954, it remained until the middle and late 1979's for this phenomenon to attract renewed attention. After confirming the impaired thermogenesis in the obese mouse, Joosten and Van Der Kroon [54], tested the hypothesis that hypothyroidism might be the cause of the hypothermia, and concluded that the ob/ob mouse might be hypothyroid thus providing a basis for their diminished thermogenesis. Ohtake, *et al.* [83] reexamined this question and could find no major abnormality in the hypothalamic-pituitary-thyroid axis. Normal circulating levels of thyroid hormones have been reported by them [83] and by two other groups [127, 76]. Ohtake and Bray [83] did, however, suggest that the response to thyroid hormone might be reduced, but this has not been confirmed by Lin *et al* [65]. Ismael-Beigi and Edelman have suggested that thyroid induced caloriegenesis might result from increased activity of the ($Na^+ + K^+$)ATPase (sodium pump) [52]. With this in mind, York, Bray and Yukimura [125] examined the possibility that the decreased thermogenesis in the obese (ob/ob) mouse might result from an impaired response of the sodium pumping enzyme [($Na^+ + K^+$)ATPase] to thyroid hormones. In these studies, hypothyroid obese (ob/ob) and lean animals were treated with triiodothyronine. Lean animals which became obese after treatment with gold thioglucose and the lean controls showed the expected rise in activity of the sodium pumping enzyme (ATPase), but the obese (ob/ob) mice failed to show this response. Lin and colleagues using a different technique for measuring (NA^+ + K^+)-ATPase, reached a similar conclusion [62, 63]. With ouabain binding to APTase as an assay for this enzyme, they showed reduced quantities of enzyme in muscle and liver of ob/ob mice. One explanation of the reduced action of triiodothyronine would be reduced nuclear binding. Guernsey and Morishige [38] confirmed the low thyroid levels of (Na^+ + K^+)ATPase in ob/ob mice and also fould that the binding of triiodothyronine to nuclear receptors was impaired in ob/ob mice, providing a potential nuclear mechanism for this defect. More recent data, however, have feiled to identify any change in thyroidal receptors. Moreover, induction of hypothyroidism at a young age with either PTU or radioactive iodine, did not improve the syndrome. The impairment in (N^+ + K^+)-ATPase however is reversed by adrenalectomy. It thus seems unlikeli that a defect in the (Na^+ + K^2)-ATPase is central to the development of the obese mouse.

Trayhurn and James [115] pursuing another line of study, suggested that the diminished thermogenesis in the ob/ob mouse might reflect impaired function of brown adipose tissue. Trayhurn *et al* showed that the total oxygen consumption of the ob/ob [115], the db/db mouse [113], and lean mice were nearly comparable in the basal state, although not when expressed in terms of body surface area [64]. The stimulation of oxygen consumption by norepinephrine, however, was significantly lower in the obese mouse than in the lean animals [114]. Since norepinephrine is known to stimulate brown adipose tissue, these workers examined the function of brown adipose tissue and concluded that it was functionally impaired in the obese mouse compared to the lean animal. Himms-Hagen and Desautles [43] showed that the binding of GDP to thermogenin, a mitochondrial protein from brown adipose tissue of the obese mouse, was less than normal. Blood flow in the brown adipose tissue is also low and the heat production in brown fat after direct stimulation of its nerve supply *in vitro* is defective [112]. The finding of Thurlby and Trayhurn [111] and of Himms-Hage and Desaultes [43] suggest that faulty metabolism of brown adipose tissue may be the defect accounting for impaired thermogenesis in the obese mouse, and thus for the storage of excess fat.

A third mechanism controlling heat production is the formation and breakdown of muscle protein. Obese mice have less muscle than lean ones [118], and the quantities of protein deposited during weight gain are reduced at all ambient temperatures between 17 and 28°C [111]. Protein synthesis was similar, but breakdown rates were higher in obese mice, which receive food dispensed at the same time and in the same amount by a lean animal bar pressing for food (yoke feeding). The ob/ob mouse gains both more weight and more fat [19]. Moreover, when lean heterozygotes carrying the ob/+ or db/+ gene are fated, they survive longer than lean homozygotes (+/+) [20].

Substrate cycles, also referred to as futile cycles, are a final mechanism that might be involved in heat production and energetic efficiency. Recently,

Newsholme *et al* [79] have exploted the maximal activities of some of the enzymes in liver that might be involved in such cycles. Abnormalities in such cycles have not yet been shown to be important in the develpment of the obese mouse.

The Endocrine System. Many of the animals with genetic obesity are stunted. This may reflect a deficiency of growth hormone somatomedin, or impaired protein synthesis for other reasons [118]. Serum levels of growth hormone are normal or low in ob/ob mouse at most ages [99], and are also somewhat depressed in the fa/fa rat [74]. That a low level of growth hormones is unimportant in the genesis of this syndrome has been shown by beeding growth-homone deficient dwarf (dw/dw) mice with ob/ob mice, where the offspring are small but obese [54]. Somatomedin levels are the same in obese and lean mice [105].

Hypophysectomy effectively stops the rapid progression of obesity in the ob/ob mouse [40] and the fatty (fa/fa) [88] rat. This may result from the removal of ACTH, since adrenalectomy also stops the rapid progression of obesity in these animals [88, 77, 104, 130]. One study showed that diurnal rhythm for ACTH and corticosterone were normal in the fatty rat [39] but another study found a loss of diurnal variation and higher levels of corticosterone in these animals [73, 74]. Increased sensitivity of the fatty rat to the hyperphagic effect of corticosterone has also been demonstrated by Yukimura, Bray and Wolfsen [132], indicating that the phenotypic expression of the genetic defect in the fatty rat apparently depends on circulating corticosterone [41]. In the fatty rat Yukimura and Bray [131] demonstrated that adrenalectomy reduced the size of the adiposytes but did not prevent their increase in numbers, suggesting that some factor is operating on the adipocyte [132]. A similar picture emerges for the obese mouse. Adrenalectomy slows weight gains to normal. Food intake drops to normal. Brain weight, spleen weight and muscle weight also return to normal. In contrast to the fatty rat, plasma corticosterone is elevated in the ob/ob and db/db mouse from a very young age [27, 127].

Changes in the response to insulin in adipose tissue, liver and muscle, have formed the basis for a number of hypotheses to explain genetic obesity [26, 106]. Treble and Mayer [116] found that glycerokiinase was elevated in the adipose tissue of the ob/ob mouse and proposed that the ability of fat cells to reutulize glycerol might account for the progressive fat storage. Thenen and Mayer [110] and Ho *et al* [44] have reexamined this hypothesis and concluded that the increase glycerokiinase is probably the result of the higher levels of insulin. A similar idea has been proposed to explain the regulation of stearic acid desaturase [28].

Insulin resistance has been noted for many years [15] but varies considerably between different types of genetic obesity [15, 103]. Insulin resistance and altered insulin binding can be demonstrated using soleus muscle [70, 24, 22, 86] and adipose tissue [53, 37, 23, 10, 16,24, 107] and liver [90]. The attractive notion, that the insulin resistance could be accounted for by changes in receptor number and/or affinity, [103] has given way to more complex interpretation involving both receptor and post-receptor changes. In spite of the high insulin levels which have been con firmed many times [15] the animals may be mildly [117] or severely [15] hyperglycemic. Maintenance of normal glucose levels thus probably reflects both enhanced gluconeogenesis [15, 66, 122] as well as insulin resistance [34].

The Brain. Recent anatomic studies measuring neuronal size and brain weight have indicated a generalized reduction in most areas of the brain of the ob/ob mouse [4, 120, 35]. In one study by Bareiter and Jeanrenaud [4] the brains from male ob/ob mice were 14% smaller than in lean age-matched controls. The cross-sectional area of neurons in the ventromedial nucleus, cingulate cortex, medial amydaloid nucleus, ventrobasal nucleus of the thalamus, dorsomotor nucleus of the vagus, and the motor nuclei of the VII and XII nuclei were significantly smaller in tissues from the ob/ob mice. Only the lateral hypothalamic neuronal areas were the same in these two types of animals. This generalized reduction in volume of neuronal tissue may be the anatomic substrate for hypothalamic defects.Data from Van der Kroon and Speijers [120], from Garthwaite *et al* [35] and from our laboraory have confirmed the smaller brain size of the ob/ob mouse. Van der Kroon and Speijers reported that DNA content and cerebroside content (measured as µg of galactose/brain) were reduced. Additional studies are needed to enlarge on these reports and to provide a picture of brain development and other possible abnormalities.

Studies on brain neurotransmitters in genetic obesity have been reported from several laboratories [67, 30, 82, 68, 60, 9]. Lorden *et al* [68] reported inreased concentrations of norepinephrine in the hypothalamus of 2-and 5-month old ob/ob mice of both sexes. Turnover of these catecholamines, however, did not differ in the two groups of animals. Using older animals, Nemeroff *et al* [78] could find no difference in the hypothalamic levels of norepinephrine or dopamine. By 8 months of age the ob/ob mouse is no longer rapidly gaining weight, however, suggesting that the findings in the younger animals may be more important for the development of this syndrome. Feldman and Blalock [30] on the other hand have reported decreased levels of brain norepinephine. They also find that increasing the level of norepinephrine in the brain by treatment with monopamine oxidase inhibitors does not prevent the obesity. Dopamine seems to be normal except in the pituitary where it is reduced.

Pharmacologic studies have shown that reserpine lowers the norepinephrine levels in brain more slowly in ob/ob mice [82]. The antagonist, 6-hydroxy-dopamine, reduced brain norepinephrine and dopamine in ob/ob mice, but did not reduce the gain in weight or the hyperglycemia [67]. In db/db mice 6-hydroxydopamine did lower glucose and weight gain as well as brain norepinephrine. This effect was moderated by simultaneous blockade of monoamine oxidase (MAO) with desmethylimipramine [67]. Brain norepinephrine is also altered in the fatty rat [6]. In this animal, tyrosine hydroxylase, dopamine β-hydroxylase and phenethanolamine-N- methyl transferase have all been measured [61]. The changes between the 3 ages at which enzyme measurements were made were greater than the differences at one age between lean and fatty rats, raising doubts about the importances of brain norepinephrine in the pathogenesis of genetic obesity.

Serotonin and the neurons which contain this neurotransmitter compose a second neural pathway which is involved in feeding [9]. In the obese (ob/ob) mouse brain with the ones on norepinephrine makes studies on putative brain neurotransmitters a fruitful basis for further explorations.

Several brain peptides have also been measured in genetic obesity. Margules and his colleagues [72] have reported that *beta*-endorphin is significantly increased in the pituitary but not the hypothalamus of the obese mouse and of the fatty rat. MSH [85] and ACTH [35] two other parts of the pro-opio melanocortin molecule from which *beta*-endorphin comes, are also increased in pituitaries of ob/ob mice. These increased concentrations of opiate-like peptides might be important in the development of this syndrome, since naloxone, a drug which blocks the opioid receptors, acutely suppressed food intake in the obese (ob/ob) mice more than in lean controls. Data from our laboratory confirmed this observation [98]. We used an eight hour feeding period with two injections of naloxone at the beginning and middle of each treatment day, which was comparable in ob/ob and lean animals. As the eight hour feeding wore one, even with the second injection of naloxone, food intake returned to or increased above control levels. By the second, third and fourth day the food intake during the eight hour period in naloxine-treated lean mice was significantly above that of the vehicle-treated controls. Levels two hundred percent higher than in the lean, vehicle-treated mice were found. The ob/ob mice also increased their food intake significantly during treatment with naloxone. The importance of the *beta*-endorphin system in the genetic obesity thus remains uncertain. However, endorphins may well be involved in the regulation of body fat.

The observations that cholecystokinin is lower in the brain tissue from ob/ob mice than in the control, was first reported by Straus and Yalow [109]. These observations aroused considerable scientific interest, because cholecystokinin has been shown to produce satiety in animals and in man [36, 100]. The possibility existed that reduced leveles of the octapeptide form of the hormone in brain, might be responsible for the overeating and potentially for the other defects in these animals. Recent studies by Schneider, Monahan and Hirsch [96] using a different antibody to cholecystokinin failed to find and differences between obese and lean animals under any of the experimental conditions which were studied. We have likewise failed to find any differences. This difference between several laboratories in measurements of CCK leveles in ob/ob and lean animals leaves the issue of peptides in the ob/ob mouse open to further investigation. Other peptides including calcitonin [71] and somatostatin [84] may also be different.

Circulating and cellular mechanisms in genetic obesity. The use of parabiotic animals has been one approach to test the possibility that circulating factors may be involved in some of the experimental obesities [15]. When a fat animal is parabiosed to a lean animal the fat animal, bet in an ob/ob, fa/fa or (A^{y}a) animal, remains the same weight or becomes fatter [15]. The lean partner may become thinner. When a db/db mouse was parabiosed to either a lean or fat ob/ob mouse, the db/db partner survided the union whereas both the lean and ob/ob partners died [18]. This experiment has been interpreted as indicating that the db/db mouse produces excessive quantities of a satiety factor to which its hypothalamus presumably cannot respond, but which is transferred through the parabiotic union and inhibits food intake in both the lean and ob/ob mouse. The ob/ob mouse, on the other hand, while able to respond to this satiety factor is apparently unable to secrete sufficient quantities to suppress its own food intake. The nature of this satiety factor is presently unknown.

A second approach to the question of whether there are primary cellular abnormalities in the experimental forms of obesity has used fat cell transplants. Ashwell, Meade and their colleagues [2, 75] have transplanted adipose tissue from ob/ob and lean animals to appropriate lean or ob/ob animals and observed the changes in size of the adipocytes during the weeks following transplantation. In all of the experimental situations the adipose tissue takes on the characteristics of the recipient animal. That is, large fat cells from the ob/ob mouse become smaller when transplanted into a lean animal. Conversely small fat cells from lean donors become large when transplanted into corpulent ob/ob recipients. The intepretation of these data is that the defect in genetic obesity is in the internal millieu in which the cells reside and not to innate changes in the fat cells of obese mice.

REFERENCES

1. Anand, B.K. and J.R. Brobeck. Hypothalamic control of food intake in rats and cats. *Yale J. Biol. Med.* 24:123-146, 1951.
2. Ashwell, M., C.J., Meade, P. Medawar and C. Sowter. Adipose tissue. Contributions of nature and nurture to obesity of an obese mutant mouse (ob/ob). *Proc. R. Soc. London, Ser B* 195:343-353, 1977.
·3. Babinski, M.J. Tumeur du corps pituitaire sans acromegalie et avec de ceveloppement des organes genitaus. *Rev. Neurol.* 8:531-533, 1900.
4. Bareiter, D.A. and B. Jeanrenaud. Altered neuroanatomical organization in the central nervous system of the gentically obese (ob/ob) mouse. *Brain Res* 165:249-260, 1979.
5. Bernadis, L.L. and J.K. Goldman. Origin of endocrine-metabolic changes in the weanling rat ventromedial syndrome. *J. Neurosci. Res* 2:91-116, 1976.
6. Bernstein, R.S., M.D. Merville, M.C. Marshall, A.L. Carney. Effects of dietary composition on adipose tissue hexokinase II and glucose utilization in normal and streptozotocin-diabetic rats. *Diabetes* 26:770-779, 1977.
7. Berthoud, H.R. and B. Jeanrenaud. Acute hyperinsulinemia and its reversal by vagotomy following lesions of the ventromedial hypothalamus in anesthetized rats. *Endocrinology* 105:146-151, 1979.

8. Blazquez, E. and C.L. Quijada. The effect of a high fat diet on glucose, insulin sensitivity and plasma insulin in rats. *J. Endocrinol.* 42:489-494, 1968.

9. Blundell, J.E. Is there a role for serotonin (5-hydroxytryptamine) in feeding? *Int. J. Obesity* 1:15-42, 1977.

10. Boulange, A., E. Planche and P. DeGasquet. Onset of genetic obesity in the absence of hyperphagia during the first week of life in the Zurker rat (fa/fa). *J. Lipid Res* 20 (7):857-864, 1979.

11. Bray, G.A. and T.F. Gallagher, Jr. Manifestations of hypothalamic obesity in man: A comprehensive investigation of eight patients and a review of the literature. *Medicine* 54 (4):301-330, 1975.

12. Bray, G.A., M. Lee and T. Bray. Weight gain of rats fed medium-chain triglycerides is less than rats fed long-chain triglycerides. *Int. J. Obesity* 4:27-32, 1980.

13. Bray, G.A. and Y. Nishizawa. The ventromedial hypothalamus modulates fat mobilization during fasting. *Nature.* 274:900-902, 1978.

14. Bray, G.A. and D.A. York. Genetically transmitted obesity in rodents. *Physiol Rev.* 51:598-646, 1978.

15. Bray, G.A. D.A. York. Hypothalamic and genetic obesity in experimental animals: an autonomic and endocrine hypothesis. *Physiol Rev.* 59:719-809, 1979.

16. Carnie, J.A., D.G. Smith and M. Mavrisva. Effects of insulin on lipolysis and lipogenesis in adipocytes from genetically obese (ob/ob/mice) *Biochem. J.* 184 (1):107-112, 1979.

17. Carpenter, R.G., B.A. Stamouts, L.D. Dalton, L.A. Frohman and S.P. Grossman. VMH obesity reduced but not reversed by scopolamine methyl nitrate. *Physiol. Behav.* 23 (5):955-959, 1979.

18. Coleman, D.L. Effects of parabiosis of obese with diabetes and normal mice. *Diabetologia.* 6:294-298, 1973.

19. Coleman, D.L. Obesity and diabetes. Two mutant genes causing diabetes-obesity syndromes in mice. *Diabetologia* 14:141-148, 1978.

20. Coleman, D.L. Obesity genes, beneficial effects in heterozygous mice. *Science* 203 (4381):663-665, 1979.

21. Cox, J.E. and T.L. Powley. Prior vagotomy blocks VMH obesity in pairfed rats. *Am. J. Physiol.* 240:E573-E583, 1981.

22. Crettaz, M., M. Prentki, D. Zaninetti and B. Jeanrenaud. Insulin resistance in soleus muscle from obese zucker rats-involvement of several defective sites. *Biochem J.* 186 (2):525-534, 1980.

23. Cushman, S.W., M.J. Zarnowski, A.J. Franzusoff and L.B. Salans. Alterations in glucose-metabolism and its stimulation by insulin in isolated adipose-cells during development of genetic obesity in Zucker fatty rat. *Metabolism* 27 (12):1930-1940.

24. Czech, M.P. D.K. Richardson, S.G. Becker, C.G. Walters, W. Gitomer and J. Heinrich. Insulin-response in skeletal-muscle and fat-cells of genetically obese zucker rat. *Metabolism* 27 (12):1967-1981, 1978.

25. Davis, T.R.A. and J. Mayer. Imperfect homeothermia in the hereditary obese-hyperglycemic syndrome of mice. *Am. J. Physiol.* 177:222-226, 1954.

26. Dehaye, J.P., J. Winand, P. Popoczek and J. Christophe. Relationship between lipolysis and calcium in epididymal adipose tissue of obese hyperglycemic mice. *Diabetologia* 16 (6):339-408, 1979.

27. Dubuc, P. Basal cortocosterone levels of young ob/ob mice. *Horm. Metab. Res.* 9:95-96, 1977.

28. Enser, M. Role of insulin in the regulation of stearic acid desaturase activity in liver and adipose tissue from obese-hyperglycemia (ob/ob) and lean mice. *Biochem. J.* 180 (3):551-558, 1979.

29. Faust, I.M., P.R. Johnson and J. Hirsh. Noncompensation of adipose mass in partially lipectomized mice and rats. *Am. J. Physiol.* 231:538-544, 1976.

30. Feldman, J.M. and J.A. Blalock. Role of altered tissue norepinephrine concentration in the hereditary obese hyperglycemic syndrome of mice. *Res. Com. C.P.* 26 (3):479-493, 1979.

31. Fenton, P.F. and H.B. Chase, Effect of diet on obesity of yellow mice in inbred lines. *Proc. Soc. Exp. Biol. Med.* 77:420-422, 1951.

32. Frolich, A. Ein Fall von Tumor der hypophysis cerebri ohne akromegalie. *Wien Klin Rund.* 15:883-886, 1901.

33. Gale, S.K. and A. Sclafani. Comparison of ovarina and hypothalamic obesity syndromes in the female rat: Effects of diet palatability on food intake and body weight. *J. Com.Psychol.* 91:381-392, 1977.

34. Gardner, L.B., O.E. Michaelis and S. Cataland. Serum-insulin and glucagon and hepatic and adipose cyclic-AMP responses of Zucker rats fed carbohydrate diets *ad libitum* or in meals. *Nutr. Rep. Intern.* 29 (6):845-854, 1979.

35. Garthwaite, T.L., R.K., Kalkhoff, A.R. Guansgin, T.C. Hagen and L.A. Menhan. Plasma-free trytophan, brain-serotonin and an endocrine profile of the genetically obese hyperglycemia mouses at 4-5 months of age. *Endocrinology* 105 (5):1178-1182, 1979.

36. Gibbs, J. and G.P. Smith. Cholecystokinin and satiety in rats and rhesus monkeys. *Am. J. Clin. Nutr.* 30:758-761, 1977.

37. Gruen, R., E. Hietanen and M.R.C. Greenwood. Increased adipose tissue lipoprotein lipase activity during development of genetically obese rat (fa/fa). *Metabolism* 27 (12):1955-1966, 1978.

38. Guernsey, D.L. and W.K. Morishige. Na$^+$ pump activity and nuclear T$_3$ receptors in tissue of genetically obese (ob/ob) mice. *Metabolism* 28:629-632, 1979.

39. Han, P.W. and L.A. Frohman. Hyperinsulinemia in tube-fed hypophysectomized rats bearing hypothalamic lesions. *Am. J. Physiol.* 219:1632-1636, 1970.

40. Herbai G. Weight loss in obese-hyperglycemic and normal mice following transauricular hypophysectomy by a modified technique. *Acta Endocrinol.* 65:712-722, 1970.

41. Herberg, L. and H.K. Kley. Adrenal function and the effect of a high fat diet on C57BL/6J and C57BL/6J ob/ob mice. *Horm Metab. Res.* 8:410-415, 1975.

42. Hetherington, A.W. and S.W. Ranson. Hypothalamic lesions and adiposity in the rat. *Anat. Rec.* 78:149-172, 1940.

43. Himms-Hagen, J. and M. Desautels. A mitochondrial defect in brown adipose tissue of the obese (ob/ob) mouse: reduced binding of purine necleotides and a failure to respond to cold by an increase in binding. *Biochem. Biophys. Res. Comm.* 83:628, 1978.

44. Ho, R.J., C.C. Fan and L.A. Barrera. Comparison of adipose glycerol kinase of hyperglycemic obese mice and lean littermates. *Molec. Biochem.* 27:89-96, 1979.

45. Ingalls, A.M., M.M. Dickie and D.G. Snell. Obesity, a mutation in the mouse. *J. Heredity.* 41:317-318, 1950.

46. Inoue, S. and G.A. Bray. The effect of subdiaphragmatic vagotomy in rats with ventromedial hypothalamic obesity. *Endocrinology* 100:108-114, 1977.

47. Inoue, S. and G.A. Bray. An autonomic hypothesis for hypothalamic obesity. *Life Sci.* 25:561-566, 1979.

48. Inoue, S. and G.A. Bray. Role of autonomic nervous system in the development of ventromedial hypothalamic obesity. *Brain Res. Bull.* 5:109-117, 1980.

49. Inoue, S., G.A. Bray and Y. Mullen. The effect of transplantation on the pancreas on the development of the obese-hyperglycemic syndrome in mice (ob/ob). *Metabolism* 23:435-436, 1977.

50. Inoue, S., G.A. Bray and Y. Mullen. Transplantation of pancreatic betacells prevents the development of hypothalamic obesity in rats. *Am. J. Physiol.* 235:E266-E271, 1978.

51. Inoue, S., L.A. Campfield and G.A. Bray. Comparison of metabolid alterations in hypothalamic and high-fat diet induced obesity. *Am. J. Physiol.* 233:R162-R168, 1977.

52. Ismael-Beigi, F. and I.S. Edelman. The mechanism of the calorigenic action of thyroid hormone. Stimulation of Na$^+$ and K$^+$ activated adenosine triphosphatase activity. *J. Gen. Pshysiol.* 57:710-722, 1971.

53. Johnson, P.R., J.S., Stern, M.R.C. Greenwood and J. Hirch. Adipose tissue hyperplasia and hyperinsulinemia in Zucker obese female rats: development study. *Metabolism* 27 (12):1941-1954, 1978.

54. Joosten, H. and P. van der Kroon. Role of the thyroid in the development of the obese-hyperglycemic syndrome in mice (ob/ob). *Metabolism* 23:435-436, 1974.

55. Kanarek, R.B. and E. Hirsch. Dietary-induced overeating in experimental animals. *Fed. Proc.* 36:154, 1977.

56. King, B.M., R.G. Carpenter, B.A. Stamoustsos, L.A. Frohman and S.P. Grossman. Hyperphagia and obesity following ventromedial hypothalamic lesions in rats with sub-diaphragmatic vagotomy. *Physiol Behav.* 20:643-651, 1978.

57. Lavau, M. and C. Susini. [U-^{14}C] glucose metabolism *in vivo* in rats rendered obese by a high fat diet. *J. Lipid. Res.* 16:134-142, 1975.

58. Lavau, M., S.K., Fried, C. Susini and P. Freychet. Mechanism of insulin resistance in adipocytes of rats fed a high fat diet. *J. Lipid. Res.* 20:8-16, 1979.

59. Leveille, G.A., R.S. Pardini and J.A. Tillotsan. Influence of medium-chain triglycerides on lipid metabolism in the rat. *Lipids* 2:287-294, 1967.

60. Levin, B.E. and A.C. Sullivan. Catecholamine levels in discrete brain nuclei of 7 month old genetically obese rats. *Pharm. Biochem. Behav.* 11 (1):77-82, 1979.

61. Levin, B.E. and A.C. Sullivan. Catecholamine synthesizing enzymes in various brain regions of the genetically obese zucker rat (technical note). *Brain Res.* 171 (3):560-566, 1979.

62. Lin, M.H., D.R. Romsos, T. Akera and G.A. Leveille. (Na$^+$ + K$^+$) ATPase enzyme units in skeletal muscle from lean and obese mice. *Biochem. Biophys Res Comm* 80:398-404, 1978.

63. Lin, M.H., D.R. Romsos, T. Akera and G.A. Leveille (Na$^+$ + K$^+$) ATPase enzyme units in skeletal muscle and liver of 14 day old lean and obese (ob/ob) mice. *Proc. Soc. Exptl. Med.* 161 (3):235-238, 1979.

64. Lin, P.Y., D.R. Romsos, J.G. Vendertuig and G.A. Leveille. Maintenance energy requirements, energy retention and heat-production of young obese (ob/ob) and lean mice fed a high fat or a high carbohydrate diet. *J. Nutr.* 109 (7):1143-1153, 1979.

65. Lin, M.H., J.G. Vandertuig, D.R. Romsos, T. Akera and G.A. Leveille. (Na$^+$ + K$^+$) ATPase enzyme units in lean and obese (ob/ob) thyronine injected mice. *Am. J. Physiol.* 237 (3):E265-E272, 1979.

66. Lombardo, Y.B. and L.A. Menahan. Gluconeogenesis in perfused livers of gentically obese hyperglycemic (ob/ob) mice. *Horm. Metab.* 11 (1):9-14, 1979.

67. Lorden, J.F. Differential effects on body-weight of central 6-hydroxy-dopamine lesions in obese (ob/ob) and diabetes (db/db) mice. *J. Comp. Physiol Psychol.* 93 (6):1085-1096, 1979.

68. Lorden, J.F., G.A. Oltmans and D.L. Margules. Central catecholamine levels ls in genetically obese mice (ob/ob and db/db). *Brain Res.* 96:390-394, 1975.

69. Mailaisse, W.J., D. Lemonnier, F. Mailaisse-Legae and I.M. Mendel Brum. Secretion of and high sensitivity to insulin in obese rats fed a high fat diet. *Horm. Metab. Res.* 1:9-13, 1975.

70. Marchand, Y.L. and P. Freychet. Studies of insulin insensitivity in soleus muscles of obese mice. *Metabolism* 27 (12):1982-1993, 1978.

71. Margules, D.L., J.J. Flynn, J. Walker and C.W. Cooper. Elevation of calcitonin immmono-reactivity in the pituitary and thyroid gland of genetically obese rats (fa/fa). *Brain Res.* 4 (5):589-591, 1979.

72. Margules, D.L., B. Moisset, M.J. Lewis, H. Shibuya and C.B. Pert: B-endorpin in associated with overeating in genetically obese mice (ob/ob) and rats (fa/fa). *Science* 202:988-991, 1978.

73. Martin, R.J. and H.J.H. Gahagan. The influence of age and fasting on serum hormone levels in the lean and obese Zucker rat. *Proc. Soc. Exp. Biol. Med.* 154:610-613, 1977.

74. Martin, R.J., P.J. Wangness and H.J. Gahagan. Diurnal changes in serum metabolites and hormones in lean and obese Zucker rats. *Horm. Metab. Res.* 10:187-192, 1978.

75. Meade, C.J., M. Ashwell and C. Sowter. Is genetically transmitted obesity due to an adipose-tissue defect? *Proc. Roy. Soc.* B 205 (1160):395.

76. Mobley, P.W. and P.U. Dubic. Thyroid hormone levels in the developing obese hyperglycemic syndrome. *Horm. Metab.* 11 (1):37-39, 1979.

77. Naeser, P. Effects of adrenalectomy in the obese-hyperglycemic syndrome in mice (gene symbol. ob). *Diabetologia* 9:376-379, 1973.

78. Nemeroff, C.B., G. Visette and S.J. Kizer. Reduced hypothalamic content of immunoreactive LR-RH activity in genetically obese (ob/ob) mice. *Brain Res* 146:385-387, 1978.

79. Newsholme, E.A., K. Braind, J. Lang, J.C. Stanley and T. Williams. Maximum activities of enzymes that are involved in substrate cycles in liver and muscle of obese mice. *Biochem. J.* 182 (2):621-624, 1979.

80. Nishizawa, Y. and G.A. Bray. Ventromedial hypothalamic lesions and the mobilization of fatty acids. *J. Clin. Invest.* 61:714-721, 1978.

81. Ogundipe, O.O. and G.A. Bray. The influence of diet and fat cell size on glucose metabolism, lipogenesis and lipolysis in the rat. *Horm. Metab. Res.* 6:351-356, 1974.

82. Oltmans, G.A., R. Olsauskas and J.E. Comaty. Hypothalamic catecholamine systems in genetically obese mice (ob/ob): decreased sensitivity to reserpine treatment. *Neuropharm.* 19 (1):25-33, 1980.

83. Ohtake, M., G.A. Bray and M. Azukizawa. Studies on hypothermia and thyroid function in the obese (ob/ob) mouse. *J. Physiol.* 233:R110-R115, 1977.

84. Patel, Y.C., D.P. Cameron Y. Stefan, F. Malaisse-Legae and L. Orri. Somatostatin: widespread abnormality in tissues of spontaneously diabetic mice. *Science* 198:930-931, 1977.

85. Peaslee, M.H., B. Moisset, H. Shibuya and C.E. Pert. Increase in pituitary melanocytestimulating hormone-activity of genetically obese (ob/ob) mice. *Experientia* 36:(1):133-134, 1980.

86. Poggi, C., Y. Lemarchand, J. Zapf, E.R. Froesch and Freychet. Effects and binding of insulin-like growth factor I in the isolated soleus muscle and of lean and obese mice - comparison with insulin. *Endocrinology* 105 (3):723-730, 1979.

87. Powley, T.L. The ventromedial hypothalamic syndrome, satiety and a cephalic phase hypothesis. *Psychol. Rev.* 84:89-126, 1977.

88. Powley, T.L. and S.A. Morton. Hypophysectomy and regulation of body weight in the genetically obese Zucker rat. *Am. J. Physiol.* 230:982-987, 1976.

89. Powley, T.L. and C.A. Opsahl. Ventromedial hypothalamic obesity abolished by subdiaphragmatic vagotomy. *Am. J. Physiol.* 226:25-33, 1974.

90. Richards, D.K. and M.P. Czech. Diminished activities of fatty acid synthesis enzymes in insulin-resistant adipocytes from spontaneously obese rats. *Horm. Metab. Res.* 11 (7):427-431, 1979.

91. Rothwell, N.J. and M.J. Stock. Mechanism of weight gain and loss in reversible obesity in the rat. *J. Physiol.* 276:60P-61P, 1978.

92. Rothwell, N.J. and M.J. Stock. A role for brown adipose tissue in diet-induced thermogenesis. *Nature* (2821):31-35, 1979.

93. Rowe, E.A. and B.J. Rolls. Dietary obesity: permanent changes in body weight. Paper presented at the Sixth International Conference on the Physiology of Food and Fluid Intake, Jouy en Josas, France., 1977.

94. Schemmel, R. Physiological considerations of lipid storage and utilization. *Amer. Zool.* 16:661-670, 1976.

95. Schemmel, R., O. Mickelsen and J.L. Gill. Dietary obesity in rats: body weight and body fat accretion in seven strains of rats. *J. Nutrition* 100:1041-1048, 1970.

96. Schneider, B.A., J.W. Monahan and J. Hirsch. Brain cholecystokinin and nutritional status in rats and mice. *J. Clin. Invest.* 64:1348-1356, 1979.

97. Sclafani, A. and D. Sprienger, Dietary obesity in adult rats: similarities to hypothalamic and human obesity syndromes. *Physiol. Behav.* 17:461-471, 1976.

98.   Shimomura, Y., J. Oki, Z. Glick and G.A. Bray. Opiate receptors, food intake and obesity. *Pysiol. Behav.* 28:441-445, 1982.

99.   Sinha, Y.N., C.B. Salocks and W.P. Vanderlaan. Prolactin and growth hormone secretion in chemically induced and genetically obese mice. *Endocrinology* 97:1386-1393, 1975.

100.   Smith, G.P. and J. Gibbs. Cholecystokinin and satiety: Theoretic and therapeutic implications. *In*: Hunger, Basic Mechanisms and Clinical Implications. (D. Novin, W. Wyrwicka and G.A. Bray, Eds); New York, Raven Press. pp. 349, 355, 1976.

101.   Smith, P.E. The disabilities caused by hypophysectomy and their repair. The tuberal (hypothalamic) syndrome in the rat. *JAMA* 88:158-161, 1927.

102.   Smith, U., J. Kral and P. Bjorntorp. Influence of dietary fat and carbohydrate on the metabolism of adipocytes of different size in the rat. *Biochem. Biophys. Acta.* 337:278-285, 1974.

103.   Soll, A., C.R. Kahn, D. Neville and J. Roth. Insulin binding to liver plasma membrane in obese hyperglycemic (ob/ob) mouse. Demonstration of a decreased number of functionally normal receptors. *J. Biol. Chem.* 250:4702-4707, 1975.

104.   Solomon, J. and J. Mayer. The effect of adrenalectomy on the development of the obese-hyperglycemia syndrome in ob/ob mice. *Endocrinology* 93:510-513, 1973.

105.   Spencer, G.S.G. and M.B. Enzer. Plasma somatomedin activity in obese hyperglycemia mice (technical note). *Horm. Metab.* 11 (9):528-530, 1979.

106.   Stauffer, W. and A.E. Renold. Effect of insulin *in vivo* on diaphragm and adipose tissue of obese mice. *Am. J. Physiol.* 216:98-105, 1969.

107.   Steele, N.C., R.J., Martin and C.A. Baile, Insulin receptor characteristics and insulin degradation by Zucker lean and obese rats. *Horm. Metab. Res.* 11 (9):525-526, 1979.

108.   Stellar, E. The physiology of motivation. *Psychol. Rev.* 61:5-22, 1954.

109.   Straus, E. and R.S. Yalow. Cholecystokinin in the brains of obese and nonobese mice. *Science* 2-3:68-69, 1979.

110.   Thenen, S.W. and J. Mayer. Hyperinsulinemia and fat cell glycerokinase activity in obese (ob/ob) and diabetic (db/db) mice. *Horm. Metab. Res.* 8:80-81, 1976.

111.   Thurlby, P.L. and P. Trayhurn. Role of thermoregulatory thermogenesis in the development of obesity in genetically-obese (ob/ob) mice pair-fed with lean siblings. *Blit. J. Nutr.* 42 (3):377-385, 1979.

112.   Thurlby, P.L. and P. Trayhurn. Regional blood flow in genetically obese (ob/ob) mice -the importance of brown adipose tissue to the reduced energy expenditure on nonshivering thermogenesis. *Pflugers Arch.* 386 (3):193-201, 1980.

113.   Trayhurn, P. Thermoregulation in the diabetic obese (db/db) mouse role of nonshivering thermogenesis in energy balance. *Pflugers Arch.* 38- (3):227-232, 1979.

114.   Trayhurn, P., P.L. Thurlby, A.E. Goodbody and W.P.P. James. Brown adipose tissue and thermogenesis in obesity. *In*: Obesity: Pathogenesis and treatment. Serono Symposium. Academic Press. 28:73-86, 1981.

115.   Trayhurn, P. and W.P. James. Thermoregulation and non-shivering thermogenesis in the genetically obese (ob/ob) mouse. *Pflugers Arch.* 373:189-193, 1978.

116.   Treble, D.H. and J. Mayer. Glycerokinase activity in white adipose tissue of obese hyperglycemic mice. *Nature* 200:363-364, 1963.

117.   Triscari, J., J.S. Stern, P.R. Johnson and A.C. Sullivan. Carbohydrate metabolism in lean and obese Zucker rats. *Metabolism* 28 (2):183-189, 1979.

118.   Trostler, N., D.R., Romsos, W.G. Bergen and G.A. Leveille. Skeletal muscle accretion and turnover in lean and obese (ob/ob)mice. *Metabolism* 28 (9):928-933, 1979.

119.   Ungerstedt, U. Adipsia and aphagia after 6-hydroxydopamine induced degeneration of the nigro-striatal dopamine system. *Acta Physiol. Scand. Suppl.* 367:95-112, 1971.

120.   Van der Kroon, P.H.W. and G.J.A. Speijers. Brain deviations in adult obese-hyperglycemia mice (ob/ob) mice. *Metabolism* 28 (1):1-3, 1979.

121.   Vander, Tuig, J.A., A.W. Knehans and D.R. Romsos. Reduced sympathetic nervous activity in rats with ventromedial hypothalamic lesions. *Life Sci.* 30:913-920, 1982.

122. Wade, A.J. Glucose metabolism and recyclicing of radiactively labelled glucose in the Zucker genetically obese rat (fa/fa). *Biochem. J.* 186 (1):161-168, 1980.

123. Wampler. R.S. and C.T. Snowden. Development of VMH obesity in vagotomized rats. *Physiol. Behav.* 22:85-93, 1979.

124. Wiley, J.H. and G.A. Leveille. Metabolic consequences of dietary medium-chain triglycerides in the rat. *J. Nut.* 103:829-835, 1973.

125. York, D.A. G.A. Bray and Y. Yukimura. An enzymatic defect in the obece (ob/ob) mouse. Loss of the thyroid induced sodium potassium dependent andenonotriophosphatase. *Proc. Natl. Acad. Sci.* 75:477-481, 1978.

126. York, D.A. and V. Godbole. Effect of adrenalectomy on obese fatty rats. *Horm Metab. Res.* 11 (11):646, 1979.

127. York, D.A., W. Otto and T.G. Taylor. Thyroid status of obese (ob/ob) mice and its relationship to adipose tissue metabolism. *Comp. Biochem. Physiol.* B 59:59-65, 1978.

128. Young, J.B. and Landsberg. Effect of diet and cold exposure on norepinephrine turnover in pancreas and liver. *Am. J. Physiol.* 236:E524-E533, 1979.

129. Young, J.B. and L. Landsberg. Impaired suppresion of sympathetic activity during fasting in the gold thioglucose treated mouse. *J. Clin. Invest.* 65:1086 1094, 1980.

130. Yukimura, Y. and G.A. Bray. Effects of adrenalectomy on thyroid function and insulin levels in obese (ob/ob) mice. *Proc. Soc. Ecp. Biol. Med.* 159:364-367, 1978.

131. Yukimura, Y. and G.A. Bray. Effects of adrenalectomy on body weight and the size and number of fat cells in the Zucker (fatty) rat. *Endo. Res Comm.* 5 (3):189-198, 1978.

132. Yukimura, Y., G.A. Bray and A.R. Wolfsen: Some effects of adrenalectomy in the fatty rat. *Endocrinology* 103:1924-1928, 1978.

133. Zaragosa-Hermans, N. and J.P. Felber. Studies on the metabolic effects induced in the rat by a high fat diet. I. Carbohydrate metabolism *in vivo*. *Horm. Metab. Res.* 2:323-329, 1970.

DISCUSSION[1]

Neel commented on the irony of the Prader-Willi syndrome as a genetic paradigm, since these individuals (many of whom have a cytological deletion) are sterile and so do not lend themselves to the usual genetic studies. Coleman suggested that from this experience, hypothermia probably did not play the critical role in obesity in obese mouse strains. Rosenberg suggested that the characteristics of genetically obese mice and rats as described by Bray would qualify them for the diagnosis of amilial Cushing's disease, to which Bray, with qualifications, agreed. Waterlow, referring to the clinical phenomenon of obesity in middle-aged women, wondered if hormonal factors in obesity had been given their due. Blackburn broadened the discussion with several slides suggesting that despite prevailing opinions, there really is no hard evidence that, in many cultures, a little obesity is deleterious. Garby commented that the kinds of associations (or non-associations) presented by Blackburn did not indicate causality; Blackburn agreed, but noted that neither did they exclude causality.

[1]*Summary of the discussion prepared by J. Neel.*

Blackburn further suggested that in the total complex nutritional picture, there had been too much emphasis on single indicators, such as coronary heart disease, as to the value of a diet, and at the same time, over-emphasis on regulation of single components in the diet. Frenk asked two questions: why do some people respond to anxiety with hyperphagia, and to what extent does subcutaneous fat alter metabolic requirements by its insulating properties. No one offered significant new insights to these questions. Martorell wondered whether under-nutrition in childhood predisposed to hyperphagia if food became available in more than adequate quantities in later life; Nesheim allowed that this was not observed in rats who were severely undernourished when young. Waterlow commented that whereas nutritionists tended to be 'community-minded', perhaps a principal thought emerging from the conference was the need to be more 'individual-minded'. Nesheim asked Bray to comment on the genetic-environment interaction in 'middle range' (rather than extreme) obesity; Bray responded by suggesting that although there were differences between rodent strains in apparent susceptibility to middle-range obesity, clearly the environment could be manipulated to play a contributing role. Ward suggested we should be much more specific in our use of the term 'obesity', that even by the simple criterion of distributions of fat, there were several kinds. Cederbaum, returning to the earlier discussion of genetic differences between individuals in nutritional requirements, pointed out that there were still many studies to be done on just how the heterozygotes for known biochemical disorders differ from normal. Hillman attempted to brige the difference between the 'genetic' and 'environmental' viewpoints by suggesting that where nutrition is grossly inadequate, or, at the other extreme, very comfortably adequate for all, genetic differences between individuals in nutritional needs were not apt to sufarce, but that such differences (other than the extreme, monogenic disorders) were best studied in populations on "just adequate" diets. Cravioto noted that in his presentation he had appeared to some to ignore genetic factors in susceptibility to malnutrition, whereas in fact he was directing work on that very point in his Institute. Frenk drew attention to the difference in obesity in U.S. and Mexican Papago Indians, and the studies this might make possible. Cohen thought that for all the discussion, the group had still not done well at generating the important questions for future study. Lisker and Payne felt that first emphasis still had to be on malnutrition, predominantly environmental, due at present more to a maldistribution of food than to any world-wide shortages. Scrimshaw and Neel, agreeing, nevertheless felt the group should pass from the obvious to a more detailed agenda. Payne closed the discussion by reminding the group of the need for restraint in nutritional recommendations based upon half-knowledges.

PART V

ASSESSMENT OF NUTRITIONAL STATUS

LIMITATIONS OF METABOLIC STUDIES

Benjamin Torún

Division of Human Nutrition and Biology
Institute of Nutrition of Central America and Panama (INCAP)
Guatemala City, Guatemala

INTRODUCTION

Metabolic studies are those related to the processes by which living cells or tissues undergo chemical change. In the context of nutrition, "metabolic studies" refer to the processes by which proteins, fats, carbohydrates, minerals, vitamins and water, of either exogenous or endogenous origin, participate in the chemical changes of an organism. In a narrower sense, and mainly for operational purposes, nutritional metabolic studies are usually defined as those that take place within the confines of a so-called *metabolic ward,* or those that define the fate of a nutrient ingested by a man or an animal. A variety of the latter are the *metabolic balance studies,* which measure and *compare* the amount of a nutrient that enters the body—usually by the gastrointestinal tract—and the amount that is excreted by that body.

This paper gives an overview of the characteristics of a metabolic ward and of various nutritional metabolic studies in humans. Emphasis is made on their applications, pitfalls and limitations.

The Metabolic Ward in Nutritional Studies

One of the major applications of a metabolic ward is research related to dietary studies and the consequences of eating —or of not eating— certain foods or nutrients. In contrast to experiments with isolated cells or subcellular fractions, man responds simultaneously to many factors in his environment, such as diet, climate, physical surroundings and emotional stimuli. These multifactorial responses are further influenced by circumstancial conditions such as exercise, feeding patterns, sleeping habits and behavioral changes. A meta-

361

bolic ward provides a suitable environment to control many of those factors and circumstances, thereby limiting the experimental variables to those of interest for a specific investigation. This allows a better evaluation and interpretation of the results.

Hodges (11) cited the work of James Lind in 1747 (16) as one of the earliest descriptions of a controlled dietary study, done in an environment that preceded by more than a century the establishment of metabolic wards. Twelve sailors on board of the British ship, "Salisbury", developed scurvy with "putrid gums, spots, lassitude and weakness of their knees". They were placed in an apartment for the sick in the ship's forehold, and received the same diet: water-gruel sweetened with sugar in the morning, fresh mutton broth, puddings and boiled biscuits for dinner, and for supper barley and raisins, rice and currents or sago and wine. Six different treatments were given to each of 2 patients: a quart of cider a day; 25 drops of "elixer vitriol" three times a day; two spoonfuls of vinegar three times a day; half a pint of sea water every day; two oranges and one lemon every day; or a purgative made of garlic, mustardseed, raphon, balsam of Peru and gum myrrh, three times a day. The "most sudden and visible good effects" were perceived from the use of the oranges and lemons; one of the sailors who had taken them was fit for duty at the end of six days, and the other, who was the best recovered, was appointed nurse to the rest of the sick.

Facilities gradually developed in various hospitals and they evolved in this century from relatively simple research wards [e.g., 2] to elaborate, modern metabolic units. But these present-day metabolic wards, with all their sophisticated equipment and computerized facilities, still require the essential elements included in Lind's work aboard the "Salisbury", in order to conduct adequate research: a hypothesis to be tested, a group of individuals willing to participate as experimental subjects, a controlled environment, a uniform diet, well defined variable treatments, and an objective evaluation of the results. Another essential requirement is a well-trained, highly-motivated staff. A metabolic ward is designed to standardize procedures, reduce the possibility of errors and keep a detailed record of the events that might influence the experimental subjects. All these require a strict discipline of the attending staff.

The metabolic ward must have adequate facilities to house the patients or healthy subjects, deal with therapeutic or emergency conditions, provide indoor-and outdoor-recreation and leisure activities, prepare and serve the diets, perform the experimental tests, handle and store biological specimens, and process or relay the specimens to the laboratory.

The attending staff must be well-trained, conscious about the importance of their work, highly motivated in its performance, tolerant and absolutely honest. They must be aware of the importance to establish a good rapport with the experimental subjects, to record all events meticulously, since even trivial details might later be significant, and to admit and report errors and departures from the experimental protocol.

All studies involving humans as experimental subjects, must be critically assessed by a committee of persons who are not related to the investigation, in order to protect the subjects, establish the safety or potential risk of the procedures and decide upon the relevance of the research in relation to the discomfort of the subjects. Guidelines for such committees, including the considerations of studies on children and mentally incapacitated persons, have been published.

It is essential that the persons who act as experimental subjects are willing to cooperate: an uncooperative subject can ruin any project, either by intent or neglect. These persons can be either patients who have a disease or condition of particular interest, or healthy volunteers. They should understand the purpose of the investigation, the nature of the procedures and the importance of the results. They should have a feeling of participation and must understand that their role in the project is of utmost importance. Children must be kept comfortable and happy at all times; whenever possible, the experimental procedures should be dealt as games and provide a pleasant experience.

Advantages of the Metabolic Ward

The main advantages are the collection of carefully controlled information and the reduction of interfering variables. The detailed and careful recording of all observations, whether part of the experimental protocol or due to unexpected circumstances, may give results of great importance in the short-and long-term. Important, and sometimes serendipitous, discoveries can result from well-kept records. For example, the occurrence of infections during the investigation of nutritional requirements can provide useful information about metabolic alterations of a nutrient during the disease, or about the change in requirements during and after the disease.

Limitations of Metabolic Ward Studies

One of the main limitations is the small number of subjects in most studies, usually due to high costs or to a scarcity of appropriate subjects. This can be compensated by the high precission, accurancy and number of metabolic measurements: we can sometimes learn as much from a large number of detailed observations obtained in a small number of persons, as from a small number of less rigorous observations in a large number of persons. But if the inter-individual variability is too large, it may not be possible to draw definite conclusions from a small number of subjects. Nevertheless, the results may suggest phenomena that can be tested or confirmed out of the metabolic ward with a larger number of individuals.

Another limitation may be the artificial conditions of the metabolic ward, as compared with the so-called "field" or "real life" environment. Before generalizing the conclusions drawn from a study, one must consider the characteristics within the metabolic ward that often contrast with those of the outside world, such as: 1) the hygienic environment with low infectious morbidity; 2) the rigid scheduling of activities such as arising, eating meals, engaging in exercise and going to bed; 3) the homogeneity and monotony of the diet, sometimes eaten in the same amounts day after day and divided into identical servings; and, 4) the confinement to the metabolic ward facilities. These limitations may be of little importance for studies such as the evaluation of a specific treatment for bed-ridden patients, but they may be of great importance for other investigations, such as the establishment of certain nutritional requirements for a population. In the latter case, some crucial field conditions may be mimicked in the metabolic ward by a programmed modification of schedules, provision of varied diets that can be freely chosen by the subjects, and physical activities similar or equivalent to those of the general population, including supervised walks and out-of-doors games. All these conditions must be under strict control of the investigators and quantitatively measured. This can be done, [e.g., 22], although it complicates the design of the experimental protocol and taxes the efforts of the investigators and attending staff. However, some field conditions, such as poor environmental hygiene or high risks of infection, cannot be mimicked for obvious ethical reasons and others cannot be technically reproduced.

The duration of studies that require longitudinal observations can also be a limiting factor in the interpretation and generalization of the results. Long term investigations are expensive and it is often difficult to find healthy subjects who are willing to live in the metabolic ward for extended periods of time. Some researchers have succeeded in recruiting highly motivated individuals who otherwise would be confined to prisons or orphanages. They must be provided with an environment at least as good as that of the institution from where they come, and there must be strict adherence to their human rights and privacy.

Metabolic Balance Studies

The name of these studies derives from the maxim that "input minus output equals balance". They compare the amounts of a nutrient that enters the human body with the amounts of the nutrient or its metabolites that are excreted. This can be expressed by the equation $B = I - E$, where B is balance, I is intake and E is excreta.

The usefulness and uncertainties of metabolic balance studies have been objects of discussions for many years, strongly expressed by critics and supporters alike [3, 9, 11, 12, 25], but are still the keystone of many nutritional investigations. Depending on the cooperation and reliability of the experimental subjects and on the nature and duration of the investigations, metabolic balance studies can be done on an inpatient or outpatient basis, although it is preferable to do them in a metabolic ward. Subjects who are not confined to the ward can eat their meals there or can perform the whole study in their home environment. However, the lack of supervision may lead to errors, unless the experimental subject is highly motivated, understands perfectly the procedure and the investigation, and is honest and reliable.

Requirements and Sources of Error in Metabolic
Balance Studies

Accurate balance calculations require precise weight or volume measurements of foods and body excreta, accurate timing of the beginning and end of the measurements, adequate homogenization and aliquoting of representative samples for analysis, and detailed recording of the conditions surrounding the experimental subjects. Most balance studies also require attaining a steady state, specially after introducing dietary changes.

The intake portion of the balance equation usually refers to food, but the ingestion, and parenteral administrations of drugs and other substances are also part of the intake. Foods must be prepared in a metabolic kitchen under standardized conditions, using sensitive and accurate weighing instruments and, whenever possible, the same batch of raw materials. When the nutrient being assayed is a trace mineral, special attention must be payed to the water and the utensils used to prepare and feed the meals; for example, tap water contains variable amounts of zinc and ironware can give off relatively large amounts of iron when cooking or storage conditions are favorable. Therefore, the water source and utensils must be standardized and, if necessary, the chemical contribution made to the foods must be assayed frequently.

Liquid formulas allow a better quantitation of intake, but they are less well accepted by older children and adults and they may result in a gastric emptying pattern different from that with solid foods, which might influence the digestion and absorption of certain nutrients. Each food component of a meal must be served in a separate container and the exact amount eaten by the subject must be assessed by differential weighing of the container before and after the meal. Children must be helped to eat, as needed. Losses through spillage or spitting must be determined by weighing tared clothes used to pick the spillage. Young children should wear tared clothes and bedding.

It is more accurate to weigh than to measure the urine voided in a large sized volumetric container; the exact volume can be calculated from the specific gravity. The beginning and end of the collection period should be timed after voluntary emptying of the bladder or, in small children, after spontaneous voiding. If the period is near 24 hours, mathematical corrections may be used to calculate the exact 24-hour output.

The deviation of fecal collection periods is usually determined by the appearance of a non-absorbable colored marker fed at the beginning and end of the period. The timing, however, may not be accurate in individuals with constipation or irregular bowel movements. Most investigators recommend collection periods of at least 7 days in adults to minimize the errors. Three or four days may be adequate for children who defecate more than once each day. A better, but more complex timing can be done by measuring the amount recovered in feces of a non-absorbable marker fed throughout the collection period in a constant proportion to the nutrient under assay. The marker must not interfere with gastrointestinal motility or chemical processes, and must progress along the gastrointestinal tract at the same rate as the nutrient being assayed.

Collections are more difficult in children, specially girls, who do not yet control urination and defecation. They are frequently confined to metabolic beds with collecting systems. The limited physical activity influences bowel movements and, if long enough, may influence the urinary excretion of some substances such as calcium. Consequently, inactivity must be reduced to a minimun, stimulating the children to move as much as possible in the metabolic bed, and allowing them to walk wearing self-adhesive urine collection bags after they defecate.

Vomitus is part of the excreta. Its weight can be quantified in a similar fashion as food spillage. Whenever possible, vomitus must be chemically analyzed to determine the exact amount of lost nutrient. If not, its nutrient concentration must be estimated from the food contents and the time of vomiting, relative to food intake. At best, this is an approximation and frequent or voluminous vomiting may invalidate the balance study.

Milk secretions must also be considered as "excreta" in lactating women.

Other losses of body constituents include visible and insensible sweat, desquamated skin, sputum, menstural bleeding, clinical blood sampling, etcetera. The role of these miscellaneous losses in balance studies was discussed by Calloway and coworkers [6]. They can sometimes account for large losses of nutrients (for example sodium excretion through sweat in cystic fibrosis or in hot environments). The miscellaneous losses of some nutrients can be calculated from data reported in the scientific literature.

Foods and excreta must be thoroughly homogenized to obtain truly representative aliquots for chemical analysis. When using mixed diets, it is best to analyze each food separately.

Some studies introduce a consistent bias in metabolic balance calculations. If it is assumed that all food is eaten, intake may be overestimated when the exact amount is not measured; excreta can be underestimated due to small losses in collection or neglect to include miscellaneous losses. The end-result is an overestimation of positive or an underestimation of negative balances.

Limitation of Metabolic Balance Studies

Some limitations of metabolic balance studies are universal but others are related to the proposed applications of the metabolic balance.

The limitations of metabolic ward studies apply to balance studies, but the duration of the balance period merits additional comments. Balance studies carried out during 3 to 7 days do not necessarily represent the long-term balance of a nutrient. In fact, the normal day-to-day variations in food intake end the short periods of augmented or decreased losses, suggest that days of negative and positive balance alternated to produce, in the long-rum, zero or nearzero balance in adults and a positive balance in growing children and pregnant women.

Another problem of short-term metabolic balance studies is the time required to reach a steady state after a dietary change. If the excreta are expected to indicate the metabolic fate of substances ingested under habitual conditions, the experimental subject must reach a new equilibrium after the transition from one pattern of intake to another. The duration of this equilibration period varies and may be long for some substances [17]. Furthermore, Sukhatme and Margen [21] postulated an autoregression process that serially correlates the fluctuations in nitrogen balance with the values of the previous days.

Pathological or physiological alterations in metabolism can invalidate the comparisons of short-term balance studies. Infections and fever influence the subject's appetite and the intermediary metabolism of absorbed nutrients; there may be an increase in catabolism and augmented urinary losses of the nutrient or its metabolites. Periodic metabolic changes can influence balance data, as is the case with the fluctuations in urinary nitrogen during the mestrual cycle [14].

On the other hand, changes in physical activity or body composition can influence the results of long-term balance studies, and they should always be considered. Another potential problem with long-term balance studies is that small errors with a consistent bias (e.g., overlooking integumental losses) can have a large cumulative effect.

A major limitation of metabolic balance studies is that they only indicate the total net change of a substance in the body, but do not provide information about internal body distributions, turnover rates, pool sizes or intermediary metabolic fate of the substances. Furthermore, they do not indicate the amounts of endogenous substances excreted by urine or feces, nor of the bacterial contribution to fecal matter. The true absorption of a nutrient can be determined with the ingestion of isotopically labeled substances that can be differentiated from endogenous and bacterial products, or correcting from the calculations of fecal excretion with data from experiments done with a diet free of the nutrient.

The interpretation of metabolic balance data can be complicated by the yet unexplained phenomenon that high intakes of many substances produce apparently high retentions that are not confirmed by carcass analysis of animals nor by body composition measurements in humans [7, 9, 10, 13, 23]. The explanations offered for these findings include consistent errors in the measurement of losses, respiratory excretion of volatile substances and changes in body composition. None of them, however, are satisfactory and we must conclude that, for most nutrients, the assessment of retentions with high intakes give fallacious results.

Balance studies of some nutrients or of their metabolic results, can only be done if other methods are used simultaneously with the measurements of intake and excreta. Foremost among them is dietary energy balance. A very large component in the balance considerations is energy expenditure (Exp), such that the balance equation becomes: $B = I-E-Exp$. Energy expenditure must be measured by direct or indirect calorimetry, or estimated from heart rate or time-and-motion observations [1]. The errors inherent to these methods must be added to those of the metabolic balance technique.

Application of Metabolic Balance Studies

Metabolic balance data have useful applications in spite of their recognized limitations and technical uncertainties. Among them, the following can be mentioned:

1. Definition of the minimal daily requirements of a nutrient.

2. Evaluation of changes in nutritional requirements due to physiological conditions (e.g. age, pregnancy, lactation, exercise, genetic characteristics, infections, endocrine disorders, etc.)

3. Definition of the nutritional needs of hospitalized patients with acute or chronic diseases, or with increased nutrient losses (e.g., burns, protracted diarrhea, trauma, prolonged immobilization, etc.).

4. Study of dietary, metabolic and environmental factors that influence absorption, excretion or retention of a nutrient.

5. Evaluation of long-term trends of change in body composition.

6. Complementary information for other metabolic, physiological or diagnostic studies (e.g., total energy requirements, malabsorption syndromes, nutritional impact of environmental contamination, etc.).

Dietary energy metabolism

It is now accepted that energy requirements are determined by energy expenditure and not by energy intake [8]. Hence the importance of its measurement, as well as that of total energy balance. Energy expenditure can be measured by direct calorimentry, indirect calorimetry or physiological measurements that correlate with oxygen uptake, such as heart rate monitoring. All these techniques have physiological or practical advantages and limitations.

Direct calorimetry is the most precise of the currently available methods. Its main limitations are the costs of building a calorimetric chamber and the confinement of the experimental subject to such restricted quarters for the duration of the studies.

Indirect calorimetry is based on measurements of inhaled and exhaled oxygen and carbon dioxide, and on the energy equivalence of the oxygen consumed. The energy cost of various activities can thus be measured. The summation of the periods of time that a person spends in each activity, multiplied by the corresponding energy costs, gives an estimate of total energy expenditure; these are the so-called time-and-motion studies [24]. Their main advantages are that they can be done in free-ranging individuals, either in a metabolic ward or in the field. Their main limitations are: 1) when the energy cost of activities cannot be measured in the experimental subjects, it is necessary to rely on data published by other investigators and to assume that they apply to our subjects; 2) it must be assumed that the energy cost of an activity is constant throughout its performance, although there may be wide variations in performance efficiency; 3) the activities must be accurately timed by an external observer who can observe only one subject at a time; 4) the presence of the observer may induce behavioral changes and modify the subject's habitual activities.

Heart-rate monitoring is based on its linear relationship with oxygen consumption [4]. Its main advantage is that the subject wears a heart-beat monitoring device and an observer need not be in the proximity. Its main limitations are: 1) the correlation between heart-rate and oxygen consumption must be assessed in each subject due to large inter-individual variability; 2) the correlation is linear within certain limits and is lost during rest periods; 3) frequent assessments of heart-rate must be made, since the correlation with oxygen consumption may vary at high and low levels of energy expenditure; 4) the correlation may be influenced by various physiological, pathological and environmental conditions.

Water with a double isotope label of ^{2}H and ^{18}O has been recently used to assess energy expenditure in man [18]. It is based on assessments of body composition, CO_2 production and respiratory quotient. It seems to be a promising method for metabolic ward and field applications, but it must be further tested and validated. One of its main current limitations are the high costs of the doubly-labeled water and the analysis of the stable isotopes.

Hydrogen Breath Test

This is another useful test in nutritional metabolic studies. It is based on the observation that certain bacteria of the normal human colonic flora will ferment unabsorbed carbohydrate with evolution of hydrogen gas [5, 15]. The gas is absorbed into the blood by the colonic mucosa, and excreted through the lungs. Thus, an increase in the concentration of exhaled H_2 is stoichiometrically related to the amount of unabsorbed carbohydrate. Its major applications are in the study of intestinal carbohydrate absorption, diagnosis of lactose malabsorption, study of gastrointestinal transit time, and diagnosis of bacterial overgrowth of the small intestine. The method, however, has a series of pit falls and limitations that must be considered in its application and in the interpretation of its results. The Table, adapted from studies and reviews by Solomons [19, 20] summarizes the main pitfalls and limitations of the method.

SUMMARY

Metabolic studies are essential for nutritional research. However, all techniques have pitfalls and limitations that must be taken into account to apply them correctly and, more important, to interpret their results adequately. We have discussed in detail the limitations related to the metabolic ward and metabolic balance studies, and commented briefly on other techniques frequently used in our metabolic ward and field studies. The potential, limitations and applications of other methods are discussed in other sections of this Workshop.

LIMITATIONS AND PITFALLS IN THE APPLICATION AND INTERPRETATION OF THE HYDROGEN BREATH TEST*

Idiopathic absence of appropriate flora
   Consequence: No H_2 response to nonabsorbed carbohydrate

Use of oral antibiotics prior to the hydrogen breath test
   Consequence: Reduction in the mass of fermenting bacteria in the colon

Cigarette smoking during the hydrogen breath test
   Consequence: Abrupt increase in breath H_2 concentration not related to carbohydrate

Active diarrhea at the time of the hydrogen breath test
   Consequence: Reduced H_2 response to a given amount of nonabsorbed carbohydrate

Sleeping during the hydrogen breath test
   Consequence: Increased concentration of breath H_2

Incorporation of the test carbohydrate into a fiber-containing meal
   Consequence: Excess of excretion of breath H_2 not related to malabsorption of the test carbohydrate

Acidic colonic pH due to recent fermentation of carbohydrates
   Consequence: Reduced H_2 production (pH optimum. 7.2)

Use of enemas prior to the hydrogen breath test
   Consequence: Wash-out of fermenting flora

Delayed gastric emptying
   Consequence: Alterations in the kinetic characteristics of the H_2 response curve

Hyperventilation or crying during collection of breath specimen
   Consequence: Dilution of pulmonary H_2 with air of the anatomic dead space.

Adapted from Solomons, NW, references 19 and 20.

REFERENCES

1. Astrand, P.O., and Rodahl, K. "Textbook of Work Physiology", 669 pp. McGraw-Hill, New York, 1970.
2. Bauer, W., and Aub, J.C. Studies in inorganic salt metabolism: ward routine and methods. *J. Am. Dietet. Assn.* 3:106, 1927.
3. Beisel, W.R. Metabolic balance studies - their continuing usefulness in nutritional research (Editorial). *Am. J. Clin. Nutr.* 32:271, 1979.
4. Bradfield, R.B. A technique for determination of usual daily energy expenditure in the field. *Am. J. Clin. Nutr.* 24:1148, 1971.
5. Calloway, D.H., and Murphy, E.L. The use of expired air to measure intestinal gas formation. *Ann. N. Y. Acad. Sci.* 150:82, 1968.
6. Calloway, D.H., Odell, A.C.F., and Margen, S. Sweat and miscellaneous nitrogen losses in human balance studies. *J. Nutr.* 101:775, 1971.
7. Duncan, D.L. The interpretation of studies of calcium and phosphorus balance in ruminants. *Nutr. Absts. Rev.* 28:695, 1958.
8. FAO/WHO/UNU. Report of the Joint FAO/WHO/UNU Meeting of Experts on Protein and Energy Requirements. Rome, FAO, 1981 (in press).
9. Forbes, G.B. Another source of error in the metabolic balance method. *Nutr. Rev.* 31:297, 1973.
10. Hegsted, D.M. Balance studies (Editorial). *J. Nutr.* 106:307, 1976.
11. Hodges, R.E. The role of a metabolic ward in nutritional studies. *Am. J. Clin. Nutr.* 24:930, 1971.
12. Isakson, B., and Sjogren, B. A critical evaluation of the mineral and nitrogen balances in man. *Proc. Nutr. Soc.* 26:106, 1967.
13. King, J.C., Calloway, D.H., and Margen, S. Nitrogen retention, total body 40_K and weight gain in teenage pregnant girls. *J. Nutr.* 103:772, 1973.
14. Kurzer, M.S., and Calloway, D.H. Urinary nitrogen cycles and the protein requirements of healthy young women, 12 Internat. Congr. Nutr., San Diego, California, 1981.
15. Levitt, M.D. Production and excretion of hydrogen gas in man. N. Engl. *J. Med.* 28:122, 1969.
16. Lind, J. "A treatise on the Scurvy". Sands, Murray and Cochran, Edinburgh, 1753.
17. Malm, O.J. Calcium requirement and adaptation in adult men. *Scand. J. Clin. Lab. Invest.* 10 (Suppl. 36):1, 1958.
18. Schoeller, D.A., and van Santen, E. Measurement of energy expenditure in man by the doubly labeled water method. *J. Appl. Physiol.* (in press).
19. Solomons, N.W. Diagnosis and screening techniques for lactose maldigestion: Advantages of the hydrogen breath test. In "Lactose Digestion" (D.M. Paige and T.M. Bayless, eds.), pp. 91-109. Johns Hopkins Univ. Press, Baltimore, 1981.
20. Solomons, N.W. The use of H_2 breath-analysis tests in gastrointestinal diagnosis. In "Current Concepts in Gastroenterology", 1982 (in press).
21. Sukhatme, P.V., and Margen, S. Models for protein deficiency. *Am. J. Clin. Nutr.* 31:1237, 1978.
22. Torun, B., and Viteri, F.E. Capacity of habitual Guatemalan diets to satisfy protein requirements of pre-school children with adequate dietary energy intakes. *Food Nutr. Bull.,* suppl. 5:210, 1981.
23. Torun, B., Scrimshaw, N.S., and Young, V.R. Effect of isometric exercises on body potassium and dietary protein requirements of young men. *Am. J. Clin. Nutr.* 30:1983, 1977.
24. Viteri, F.E., Torun, B., Galicia, J.C., and Herrera, E. Determining energy costs of agricultural activities by respirometer and energy balance techniques. *Am. J. Clin. Nutr.* 24:1418, 1971.
25. Walker, A.R.P. Uncertainties in the interpretation and validity of long-term balance studies (Editorial). *Am. J. Clin. Nutr.* 10:95, 1962.

DISCUSSION[1]

Sonya Connor asked if the hydrogen breath test might be useful in the measurement of dietary fiber intake. Torún was cautious in his response pointing out that the efficacy depended upon the type of fiber and the type of intestinal flora. He thought it might be adequate as a semiquantitative measurement in certain defined situations. Solomons concurred, mentioning studies by Eastwood et al. in which hydrogen levels were very slow to increase when high levels of hemicellulose and pectins were fed. The ingestion of other hydrogen producing carbohydrates would complicate this further. Scrimshaw raised the question of psychological as well as infectious factors complicating the interpretation of metabolic studies. He noted that when students were used for long-term balance studies, exams or other periods of stress caused them to deviate from the stable pattern they had shown before and afterward. Other examples were offered as well. He emphasized the importance of having the staff versed in the study so that unrecorded food intake was eliminated. He emphasized that whenever an outlier is detected, it is vital to be certain that this was not merely an error in the study. Harper commented that changes in pool size are measured by balance procedures and that with some additional studies determining the original pool size, a relationship between pool size and the development of symptoms can be made.

[1]*Summary of the discussion prepared by S. Cederbaum.*

GENETICS, ENVIRONMENT, AND GROWTH: ISSUES IN THE ASSESSMENT OF NUTRITIONAL STATUS

Reynaldo Martorell

Food Research Institute
Stanford University
Stanford, California

Some have suggested that where malnutrition is endemic, children with high protein requirements are more likely to develop kwashiorkor and therefore die [18]. If true, mean protein requirements would be lower in populations with a very long history of malnutrition. Unfortunately, research on the issue of ethnic differences in nutrient requirements is limited and the data at hand may not be satisfactory for testing this or similar hypothesis about other nutrients. What research has been done, however, has failed to show differences between populations in requirements for protein and calories once body mass differences and environmental factors are taken into account [14].

A related hypothesis is that malnutrition exerts selective pressures against children with the genetic potential for greater growth [15]. Such children would have greater nutritional requirements than average children due to the added metabolic cost of growth and the increased needs for maintenance of a larger body mass. In time of famine, large children and adults would perhaps succumb sooner to the effects of undernutrition. Again, populations long subjected to chronic undernutrition would be made up of individuals who are small for genetic reasons. It has been suggested that the native peoples of Meso America are examples of such populations. A sedentary agricultural type of life dependent on corn can be documented for several millenia [50]. The Mayan population ranks as one of the shortest in the American continent and there is some evidence from the archaelogical record that Mayan adults were once taller [47]. Though it is possible that genetic factors account in part for the small size of the Mayan population, for reasons that will become clearer shortly, it is more likely that the principal causes are environmental. The Mayan population suffers from chronic undernutrition and high rates of infection and their small body size may be largely a phenotypic reflection of these sad realities.

Frisancho and colleagues [15] claim that in the shanty towns of Peru, the children of smaller mothers had a greater probability of survival. This was interpreted as evidence of natural selection operating in favor of small body sizes. These are unusual findings which run contrary to what many studies have found in developing countries. Greater height in women is usually associated with enhanced capacity to conceive and deliver a baby more likely to survive and to have better growth and development [44, 45].

Illustrative of these findings are the data shown in Table I. We studied the reproductive histories of 460 Mayan women and related maternal stature to infant mortality, parity, and number of surviving children [40]. Variations in socioeconomic status were minimal as all families lived in and were employed by coffee plantations, and as all received the same low salaries and limited supplies of corn. Poverty and malnutrition were salient characteristics of the families. Mothers were very short; in fact, this population appears to be among the shortest in the world. The mean height was 142.4 cm [S.D. = 5.3] and the tallest woman was only 158.6 cm or 5 feet 2 inches. In the analysis in Table I, the variation in maternal height was divided into terciles and the groups were compared in terms of infant mortality, parity, and number of surviving children. The relationship between maternal stature and infant mortality was very clear. Rates were 205 deaths per 1,000 live born for the shortest group, 150 for the middle group, and 101 for the taller mother [p < .001]. These was a tendency for shorter mothers to have greater parities. Perhaps this reflects conscious efforts by shorter women to have more children to compensate for greater child losses. Or, it may also be the case that the cessation of breast feeding brought on by the death of an infant may have hastened the re-

TABLE I

Maternal stature, infant mortality, party, and number of surviving children in Mayan women [b]

	Terciles of height			Analysis of variance Main effects	
	Lower (n = 127)	Middle n = 124)	Upper (n = 129)	F	P
Stature (cm)					
Mean	137.7	142.0	148.2		
Range	123.3-140.2	140.3-144.7	144.8-158.6		
Infant mortality [b]	205	150	101	7.9	<.001
Parity [b]	4.75	4.10	4.22	2.1	.12
Surviving children [b]	2.83	3.02	3.15	1.7	.18

[a] *After Martorell et al. (40).*
[b] *Values standardized for age by analysis of covariance. Adjusted to the mean age of 28.4 years.*

turn of menstruation, shortened the interval between births, and thus increased parity [40]. However, the greater parities observed in the shortest mothers did not result in a greater number of surviving children. In fact, the opposite was the case; there was a clear tendency for taller women to contribute more children to the next generation. This analysis therefore does not support the hypothesis that there is differential fertility in favor of short mothers in malnourished populations.

Perhaps the principal adaptive mechanisms to malnutrition have been physiological rather than genetic *per se*. Some of the adaptations which enable individuals to tolerate poor nutritional intakes are well-known. Protein catabolism is diminished, nitrogen excretion in urine and sweat is reduced, and the efficiency of protein utilization is enhanced in individuals with low protein intakes [20]. Adaptation to low energy intakes entails a decrease in physical activity and in severe undernutrition, the basal metabolic rate also decreases. More pertinent to our paper, is how children modify their patterns of growth to cope with undernutrition. When faced with chronic but moderate deficiencies of nutrients, children grow less in height and weight but do seem to manage to maintain normal weight to height ratios [39]. As the severity and the duration of the nutritional deficiency increases, children cease to grow altogether and the process of body wasting begins. In wasting, tissue reserves are broken down to provide for basal metabolic needs. Death follows this last stage unless the underlying deficiencies are corrected.

According to Gopalan, a noted Indian nutritionist, the term "adaptation" in its strictest sense can only be applied to a situation in which an organism (or a population) responds to an environmental stress in a manner which not only ensures survival but which retains optimal functional capacity [20]. In this sense, the reponses to malnutrition which we have detailed above are not adaptations because the involve varying degrees of functional impairment. Health practitioners in developing countries are well aware that when young children show poor gains in weight and length or worse yet, that when they lose weight, they are in grave danger of dying [10]. Growth retardation frequently precedes episodes of kwashiorkor and marasmus [48]. Immunocompetence is diminished in children who are growing poorly and otherwise mild infections in well-nourished children will become severe, complicated, and often fatal in poorly nourished children [8].

Growth norms derived from data from developed countries have been and continue to be used in developing countries to define "adequate" growth. The Iowa-Harvard standards [57] were widely used for many years and it is only recently that WHO has promulgated the use of the NCHS (National Center for Health Statistics) norms derived from data from the United States [64, 68]. These data are based on large representative samples of caucasian and black children but they do not differ much from the Iowa-Harvard or other norms and their adoption will not lead to different estimates of the extent of malnutrition in developing countries.

The use of growth norms from children of European origin has not gone uncriticized by those who question their appropriateness for the myriad of ethnic groups in developing countries [19]. Because the severity of malnutrition is greatest in the preschool period, ethnic differences in this period are of greater interest than those which might exist later in life.

Secular changes in height

Discussions of the appropriateness of standards derived from European children might start by considering that nineteenth century European children were as short as children from developing countries are today. Children and adults in the industrialized countries are now bigger than they used to be [59, 65]. Children also mature faster. Menarche is reached two to four years earlier and growth is completed by 17 to 18 years of age instead of during the mid-20s [59].

Figure 1 illustrates the small size of lower class nineteenth century British children in comparison to the NCHS norms. The nineteenth century data are taken from Tanner [61] and were collected in the Manchester Stockport area as part of parliamentary inquests into the conditions of working children. Though conditions in these infamous workhouses were deplorable, factory children were only half a centimeter shorter than nonworking children of the area. Figure 1 shows that the mean heights to these children were below the fifth percentile of the NCHS norms. These British data are not unlike modern data from lower class children from such diverse countries as Guatemala and India.

Environmental and genetic hypotheses have been advanced to explain the secular changes in stature. The environmental explanation attibutes the changes to improvements in the standard of living, particulary in nutrition and environmental sanitation. The genetic hypothesis attributes the changes to heterosis or hybrid vigor resulting from the breakdown of breeding isolates brought about by increased social and geographical mobility. Most authors conclude that the effect of heterosis, in any, is bound to be small and attribute the changes to improvements in the quality of life [11, 65].

Further proof that the secular changes are due to environmental causes comes from analysis showing the adverse effect of times of was on the secular trend. Figure 2 shows the trends in height from 1910 to 1953 for German school children 7 to 18 years of age. The data on the left are for boys and that on the right for girls and each line connect cohorts of the same age. The first line at the bottom, for example, refers to the 7-8 year old group while the last at the top is for the 17 to 18 year old group. Shown clearly in Figure 2 is how the two World Wars interrupted the upward trend in height.

The secular trend in height appears to have ceased in areas of Europe, North America, and Japan suggesting that these populations may be as tall as

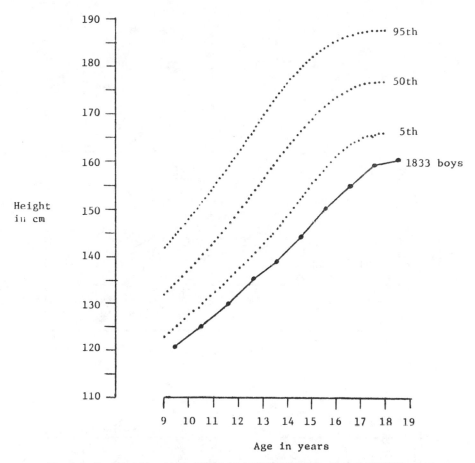

Figure 1. Size of nineteenth century British children compared to the NCHS norms.

they will ever be [4, 7, 12, 23]. An interesting feature of the secular trend is that changes in body proportions have been minimal. According to Tanner [60, p. 129], "There is some slight evidence that the secular trend towards larger size includes a faint tendency towards increasing linearity of build, but the change is a very minor one."

Comparison of well-to-do children from around the world

The phenomenon of secular changes informs us about the variance in growth which can be ascribed solely to the environment since genetic explanations are unlikely. The analysis shown in Figure 3 attempt to do the opposite, namely, to show the portion of the variance in growth which can be said to be

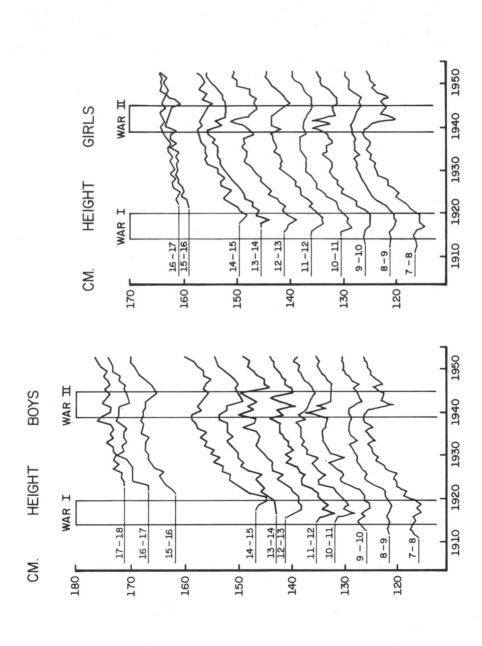

largely genetic. Figure 3 shows mean heights for samples of 7 year old children from industrialized countries and from the highest socioeconomic groups of developing countries. Preasumably, growth and development in these samples is not limited by malnutrition and disease but is instead a reflection of genetic differences. Data for the children of European origin include studies carried out in Europe and the United States. The European studies are those carried out in Czechoslovakia [51], Germany [25], Switzerland [6], and England [62] under the coordination of the International Children's Centre. All of these European data, as well as most of that for other areas, are conveniently summarized in table form in the work of Eveleth and Tanner [13]. The North American data come from the major longitudinal studies carried out in Berkeley [63], Boston [54], Cleveland [55], Denver [46], Iowa [57], and Ohio [16]. The studies selected from Latin America, as well as those from other developing countries, are those carried out among the countries' elites and represent Brazil [49], Guatemala [29, 30], Costa Rica [67] and Puerto Rico [33]. The children of African origin are represented by samples from Nigeria [13, 28], Haiti [32], Jamaica [1, 2], and five studies of black children from the United States [5, 26, 27, 35, 53, 66]. The Asian group includes samples from Formosa [31], Hong Kong [9], Jamaica [1, 2], Japan [13], and the United States [22, 34]. The Indian sample is from Hyderabad [56].

To put the data in perspective, the 75th, 50th, 25th, and 10th percentiles of the NCHS standards [64] are indicated in the far right. Seven of the European samples are above the 50th percentile but some are below, the lowest representing the study from which the British norms were derived. Many growth studies of European children have been published [13] and mean values for these, if plotted, would range from the NCHS 25th to the 75th percentile. Mean values of well-to-do children of Latin American, African, or East Indian origin hover around the NCHS 50th percentile. Similar conclusions are obtained from studies carried out in younger and older samples [21, 24, 44]. Though not apparent in Figure 3, some researchers in the United States argue that black children are genetically taller and call for separate growth standards though the differences in question are rather small [17]. The one group that does appear to be shorter than the rest is the Asian. Children of Japanese or Chinese origin, whether growing up in California, Hawaii, or in Taiwan, Hong Kong or Japan, have mean height values at 7 years of age that approximate the NCHS 25th percentile. Since the secular increases in children of Japanese origin in California and in Japan appear to have ceased [23], it is likely that the differences between Asiatic and other children are indeed genetic.

As there are many groups around the world that are not represented in Figure 3, there may well be other ethnic groups who are small for genetic reasons.

Figure 2. Trends in height from 1910 to 1953 for German school children 7 to 18 years of age. Note the interruption in the upward trend in height caused by the two World Wars.

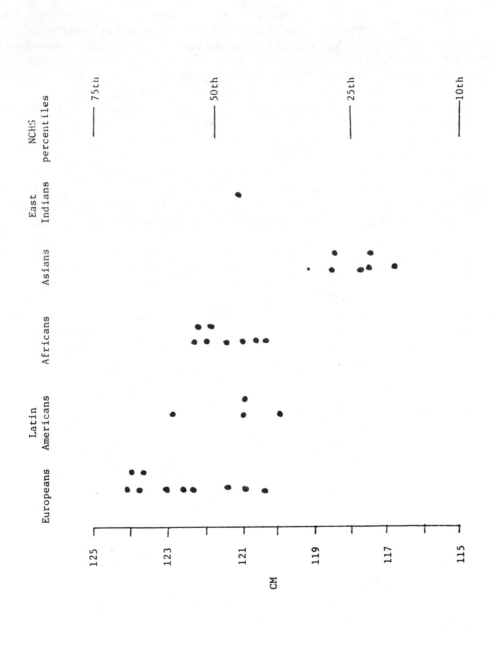

Perhaps the Meso-American Indian population, if one day it is well fed and healthy, will be tall like the Japanese but not as tall as the Europeans. If should be noted that one of the Latin American samples included in Figure 3 is from Guatemala [29,30] and that this sample was of European-Mayan ancestry. These Guatemalan children were as tall as Europeans at 7 years of age. Studies in Colombia [37, 69] and Chile [3] also show that preschool children of mixed European-Indian ancestry and of high socioeconomic status grow like European children.

Data from India [52] and Guatemala [29] suggest that the similarity in growth patterns with European children end with adolescence. Clear differences surface during the adolescence period for both sexes and Guatemalan and Indian children who were near the 50th percentile prior to puberty ended up near the 25th percentile at the end of adolescence. These data suggest that ethnic differences in growth potential are minor prior to puberty and that it is during this stage that major differentiation between ethnic groups takes place. These ideas reinforce WHO'S recomendation not to use the NCHS standards to evaluate children older than 10 years of age [69]. Malnutrition, as stated earlier, is a problem of great magnitude only in the preschool period and the use of anthropometry to evaluate the nutritional status of groups of older children is not recommended.

Social class comparisons

We are now ready to compare the relative importance of the environment and genetics as explanations of the differences in the sizes of children from around the world. This is done in Figure 4 by comparing the heights of 7 year old children from high and low socieconomic groups for a number of countries. Samples are available from Brazil [49], Costa Rica [67], Guatemala [20, 30, 70], Haiti [32], Jamaica [black children: 1, 2], Nigeria [13, 28], India [56], and Hong Kong [9]. The variance due to genetics can be ascertained by looking at the differences between the dark circles which represent children of high socioeconomic status. As was also evident in Figure 3, differences between the well-to-do samples in Figure 4 are very small and amount to no more than a few centimeters. The differences associated with social class, on the other hand, are very large. A number of the lower class samples in Figure 4 have mean values that are near the 10th percentile and lower class children from India and Guatemala have mean heights that lie beyond the range of variation of the NCHS norms. Clearly, the variation which can be attibuted to the environment is several times greater than that which can be said to be due to genetics.

Figure 3. Mean heights for samples of 7 year old children from industrialized countries and from the highest socioeconomic groups of developing countries.

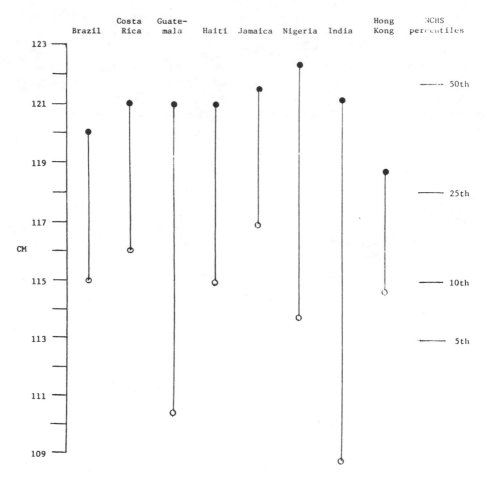

Figure 4. Heights of 7 year old children from high and low socioeconomic groups for several countries.

Experimental studies

To complete our discussion we now turn to experimental studies which allow us to examine how malnourished populations respond to improvements in nutritional intakes. One such study was the food supplementation experiment conducted by the Division of Human Development of INCAP in four poor and malnourished Guatemalan villages [43]. Two types of supplements were offered *ad libitum* twice daily and consumption of these supplements was carefully recorded on every occasion. One was a high-protein calorie drink called *atole* and the other, the control, a low-calorie drink. The low calorie drink turned out to have affected growth and development [36,42, 43] but its low concentration meant its caloric contribution to the diet of children was minimal. The data in Table II refer only to the children receiving *atole,* the protein-calorie drink, and show supplement and home diet consumption data for 3 year old children. The intent here was to create groups of children who clearly had different histories of nutritional intakes. As explained at the bottom of the table, four categories were defined based upon the average amount of supplement consumed by the child in the first 3 years of life: 1 was less than 50 kcal/day, 2 was 51 to 100 kcal/day, 3 was 101 to 200 kcal/day, and 4 was over 200 kcal/day. These calories were also accompanied by protein as indicated in the footnote. Data are shown for boys on the left and for girls on the right. Shown here are mean values for home diete energy and protein intake, mean energy and protein intake from the *atole,* and total energy and protein intake. The home diet values are means of as many as eight 24-hour recall surveys. The *atole* did not significantly alter home diet intake and as a result total intake of energy and protein rises as one moves from left to right. For

TABLE II

Energy and protein intake in Atole villages by category of Atole intake [a]

Nutrient	Males				Females				Pooled S.D.
	Categories [b]				Categories				
	1	2	3	4	1	2	3	4	
Energy (kcal/day)									
Home diet	813	782	794	770	784	708	734	758	224
Atole	26	74	143	262	24	70	145	2542	78
Total	839	856	937	1032	808	778	879	1012	226
Protein (g/day)									
Home diet	21.8	20.6	19.9	19.0	21.5	19.9	19.2	19.6	6.3
Atole	1.8	5.2	10.1	18.5	1.7	4.9	10.2	17.9	5.5
Total	23.6	25.8	30.0	37.5	23.2	24.8	29.4	37.5	7.5
Sample size	23	28	44	22	32	26	41	13	

[a] *Atole was the name of the protein-calorie supplement. Atole intake is average intake from birth to 3 years of age. Home diet is average intake from 15 to 36 months of age.*
[b] *Categories of average daily intake of energy and protein from Atole during the first 3 years of life:*

Category	kcal/day	g/day
1	0- 50	0- 3.4
2	51-100	3.5- 6.7
3	101-200	6.8-13.4
4	>200	>13.5

example, total energy intakes for boys was 839 kcal for group 1, 856 kcal for group 2, 937 kcal for group 3, and 1,032 kcal for group 4. The differences between categories 4 and 1 were around 200 kcal/day for energy and 14 g. for protein. Group 4, it should be noted, had intakes that met the FAO/WHO protein-energy requirements for their body size [4].

Figure 5 compares the heights at 3 years of age of the baseline sample and of each of the four supplementation groups to the NCHS 50th percentile. The scale on the left is the actual difference between the mean height to each of the groups and the NCHS 50th percentile. The clear bars give the data for boys and the striped bars for girls. The baseline sample, a group of children born and measured before the intervention began, was around 12 cm shorter than the NCHS norm. Group 1 differs little from the baseline sample but each subsequent group is somewhat taller such that the differences with respect to the norm decrease. Group 4, for example, is 7.5 cm shorter than the norm.

The scale on the right measures the significance of the improvements in standard deviation units. The baseline sample had mean heights that were 3.3 standard deviations below the NCHS 50th percentile. In distributional terms, group 4 improved more than one standard deviation to a value of —2.0 S.D. Since the 5th percentile level is equivalent to —1.86 S.D. units below the mean, the mean height of group 4 is still below the 5th percentile of the NCHS norms. Though the diets in group 4 were improved to levels that satisfied protein-calorie requirements, heights improved, not three standard deviations as was the initial deficit, but only one. Why didn't this group grow taller than it did? Was there a ceiling imposed by genetics?

It should be clarified that previous analysis showed that the *atole* supplement had only a minimal impact on growth after 3 years of age so that Figure 5 presents the best possible test of the effects of the supplement [42]. By 3 years of age, children from Guatemalan rural areas are already destined to be short adults. The difference shown here for the baseline, 12 cm in height, is roughly that which is also found between their parents and upper-class Guatemalans.

Infectious diseases may have been one of the key factors limiting improvements in growth. Children in group 4 were just as likely to suffer from diarrheal diseases, respiratory illnesses, and other problems as children in group 1. We found that on an average day, nearly half of the children were sick for one cause or another. Elsewhere, we have shown that diarrheal diseases were a major cause of growth retardation in these children and that these effects were independent of those of the supplement [41].

The patterns of secular changes in Europe, North America, and Japan tell us that improvements are gradual and that they span over generations. The villages we studied were poor, illiterate, and lacked adequate housing and environmental sanitation. The mothers of the children grew in an environment of malnutrition and this may have affected uterine growth, lactation performance, and perhaps even child care. It is unlikely that improvements in nutritional intakes alone could ever dramatically alter the sizes of children in poor villages of developing countries in one single generation.

Implications for the assessment of nutritional status

What implications do the data presented in the various tables and figures have for the use of anthropometry for evaluating nutritional status? To best answer this question, let us first review how anthropometry is frequently used. Broadly speaking, anthropometry is useful for evaluating the nutritional status of individuals and of populations.

Monitoring of weight gain is the single best way of assessing health in indi vidual children [48]. The emphasis in weight monitoring is not on the child's size at one point in time but on his rate of progress. A small size need not always be a matter of concern. For example, the small size of the child may be the result of nutritional problems which began and ended months or years earlier. On the other hand, failure to gain weight is always a matter of concern in children in developing countries for reasons already discussed. Since the emphasis is on weight gain and since the various percentile lines are nearly parallel, all that is required is any line depicting the normal pattern of growth in weight. Whe ther the 50th or the 25th percentile best represents the genetic potential of the average local child is irrelevant in the assessment of individual children. Because most children in many developing countries will be quite small, not even the third percentile line may be useful and instead one or more growth lines at any number of desired standard deviations below the mean may need to be constructed as detailed by Waterlow et. al. [68].

Single anthropometric examinations are also used to select individuals at risk [10]. Typically, the indicators measure the extent of wasting, examples being weight for length and the famous QUAK stick (arm circumference/height) used in Biafra, Ideally, local studies are used to identify the best predictors of risk and the appropriate cut-off points. Possible ethnic differences in body composition and body proportions [13] are unimportant if local studies are the basis for the selection of indicators.

The issue of ethnic differences in growth potential, on the other hand, is very critical in the evaluation of the nutritional status of populations. A fre- quent objective of anthropometric surveys is to aid in the diagnosis of the ex- tent and severity of nutritional problems, a procedure which requires the use of growth norms. Examples of such endeavors are the series of surveys being conducted by CDC (Center for Disease Control) around the world [21]. Since NCHS norms are being used in such varied countries as Egypt, Togo, and Haiti the issue of the appropriateness of these norms is central to the whole exercise. Growth data may also be collected for different regions or social groups within the country with the view of assessing differences in nutritional

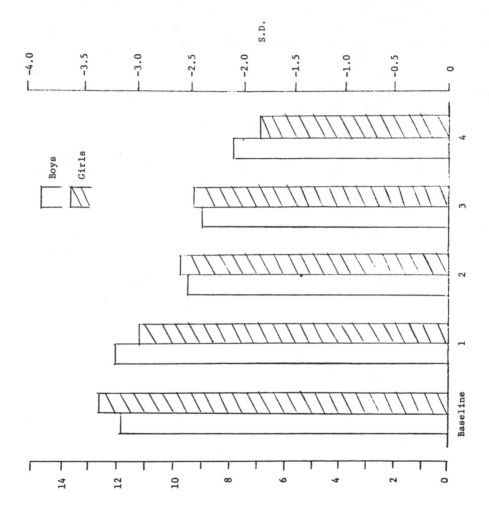

status. These data may then be used to formulate policies and allocate resources to programs. One would be particularly concerned about the validity of these comparisons if different ethnic groups inhabit the various regions of the country or if ethnic origin and social class area associated. Finally, growth data may be collected over time to monitor changes in health and nutrition in a general way or to evaluate the impact of specific programs. Because the comparison involves the same group or groups across time, norms are not in fact required to detect changes. However, it is always desirable in such cases to measure the extent of progress relative to goals and it is in the formulation of such goals (i.e., eliminating second degree malnutrition: weight for age less than 75 percent) that norms are used.

The differences in height and in other anthropometric measures that are observed between ethnic groups are, like all human characteristics, caused by differences in the gene pool, the environment and the interaction between the two. However, an analysis of the magnitude of the differences between well-to-do children of various ethnic groups and the differences within ethnic groups that are associated with social class, tell us that the variation that can be attributed to environmental factors far overshadows that which can be attributed to genetics. Asian children seem to be the known exception and norms derived from European children would not be suitable for them. However, even in the case of Asiatic children the differences are not large; if you remember, the mean difference in height at 7 years of age between U.S. and Japanese children is 3-4 cm. Mexican Zapotec Indians have a mean height of 107 cm at 7 years of age [38] making them on the average 14 cm shorter than healthy children of European origin and 11 cm shorter than healthy children of Asiatic origin. Whatever conceivable standard is used to evaluate the Zapotec Indian data, the inescapable conclusion is that for the most part their low statures are evidence of the wretched conditions of poverty, malnutrition, and disease to which they have been exposed for generations.

The complications that the issue of ethnic differences presents to nutritional assessment in multiracial societies in developing countries are therefore minor. Many ethnic groups are so uniformly poor and malnourished that large numbers of well-off children could not possibly be found and measured to generate growth norms. Till shown otherwise, one should assume that their low anthropometric values relative to other groups in the country are a reflection of their plight and not a genetic trait.

The use of international standards allows investigators to easily compare findings from various countries. But, national researchers, whether the NCHS norms are appropriate or not to their population, may choose to develop and

Figure 5. Heights at 3 years of age of the baseline sample and of each of the four supplementation groups to the NCHS 50th percentile. The scale on the left is the actual difference between the mean height of each of the groups and the NCHS 50th percentile. The clear bars give the data for boys and the striped bars for girls.

use their own standards. Very few countries, however, have been willing and able to collect the necessary data on well-nourished children to generate these norms. One conclusion from this paper, is that unless these populations are Asian, the NCHS norms are a justifiable alternative.

Whether maximal growth as has been achieved in some countries is optimal growth is not known. Studies of the secular change in growth indicate that increases in stature have been accompanied in some countries by a fall in weight for height ratios [65]. On the other hand, the children of the elite in many developing countries tend to be fatter than European and North American children [21, 29]. Thus, it is an open question whether the conditions that allow for maximal growth in height also predispose to obesity.

A final note of emphasis. The view that this presentation promotes is not that "biggest is best" but rather that "very short is bad". The interest in size is only insofar as it reflects the action of malnutrition and disease and insofar as this information can guide efforts to deal with such problems. Many point out that small people need less food. While true, this is no justification for keeping their children small. What is sometimes forgotten is that you cannot end up with populations as short as the Zapotec Indians without an environment for poor nutrition, high infectious rates, and high mortality rates.

REFERENCES

1. Ashcroft, M. T., Heneage, P., and Lovell, H. G. Heights and weights of Jamaican schoolchildren of various ethnic groups. *Am. J. Phys. Anthrop.* 24:35, 1966.
2. Ashcroft, M. T. and Lovell, H. G. Heights and weights of Jamaican children of various racial origins. *Trop. Geogr. Med.* 4:346, 1964.
3. Barja, J., Fuente, M., Ballester, D., Monckeberg, F., and Donoso, G. Weight and height of urban preschool Chilean children of three social classes. *Rev. Chilena de Ped.* 36:525, 1965.
4. Barkwin, H. and McLaughlin, S.M. Secular increase in height. Is the end in sight? *Lancet.* 2: 1195, 1964.
5. Barr, G. D., Allen, C. M., and Shinefield, H. R. Height and weight of 7,500 children of three skin colours. *Amer. J. Dis. Child.* 124:866, 1972.
6. Budliger, H. and Prader, A. Unpublished data from the Zurich Longitudinal Growth Study. May 1972. (Data published in Eveleth and Tanner, 1976).
7. Cameron, N. The growth of London schoolchildren 1904-1966: an analysis of secular trend and intra-country variation. *Ann. Human Bio.* 6:505, 1979.
8. Chandra, R. K. and Newberne, P. M. "Nutrition, Immunity, and Infections," 246 pp. Plenum Press, New York and London, 1977.
9. Chang, K. S. F., Lee, M. M. C., Low, W. D., and Kvan, E. Height and weight of southern Chinese children. *Am. J. Phys. Anthrop.* 21:497, 1963.
10. Chen, L. C., Chowdhury, A. K. M., and Huffman, S. L. Anthropometric assessment of energy-protein malnutrition and subsequent risk of mortality among preschool aged children. *Amer. J. Clin. Nutr.* 33:1836, 1980.
11. Damon A. Stature increase among Italian-Americans: environmental, genetic or both? *Am. J. Phys. Anthrop.* 23:401, 1965.
12. Damon, A. Secular trend in height and weight within old American families at Harvard, 1870-1965. I. Within 12 four-generation families. *Am. J. Phys. Anthrop.* 29:45, 1968.

13. Eveleth, P. G. and Tanner, J. M. "Worldwide Variation in Human Growth," 498 pp. Cambridge University Press, Cambridge, 1976.

14. FAO/WHO. "Energy and Protein Requirements." Food ans Nutrition Series No. 7. FAO, Rome, 1973.

15. Frisancho, A. R., Sanchez, J., Pallardel, D., and Yañez, L. Adaptive significance of small body size. *Am. J. Phy. Anthr.* 39:255, 1973.

16. Garn, S. M. "Magnitude of Secular Trends in the Fels Population," Fels Institute, Yellow Springs, Ohio, 1967.

17. Garn, S. M. and Clark, D. C. Problems in the nutritional assessment of Black individuals. *Am. J. Pub. Hlth.* 66:262, 1976.

18. Garrow, J. S. and Pike, M. S. The long-term prognosis of severe infantile malnutrition. *Lancet.* 1:1, 1967.

19. Goldstein, H. and Tanner, J. M. Ecological considerations in the creation and the use of child growth standards. *Lancet.* March 15, 1980.

20. Gopalan, C. Adaptation to low calorie and low protein intake: does it exist? In "Progress in Human Nutrition" vol. 2. (S. Margen and R. A. Ogar, eds.), pp. 132-141. AVI Publishing Company, Inc., Westport, Connecticut, 1978.

21. Graitcer, P. L. and Gentry, E. M. Measuring children: one reference for all. *Lancet.* August 8, 1981.

22. Greulich, W. W. A comparison of the physical growth and development of American-born and native Japanese children, *Am. J. Phys. Anthr.* 15:489, 1957.

23. Greulich, W. W. Some secular changes in the growth of American-born and native Japanese children. *Am. J. Phys. Anthrop.* 45:553, 1976.

24. Hafez, A. S., Salem, S. I., Cole, T. J., Galal, O. M., and Massoud, A. Sexual maturation and the growth pattern in Egyptian boys. *Ann. Human Bio.* 8:461, 1981.

   Hagen, W. Das Wachstrum in der Reifeperiode. *Der Internist.* 8:282, 1967.

26. Hamill, P. V. V., Johnston, F. E., and Grams, W. "Height and Weight of Children: United States," Vital Health Statistics Series 11, No. 104. U.S. Government Printing Office, Washington, D. C., 1970.

27. Hamill, P. V. V., Johnston, F. E., and Lemeshow, S. "Body Weight, Stature and Sitting Height: White and Negro Youths 12-17 Years, United States," Department of Health, Education and Welfare Publication, No. (HRA) 74-1608, Vital Health Statistics Series 11, No. 126. U.S. Government Printing Office, Washington, D. C., 1973.

28. Janes, M. D. Physical growth of Nigerian Yoruba children. *Trop. Geogr. Med.* 26:389, 1974.

29. Johnston, F. E., Borden, M., and MacVean, R. B. Height, weight, and their growth velocities in Guatemalan private school children of high socioeconomic class. *Human Bio.* 45:627, 1973.

30. Johnston, F. E. Wainer, H., Thissen, D., and MacVean, R. Hereditary and envirnmental determinants of growth in height in a longitudinal sample of children and youth of Guatemalan and European ancestry. *Am. J. Phys. Anthrop.* 44:469,1976.

31. Kimura, K. and Tsai, C. M. Comparative studies of the physical growth in Formosans. I. Height and weight. *J. Anthr. Soc., Nippon,* 75:11, 1967. (In Japanese with English summary.)

32. King, K. W., Foucauld, J., Fougere, W., and Severinghaus, E. L. Height and weight of Haitian children. *Am. J. Clin. Nutri.* 13:106,1963.

33. Knott, V. B. Stature, leg girth, and body weight of Puerto Rican private school children measured in 1962. *Growth.* 27:157, 1963.

34. Kondo, S. and Eto, M. Physical growth studies on Japanese-American children in comparison with native Japanese. In "Proceedings of Meeting for Review and Seminar or the U.S.-Japan Cooperative Research on Human Adaptabilities" (Japan Society for the Promotion of Science and National Science Foundation, eds.), Kyoto, 1972.

35. Krogman, W. M. Growth of the head, face, trunk, and limbs in Philadelphia white and Negro children of elementary and high school age. *Monographs Soc. Res. Child Dev.* 35:1, 1970.

36. Lechtig, A., Habicht, J.-P., Delgado, H., Klein, R. E., Yarbrough, C., and Martorell, R. Effect of food supplementation during pregnancy on birth weight. *Pediatrics.* 56:508, 1975.

37. Luna-Jaspe, H., Ariza Marcías, J., Rueda-Williamson, R., Mora Parra, J. O., and Pardo Téllez, F. Estudio seccional de crecimiento, desarrollo y nutrición en 12.138 niños de Bogotá, Colombia. *Arch. Latinoamer. Nutr.* 20:151, 1970.

38. Malina, R. M., Selby, H. A., and Swartz, L. J. Estatura, peso, y circunferencia del brazo en una muestra transversal de niños Zapotecas de 6 a 14 años. *Anales de Antropología.* 9:143, 1972.

39. Martorell, R. "Nutrition and Health Status Indicators: Suggestions for Surveys of the Standard of Living in Developing Countries," LSMS Working Paper No. 13, 97 pp. World Bank, Washington, D. C., 1982.

40. Martorell, R., Delgado, H. L., Valverde, V., and Klein, R. E. Maternal stature, fertility and infant mortality. *Human Bio.* 53:303, 1981.

41. Martorell, R., Habicht, J.-P., Yarbrough, C., Lechting, A., Klein, R. E., and Western, D. Acute morbidity and physical growth in rural Guatemalan children. *Am. J. Dis. Child.* 129:1296, 1975.

42. Martorell, R. and Klein, R. E. Food supplementation and growth rates in preschool children. *Nutr. Rep. Intl.* 21:447, 1980.

43. Martorell, R., Klein, R. E., and Delgado, H. Improved nutrition and its effects on anthropometric indicators of nutritional status. *Nutr. Rep. Intl.* 21:219, 1980.

44. Martorell, R., Lechtig, A., Yarbrough, C., Delgado, H., and Klein, R. E. Small stature in developing nations: its causes and implications. In "Progress in Human Nutrition" vol. 2 developing nations: its causes and implications. In "Progress in Human Nutrition" vol. 2 (S. Margen and R. A. Ogar, eds.), pp. 142-156. AVI Publishing Company, Inc., Westport, Connecticut, 1978.

45. Mata, L. J. "The Children of Santa María Cauqué: A Prospective Field Study of Health and Growth," 395 pp. MIT Press, Cambridge, Mass, and London, 1978.

46. McCammon, R. W. "Human Growth and Development," Charles C. Thomas, Springfield, Illinois, 1970.

47. McCullough, J. M. Secular trend for stature in adult male Yucatec Maya to 1968. *Am. J. Phy. Anthr.* 58:221, 1982.

48. Morley, D. and Woodland, M. "See How They Grow-Monitoring Child Growth for Appropriate Health Care in Developing Countries," 265 pp. Oxford University Press, New York, 1979.

49. Murillo Marques, R., Berquó, E., Yunes, J., and Marcondes, E. "Crecimiento de Niños Brasileños: Peso y Altura en Relación con la Edad y el Sexo y la Influencia de Factores Socioecómicos." Publicación Científica No. 309. Organización Panamericana de la Salud, Washington, D. C., 1975.

50. Newman, M. T. Nutritional adaptation in man. In "Physiological Anthropology"(A. Damon, ed.), pp. 210-259. Oxford University Press, New York, 1975.

51. Prokopec, M., Sachý, J., and Titlbachová, S. Results of the third whole-state investigation of the youth in 1971 (Czech countries). *Ceskoslovenska pediatrie.* 28:341, 1973. (In Czech and English summary.)

52. Rao, D. H. and Sastry, J. G. Growth pattern of well-to-do Indian adolescents and young adults. *Indian J. Med. Res.* 66:950, 1977.

53. Rauh, J. L., Schumsky, D. A., and Witt, M. T. Heights, weights and obesity in urban schoolchildren. *Child Dev.* 38:515, 1967.

54. Reed, R. B. and Stuart, H. C. Patterns of growth in height and weight from birth to eighteen years of age. *Pediatrics.* 24:904, 1959.

55. Simmons, K. The Brush Foundation Study of child growth and development. II. Physical growth and development. *Monographs Soc. Res. Child Dev.* 9:1, 1944.

56. Singh, K. V. R. D. and Swaminathan, M. S. Heights and weights of wellnourished Indian school children, *Indian J. Med. Res.* 59:648, 1971.

57. Stuart, H. C. and Meredith, H. V. The use of body measurements in the school health program. I. General considerations and the selection of measurements. II. Methods to be followed in taking and interpreting measurements and norms to be used. *Am. J. Pub. Hlth.* 36:1365,1946.

58. Tanner, J. M. "Growth at Adolescence," 2nd ed. Blackwell Scientific Publications, Ox ford, 1972.

59. Tanner, J. M. Earlier maturation in man. *Sci. Amer.* 218:21, 1968.

60. Tanner, J. M. "Foetus into Man: Physical Growth from Conception to Maturity," 250 pp. Open Books, London, 1978.

61. Tanner, J. M. "A History of the Study of Human Growth," 499 pp. Cambridge University Press, Cambridge, 1981.

62. Tanner, J. M., Whitehouse, R. H., and Takaishi, M. Standards from birth to maturity for height, weight, height velocity and weight velocity; British children 1965. *Arch Dis. Child.* 41:454, 1966.

63. Tuddenham, R. D. and Snyder, M. M. "Physical Growth of California Boys and Girls from Birth to Eighteen Years, "University of California Press, Berkeley and Los Angeles, 1954.

64. U.S. Department of Health, Education, and Welfare, Public Health Service. "NCHS Growth Curves for Children Birth-18 years United States," DHEW Publication No. (PHS) 78-1650. 74 pp. National Center for Health Statistics, Hyattsville, MD., 1977.

65. van Wieringen, J. C. Secular growth changes. In "Human Growth, Volume 2, Postnatal Growth" (F. Falkner and J. M. Tanner, eds.), pp. 445-473. Plenum Press, New York and London, 1978.

66. Verghese, K. P., Scott, R. B., Teixeira, G., and Ferguson, A. D. Studies in growth and de velopment. XII. Physical growth of North American Negro children. *Pediatrics.* 44:243, 1969.

67. Villarejos, V. M., Osborne, J. A., Payne, F. J., and Arguedas G., J. A. Heights and weights of children in urban and rural Costa Rica. *J. Trop. Ped. Environ. Child. Hlth.* 17:31, 1971.

68. Waterlow, J. C., Buzina, R., Keller, W., Lane, J. M., Nichaman, M. Z., and Tanner, J. M. The presentation and use of height and weight data for comparing the nutritional status of groups of children under the age of 10 years. *Bull. World Hlth. Org.* 55:489, 1977.

69. World Health Organization. "Measurement of Nutritional Impact," 85 pp. WHO, Gene va, 1979.

70. Yarbrough, C., Habicht, J.-P., Malina, R. M., Lechtig, A., and Klein, R. E. Length and weight in rural Guatemalan Ladino children: birth to seven years of age. *Am. J. Phys. Anthrop.* 42:439, 1975.

DISCUSSION[1]

Torun printed out that differences between high socio-economic groups in various societies could have an environmental as well as a genetic basis. He used as examples of variables, diet and patterns of exercise. A second issue he raised was that of the usefulness of local standards in highly heterogeneous populations. He implied that if one used any standard with discretion, it could be applied to populations other than those from which they derive, especially if growth rates were parallel, albeit with a lower or higher mean. Waterlow asked

[1]*Summary of the discussion prepared by S. Cederbaum.*

if genetic differences in growth potential might not express themselves in later childhood or adolescence rather than in the early years of life? This question derived from his anecdotal experience in Jamaica in which the indigenous population has a significant adolescent growth spurt in contrast to he population of oriental extraction. Martorell agreed, pointing out how fortunate this was for nutritionists interested in the impact of diet in the early years of life. Bray pursued Martorell's statement that in some studies, children of well-to-do families tended to be fatter. He cited the data of Stunkard which suggested the contrary, in a US population. Martorell responsed by emphasizing potential differences among various populations and emphasizing the possible disparity between developed and developing countries. Cederbaum asked if despite the data supporting the environmental determination of height, nutritionists would if they could, rework the experimental protocols of the last thirty years to incorporate a family design? Cravioto answered that the expected family correlation in height was seen in the upper but not the lower socio-economic stratum in both Guatamala and rural villages in Central Mexico. Cravioto went on to point out that in the lower socio-economic group there was a correlation between height and performance on the intersensory development test; this correlation was absent in the more affluent group. He feels this indicates an environmental modulation of genetic expression. Scrimshaw commented that the sibling design offered no advantage in the study of Mora, Herrera et al. in Bogatá.

GENETIC INHERITANCE AND GROWTH IN HUMAN GROUPS SUFFERING FROM CHRONIC UNDERNUTRITION

Rafael Ramos Galván

*Departamento de Investigación en Unidades
de Atención Médica,
Subjefatura de los Servicios de Investigación,
Centro Médico Nacional, Instituto Mexicano
del Seguro Social
Mexico City, Mexico*

Rosa María Ramos Rodríguez

*Instituto de Investigaciones Antropológicas
Universidad Nacional Autónoma de
Mexico City, Mexico*

From an epidemiological point of view, the main cause of undernutrition is inadequate and insufficient food consumption, which in the end causes a negative balance of nutrients [43]; it is this type of undernutrition to which the present work refers. The following definition was put forward by Gómez *et al:* "Undernutrition is a pathologic, unspecific, systemic and potentially reversible state which originates as a result of deficient utilization of adequate amounts of different nutrients by the cells of an organism, and is accompanied by various clinical manifestations ranging in different degrees of intensity according to several ecologic factors" [15].

Jolliffe's [20] etiologic classification operates as well. He refers to three categories: primary, secondary and mixed. As shall be seen further on, much evidence allows us to assert that primary undernutrition is not determined by genetic inheritance, but is mainly caused by social and cultural inheritance [38]. Therefore, its phenotypic expression will vary essentially with environmental factors.

In order to understand the natural history leading to the characteristic phenotype of an undernourished individual, it is necessary to consider some facts which by themselves might seem obvious and elementary. Nonetheless, they are usually ignored by epidemiologists, nutritionists and anthropologists, thus confusing the consequences of previous states of undernourishment with the later nutritional states.

These facts are:

—Nutrition is a dynamic and *continuing* process [19, 49]
—Nutrition occurrs in each and every cell of the organism and therefore influences greatly the size of *lean tissue mass* [19]
—Cells use nutrients, not foodstuffs [3]
—Nutrients may be obtained from endogenous or exogenous sources [3]
—Since nutrients interact with and influence each other, they may not be judged in an isolated manner as far as their use and requirements are concerned. Therefore, even though their biochemical function may be highly specific, the clinical expression of their absence is highly unspecific. In some cases, however, expressions are very specific [2, 7, 10, 14-16, 53]
—Use of nutrients depends among other factors on the previous state of nutrition

In other words, maintenance of macromolecular structures within cells and of their normal functions depends on the nutritional state. This plays an important part in the growth of tissues, organs, body parts and the organism as a whole. Physiologically regulation of these phenomena depends on the action of genetic [17], neuroendocrine [6, 28] and environmental factors [29-32] as well as on the age of the individual.

Acting teleonomically, genetic influences constitute the first decisive factor in growth. From the moment of conception when genetic sex is determined, two ontogenetic routes are established. They are similar but not equal in the two sexes, since they are inherent to the species. Females generally show slower growth than males, but develop more rapidly.

Genotype is expressed fundamentally through neuroendocrine behaviour, establishing the so-called "constitution" or "constitutional habit". The genetic-neuroendocrine interaction appears as two somatic growth bursts: the first starts at the moment of conception, reaches its highest point shortly before birth and ends at age of five or six years. It is followed by a stage of asymptotic growth and gives way to the second somatic growth burst: puberty [39, 47, 55]. Anyway, even if genetic factors grant us the ability to be, it is environmental factors which determine or model the phenotype, varying in intensity along the growth bursts.

Environmental factors which influence growth are generally known. Beginning at intrauterine growth, a peculiar phenotype is established which will have an epigenetic influence on the critical route of future growth. According to this, physical growth and nutritional state will partly depend on the genetic load of a given group, and will be translated into different growth speed and sexual dimorphism. Therefore, depending on the sex of the subject we will observe different developmental age [28], different maturity and resistance to environmental agression at the same chronological age. In turn, this will cause phenotypic differences.

Different growth speed refers not only to the sexes, but within the same sex it will vary according to the genetic load of a particular group. Greater growth speed involves greater nutritional requirements, the lack of which will lead to illness and death more frequently than in individuals growing at a lesser speed. During the first three months of life, 123 boys die for each 100 girls. In undernourished groups —particularly in undernourished pregnant mothers— the number is 132 [34], (Table I). Also, the frequency of grade III undernutrition is higher in boys than in girls. This does not occur in later years [42], (Table II). In other words; girls resist environmental agressions better during the first months of life. Therefore, due to natural selection, a group progressively ac-

TABLE I

Deaths among males for every hundred deaths ocurring among females (26)

Age periods	Group I	Group II
During the first month of life	*126*	*131*
During the first three months of life	*123*	*134*
During the first year of life	*117*	*125*

Group I. Communities in which malnutrition is less prevalent.
Group II. Communities in which malnutrition is more prevalent.

TABLE II

Frequency of severe malnutrition (second plus third degree)
in an urban underprivileged community

Age (years)	Males	Females
0	*24%*	*20%*
1	*31*	*45*
2	*31*	*34*
3	*26*	*34*
4	*10*	*36*
5	*18*	*23*
Total	*23%*	*31%*

Ramos Galván, R. et. al (23)

quires a lesser height potential, independent of the fact that the environment will diminish height even more. Whenever this phenomenon is not due to mutation it is of course reversible. If environmental conditions change, the group is capable of reaching its original genotypic height after several generations [18, 36].

Other facts appear which complicate the problem. Taking into account the multiple factors that influence nutritional status, it is not strange that Behar among others should insist that: ". . . malnutrition is not a yes or not situation but it is rather a spectrum going from adequate nutrition to severe malnutrition." He also asserts that ". . . This situation is further complicated by the fact that for many nutrients, malnutrition results from both deficiency and excess." [2]

This is partly due to the fact that from the clinical point of view and the natural history of the disease, the pathogenic process is established with varying speed and for variable periods which sometimes allow succesful homeostatic mechanisms [33, 43]. Undernutrition can therefore be pathogenically defined, after Jolliffe [20] as a process with negative balance of nutrients, in which loss reserves, biochemical changes, functional alterations and anatomic modifications follow each other.

This is essentially true and explains why pathologically undernutrition is characterized by various degrees of "dysfunction, dilution and atrophy" [43]. The adverse impact of nutritional factors on growth and development will depend on the nutritional requirements of an individual at a given time. In chronic undernutrition, endocrine glands, central nervous system and lean mass suffer less than fat, weight, height, skin or skin appendages. Similarly, cardiac muscle suffers less than skeletal muscles.

Lean body mass diminishes whenever environmental factors are not exceedingly aggressive. This is an adjustment to insufficient food ingestion, and it goes further than homeostasis (subsistence of previous equilibrium) and reaches a "homeorrhesis" (aquisition of a new equilibrium) [33]. In other cases, homeorrhesis is attained by submitted to adequate treatment. The subject experiences a period of recovery before reachig homeorrhesis (the syndrome of nutritional recovery) [13]. Anyway, homeorrhesis is usually acquired at the expense of height (nutritional dwarfism) and other anomalies of growth or physical and functional development. This agrees with the fact that ". . . as far as physical growth goes, time cannot be recovered" [43].

Sould these observations prove true, there are four clinical situations to be considered:

I.   Good previous and present status of nutrition.
II.   Good previous status of nutrition and present malnutrition.
III. Previous malnutrition but good present status of nutrition.
IV.   Previous malnutrition and present malnutrition.

All of these situations must be taken into account for diagnosis, prognosis, treatment and prevention, and also for classification of nutritional status risking confusion of physical and functional consequences of previous malnutrition with the real present status of nutrition.

The first group prevails is developed countries, but not so in underdeveloped countries. The third group is probably very significant in urban zones of the latter countries. Rural zones show a high frequency of the fourth group. Survival is achieved through the process of natural selection mentioned before with one or more periods of homeorrhesis. These adaptive mechanisms vary in importance depending on the genetic load, sex, age and intensity of environmental aggressions (food availability, infection, physical work load, climate). Unfortunately, and even though they represent four features of great significance for public health and anthropology, they have not been studied for lack of proper methodology and standards of reference.

It is not easy to interpret the complex symptoms shown by a malnourished individual. As has been said before, malnutrition is not due to purely biological reasons. It depends on psychosocial and cultural conditions of the affected; primary malnutrition must therefore be considered as a syndrome of social deprivation.

With clinical insight, Behar quotes Sandstead and refers to the problem with precision: ". . . when trying to define marginal malnutrition our difficulties actually begin with the definition of adequate nutrition". He also proposes: "Marginal malnutrition is characterized by the presence of nonspecific clinical signs and laboratory indices, while in mild malnutrition laboratory indices are specific but still with non-specific clinical signs". Clear limits can certainly not be established between a good status of nutrition and marginal malnutrition. Even less so between marginal and moderate malnutrition [56]. Signs and symptoms of malnutrition have therefore been classified in three categories as follows [41]:

1. Universal signs, always present, regardless of the etiology, intensity and clinical picture. They result from early or advanced organic depletion and of chemical changes brought about by the negative balance of nutrients. In sub jects under 18 year of age these signs are diminished growth and development. In adults they are mainly changes in body composition. They are of litte importance in life prognosis and do not change the treatment sub—stantially.

2. Circumstantial signs, not always present because they are produced by environmental or ecologic circumstances added to some related to the subject, such as skin color, hair quality, genetic load and previous nutrition. Whenever they are present, however, they simplify diagnosis.

3. Added signs, not directly caused by malnutrition but frequently present in malnourished subjects. They can be grouped as follows:

a) Those related to infections added to malnutrition.
b) Those resulting from severe electrolytic imbalance added to the peculiar balance present in chronic malnutrition.
c) Those determined by the socio-cultural environment and by affective or psychological conditions prevailing in the family [29, 32].

These symptoms form part of the social deprivation syndrome [32], which includes inadequate habitat ("folk" community according to Redfield [48]), increased sensitivity to aggressions of all types (including infections), emotional distortion, low intelectual performance and malnutrition as a nosological entity.

The "folk" community described by Redfield includes the following features: it is small, isolated, very homogeneous, illiterate, handles many magic concepts, with a profound sense of belonging and great difficulty to admit any change in cultural patterns [23], all of which favours endogamy.

Grade III malnutrition can be easily diagnosed based not only on somatometric profile but also on the signs and symptoms of malnutrition. This does not apply to marginal malnutrition, the most frequent type and of more interest to Public Health [23].

In individual cases diagnosis should be based on three items:

a) Diet
b) Somatometry
c) Analysis of clinical data obtained through questioning and exploration; and laboratory tests which confirm or deny a primary or secondary state of malnutrition.

A similar attitude should be observed in collective diagnosis (that is, of human groups) [37]; in practice, however, diagnosis is directed almost exclusively towards the phenotypic situation in these cases. That is, only the present status is considered ignoring genetic load, previous moments of possible malnutrition and their impact on physical growth and psycho-social development of the individual.

It is very useful, but also very difficult, to establish the genetic growth potential in underdeveloped communities since no somatometric record of longitudinal growth in children is kept. Also, only the present situation can be studied in adults (particulary in undernourished parents). Neither their own genetic potencial nor their children's can be established. This last one is particularly important for an evaluation of the real effect of adverse environmental factors on growth, since primary malnutrition —as has been said before— is not genetically inherited.

An interesting hypothesis has been proposed recently to solve this problem. In case it should prove right it will allow us to know the genetic potential of growth in height in undernourished groups with sufficient approximation [46].

This hypothesis stems from the fact that there are certain organs, tissues, body parts and somatometric measures which show particular resistance to ecological aggressions whereas others are very ecosensible, especially during growth crises. The latter are better represented by subcutaneous adipose tissue and to a lesser extent by the muscle mass and thus, by body weight as well as arm and leg circumference. A good example of ecoresistance is the upper body segment. Faced with environmental aggression, this magnitude will remain close to the genetically expected.

Ecoresistance of the upper segment and ecosensibility of the lower segment can be directly studied in children and adults, according to their absolute measures and calculating the standard deviation score with reference patterns of previous elaboration (Appendix I) [35]. It is of great interest to establish, always as a hypothesis, a final height potential for any given group, including in it subjects of all ages (Appendix II).

According to this the prediction of final height as calculated from the upper segment would express the minimum genetic potential of the group. The prediction made according to the lower segment would represent the maximum environmental damage which could be caused. Based on the present height it could predict maximum height to be expected from a particuar individual [46].

The magnitude of height is a matter of great importance both from a biological and an anthropological point of view. Lower weight, body surface and nutritional requirements correspond to lower height. Also, lower height brings about less growth of transversal measures, particularly of the bicrestal diameter which in turn may limit fetal growth. Furthermore, the size of the heart and major blood vessels is related to height. Hence, it can be one of the factors involved in the different capacities to resist physical exercise, particularly in extreme situations. It is thus considered that there is a critical height of 149 cms below which death rate at child bearing increases significantly, particularly when medical attention is inadequate or nonexistent. This implies orphanage for the surviving product, a great handicap to begin with. It has been observed in rural areas where 17% of the children weigh less than 2 500g at birth; communities have been studied where this percentage doubles [36]. One could conclude that malnourished communities survive at the expense of the biological future of their offspring.

Table III shows the results of a study made on 872 female students from 12 to 17 years of age. When results are grouped according to socio-economic level, the average predictions in average height considering the upper segment is always within the limits of normality [44]. It is always superior to predictions carried out according to present height or to lower segment. The average of these was significantly lower than normal. Difference of average in predictions carried out according to the segments increased as socio-economic level decre ased (4.0, 6.0 and 6.8 cms respectively). This shows that height was diminished at the expense of the lower segment, with little modification of the upper

TABLE III

Final height prediction made according to present height and upper and lower body segments in 872 females from 12 to 17 years of age, grouped according to various criteria (44)

Groups	N	Final height prediction according to:		
		Present height	Upper segment	Lower segment
According to socio-economic class				
High	202	159.5 ± 6.29	161.6 ± 5.99	157.6 ± 6.82
Middle	243	155.1 6.31	158.2 6.10	152.2 6.58
Low	427	154.5 5.78	157.8 5.83	151.0 6.70
According to present weight				
$\bar{x} + 1$ S.D.	59	161.7 ± 6.38	164.6 ± 6.10	159.2 ± 6.75
$\bar{x} \pm 1$ S.D.	393	157.8 6.49	160.7 6.42	155.2 7.10
$\bar{x} - 1$ S.D.	420	152.9 6.12	156.1 6.14	150.0 6.15
According to present height				
$\bar{x} + 1$ S.D.	38	169.5 ± 4.20	170.0 ± 4.11	168.5 ± 4.92
$\bar{x} \pm 1$ S.D.	539	158.2 5.10	161.0 5.08	155.7 4.98
$\bar{x} - 1$ S.D.	295	149.5 5.20	153.4 5.12	146.0 5.10

Socio-economic levels were established depending on area of residence, schooling and activity of parents.

segment. This hypothesis is therefore licitly used as a prediction illustrating genetic potential. To prove this, material was regrouped according to two criteria: weight and height. Results were similar, differences between the magnitude of predictions were even clearer: 5.4, 5.5 and 6.1 cms in groups made according to weight and 1.5, 5.3 and 7.1 cms in groups made according to height.

More information to support the present hypothesis is discussed in Tables IV, V and VI. Results are presented of nine different groups of men and fifteen groups of women. Average has been arranged in decreasing order of magnitude in the prediction of adult height based on present height. Furthermore, two groups were formed: one of urban origin (Mexico City), with greater hybridization and therefore less endogamy, the other of rural origin with declared endogamy.

The first three groups of men (Table IV) came from a private University (Universidad Ibero Americana); the first group consisted of 134 students whose four grandparents were of foreign origin; the second group represents the complete sample; the third group consisted of 482 students whose four grandparents were mexican by birth. The "genetic height potential" of these was slightly superior to the reference patterns (177.1, 175.9 and 175.3 cms respectively), but the average always fell within normality [50].

The second three groups correspond to boys between the ages of 9 and 15 attending public schools. The fourth group was formed by children of middle socio-economic level with "normal body weight according to height"; the fifth and sixth groups consisted of children from the orphanage (National Boarding House of the Secretary of Public Health) where they had lived from the age of six or seven. Predictions made according to the lower segment obviously lose accuracy, not so those carried out according to the upper segment [49].

The three last groups are of rural origin, with greater endogamy. The assumed genetic height potential was 160 to 166 cms (166.5, 166.3 and 159.5 cms respectively). The adult height prediction according to present height was 160.6, 158.5 and 151.3 cms. On the other hand, differences between average predictions according to upper and lower segment were very large: 11.3, 15.7 and 11.2 cms. This allows us to appreciate the intense environmental impact.

TABLE IV

Prediction of adult height (cm) in various groups of males (x)

Groups	N	According to actual height $\bar{x} \pm S.D.$	According to upper segment $\bar{x} \pm S.D.$	According to lower segment $\bar{x} \pm S.D.$
A. With minor endogamy (Urban groups)				
Students from private schools (18 to 22 years) (50)				
1. Descendants of foreign grandparents	134	174.8 $\pm$ 6.4	177.1 $\pm$ 8.6	172.7 $\pm$ 8.9
2. Mixed group	811	173.8 6.4	175.9 8.6	171.8 8.7
3. Descendants of mexican grandparents	482	173.3 6.4	175.3 8.4	171.4 8.7
Students from public schools (9 to 15 years) (12)				
4. Middle-class	72	171.6 $\pm$ 4.4	174.6 $\pm$ 5.1	168.0 $\pm$ 5.8
5. Low-class	346	164.7 8.1	168.0 7.8	160.5 9.4
6. Very low-class	87	160.7 5.2	164.0 5.9	157.0 7.9
B. With major endogamy (Rural groups)				
7. Tlapa, Gro. (Boys) (8)	164	160.6 $\pm$ 6.7	166.7 $\pm$ 6.9	155.2 $\pm$ 6.5
8. Cuentepec, Mor. (Adults) (45)	112	158.5 5.2	166.3 6.5	150.6 6.3
9. Cuentepec, Mor. (Boys) (45)	75	151.3 6.4	159.5 6.7	148.3 6.7

(x) Accepted normal height 172.8 $\pm$ 7.2 cm.

There were 15 groups of women (Tables V and VI). Table V shows nine urban groups. The first three selected from a private University (Universidad Ibero Americana) consisted of women with four foreign grandpartents and showed the higher genetic potential (170.7 ± 7.2 cms), with a present height of 162.7 ± 5.9 cms. The genetic potential in women with four mexican grandparents was estimated at 167.1 ± 7.6 cms and the present height 160.1 ± 5.6 cms, very close to the patterns of reference: 160.6 ± 7.4 cms [50]. The next six groups corresponded to girls between the ages of 12 and 18 or adults between 19 and 22, of varying socio-economical level who went to public schools. According to a decreasing socio-economic status the genetic height potential was estimated at 161.6, 158.2 and 157.8 cms as average and the adult height prediction according to present height at 159.5, 155.1 and 154.5 respectively. In women older than 18 years of age, the genetic potential was calculated at 163.8, 158.8 and 159.9 cms. Their real height was 161.1, 152.2 and 153.5 cms, respectively [44].

TABLE V

Prediction of adult height (cm) in various groups of females with minor endogamy (x)

Groups	N	According to actual height $\bar{x}$ + S.D.	According to upper segment $\bar{x}$ + S.D.	According to lower segment $\bar{x}$ S.D.
A. With minor endogamy (Urban groups) Students from private schools (18 to 22 years) (50).				
1. Descendants of foreign grandparents	105	162.7 + 5.9	170.7 + 7.2	156.1 + 7.8
2. Mixed group	717	160.6 5.8	167.9 7.6	154.1 8.1
3. Descendants of mexican grandparents	407	160.1 5.6	167.1 7.6	153.0 7.8
Students from public schools, grouped according to socio-economic level (44)				
4. Middle-class (19 to 22 years)	56	161.1 + 5.1	163.8 + 6.0	158.8 + 6.6
5. Middle-class (10 to 18 years)	202	159.5 5.4	161.6 5.8	157.6 6.6
6. Moderately low-class (10 to 18 years)	243	155.1 5.5	158.2 6.2	152.2 6.7
7. Low-class (10 to 18 years)	427	154.5 5.6	157.8 6.1	151.0 6.5
8. Low-class (19 to 22 years)	31	153.5 5.2	159.9 6.2	148.9 6.6
9. Moderately low-class (19 to 22 years)	58	152.2 4.6	158.8 4.6	144.6 6.3

(x) Accepted normal height 160.6 ± 7.4 cm.

TABLE VI

Prediction of adult height (cm) in various groups of females with major endogamy (x)

Groups	N	According to actual height $\bar{x}$ + S.D.	According to upper segment $\bar{x}$ + S.D.	According to lower segment $\bar{x}$ + S.D.
B. With major endogamy — Families emigrated from rural areas to Mexico City. Parent generation				
10. Home-servants	45	158.0 ± 6.7	161.2 ± 5.8	155.3 ± 6.2
11. Mothers of gravely undernourished children	327	151.7 6.2	158.8 6.8	142.8 7.1
— Rural areas				
12. Tlapa, Gro. (Boys) (8)	193	150.1 ± 6.8	153.3 ± 7.2	144.0 ± 6.9
13. Cadereyta, Qro. (Adult women) (57)	95	149.2 5.0	153.8 7.5	144.6 8.1
14. Cuentepec, Mor. (Adult women) (45)	150	145.5 6.3	153.2 7.1	137.3 6.2
15. Cuentepec, Mor. (Girls) (45)	86	143.2 5.1	153.3 6.9	136.8 6.1

(x) Accepted normal height 160.6 ± 7.4 cm.

Table VI refers to women of rural origin. Two very peculiar groups were studied. The tenth consisted of young women, daughters of peasants, born either in the country or in Mexico City, but who had lived in the City since they were very small; all of them servants living with middle-class urban families. Their present height was estimated at 158 ± 6.7 cms (with no significant differences in reference patterns), and prediction according to the upper segment was 161.2 ± 5.8 cms. This suggests a good growth potential. The eleventh group were mothers of clearly undernourished children hospitalized at the Hospital de Zona de Ixtacalco [58]. Their height was 151.7 ± 6.2 cms, clearly diminished, and their genetic potential was estimated at 158.8 ± 6.8 cms.

In contrast, the four last groups, studied in a rural environment suggest a very uniform genetic potential of 153 cms (153.3, 153.8, 153.2 and 153.3 cms respectively) and a final height prediction according to present height of 151.1 ± 6.8 and 143.2 ± 5.1 cms for groups 12 and 15 respectively, in agreement with the real height of 149.2 ± 5.0 and 145.5 ± 6.3 cms for groups 13 and 14 of adults.

These findings could mean that the upper segment deteriorates *in utero* for environmental reasons (which could be true and must be studied) were it not for the fact that average differences between predictions made according to upper and lower segment are larger in groups 11 to 15 of Table VI (16.0, 9.3, 9.2, 15.9 and 16.5 cms respectively) compared to group 10 where it was only 5.9 cms.

Finally, Tables VII and VIII show predictions made in various groups of sick children. The phenomenon can be appreciated in both. It is notorious in the first that the prediction made according to the upper segment does not significantly differ from normal values. Table VIII shows a comparison between predictions for six groups of patients and their siblings. The severe impact of chronic renal malfunction on the lower segment can be appreciated [54].

All of the above supports the hypothesis about the significance of the upper segment and establishes a possibility to evaluate the impact of previous episodes of deficient nutrition. The study of the cephalic perimeter which grows very rapidly during the first years of life, probably indicates the state of nutrition and growth during early years, but it must be applied to groups and not to individuals [44]. Thus, the first point (previous state of nutrition) of the four mentioned before would be clearer.

Presently, nutrition is studied through the patterns of reference related to age-weight, sometimes height-age or weight-height and the "distance" graphs

TABLE VII

Prediction of adult height in various groups of patients [1]

Disease	Males	Females
Hemophilia		
n.	21	
according to upper segment	172.7 ± 6.2	
according to present height	168.7 7.4	
according to lower segment	164.1 10.4	
Juvenile rheumatoid arthritis		
n.	6	15
according to upper segment	171.2 ± 7.5	159.1 ± 9.0
according to present height	162.7 8.1	152.4 9.5
according to lower segment	153.2 7.5	146.3 10.6
Non-cyanotic congenital heart-disease		
n.	22	38
according to upper segment	169.4 ± 9.2	158.1 ± 8.1
according to present height	160.6 ± 10.9	149.6 ± 7.4
according to lower segment	151.1 12.8	141.3 8.9
Patterns of reference	172.8 ± 7.2	160.6 ± 7.4

TABLE VIII

Predictions of adult height in various groups of patients and their siblings (1)

	Males		Females	
Disease	Patients	Brothers	Patients	Sister
Bronchial asma				
n.	24	15	9	13
according to upper segment	175.6 ± 7.4	176.2 ± 9.3	160.9 ± 6.3	167.2 ± 8.0
according to present height	170.7 8.1	171.2 6.0	155.4 4.5	161.0 7.1
according to lower segment	165.1 9.6	166.2 4.3	149.9 4.7	154.2 9.6
Diabetes mellitus				
n.	19	20	20	11
according to upper segment	169.3 ± 10.5	170.7 ± 7.5	159.6 ± 7.3	160.0 ± 9.7
according to present height	165.8 11.5	167.9 5.8	153.2 7.7	153.8 7.8
according to lower segment	161.4 10.3	165.3 6.7	147.0 9.4	149.6 9.9
Chronic renal malfunction				
n.	9	6	14	6
according to upper segment	162.4 ± 10.7	174.1 ± 5.0	150.9 ± 7.8	158.6 ± 6.3
according to upper segment	155.0 7.3	168.8 5.5	143.8 7.9	151.5 5.4
according to lower segment	148.0 6.3	163.8 7.7	137.4 8.3	144.2 7.3

Expected height (patterns of reference): Males: 172.8 ± 7.2; Females: 160.6 ± 7.4

derived from them. If we consider that episodes of malnutrition retard growth, weight-age and height-age criteria seem rather useless. It could be more indicated to relate weight with height, as has been proposed by several authors, particularly if the "antropometric segment", suggested by Quetelet many years ago, is calculated. It has the advantage of considering age, and patterns of reference of antropometric segment for each age and sex are readily available.

For similar reasons, the exclusive use of arm circumference proposed by Jolliffe is as imprecise as "weight-age". More useful is leg circumference because the muscular component in relation to fat is greater than in the arm, and muscle is a better indicator of lean tissue [35, 44].

For this reason, several indices have been proposed which take into account muscular and fatty tissue and height. These can be applied to studies of body composition of the undernourished at the time of examination [44]. Such indices would be for example:

(Arm circumference in cms)^2 × height in cms/weight in grams [25].
(Leg circumference in cms)^2 × height in cms/weight in grams [44].

Or even better,

Muscular area of the arm in cms² × 100 × height in cms/weight in grams
Muscular area of the leg in cms² × 100 × height in cms/weight in grams.

According to these formulae, a large number would indicate either a large amount of muscle or great slimness, on the contrary, a small number indicates relatively large weight at the expense of fat [40, 44].

Since exclusive knowledge of height and weight are relatively useless, they can be integrated in a somatometric profile. It must be remebered, however, that somatometry is a simple and accesible technique [2, 23, 35, 57, 60] but it only establishes deficits and excesses, and it does not *per se* diagnose malnutrition, especially the marginal type. Knowledge of the patients diet, sex, age, activity, diseases and climate must be added to give it an adequate use. Finally, as long as simple diagnostic methods are not available, we must continue searching for possibilities offered by the use of measures related to accumulated growth, body proportionality and composition [44].

A new problem arises, enlarging the possibilities of investigation. Up to now, genetic potential has not been properly considered to formulate patterns of reference nor applied to those currently available [24]. It is therefore necessary, that Anthropology and Population Genetics should help, by providing their knowledge on genic distances, to establish zones, regions and human groups where these patterns can be applied, thus avoiding groups chosen only according to political geography [5, 9, 21, 22, 26, 27, 54, 59].

The information in Appendix I and II of the present work can be applied to the population of the center, south and southeast of the Republic of Mexico, and in Central America, excluding Costa Rica and Panamá. It will probably not be useful in groups originally situated above the Tropic of Cancer, nor in South America (Colombia, Venezuela, Ecuador, Perú, and Bolivia).

REFERENCES

1. Baqueiro Rodríguez, R.A.- Crecimiento físico en niños con padecimientos crónicos. Tesis de Postgrado en Pediatría UNAM.- Hospital de Pediatría, C.M.N. México, 1981.
2. Béhar, M.- What is marginal malnutrition. *In:* Nutrition in Health and Disease and International Development. Symposia from the XII International Congreses of Nutrition (A.E. Harper and G.K. Davis Eds). pp. 237-246. Alan R. Liss. Inc. Nueva York, 1981.
3. Cahill, G.F.- Starvation in man. *N. Engl. J. Med.* 282:668, 1970.
4. Cameron, N.- The methods of auxiological anthropometry. *In:* Human Growth vol. 2, Postnatal Browth (F. Falkner and J.M. Tanner Eds) pp. 35-90 Plenum Press, Nueva York, 1978.
5. Cavalli-Sforza, L.L. y Bodmer, W.F.- The genetics of human populations. Freeman S. Fco. 1971.
6. Cheek, D.B.- Fetal and Postnatal Growth. Hormones and nutrition pp. 475-498, J. Wiley and Sons. Nueva York, 1975.

7. Cohen, E.L. and Wurtman, R.J.- Nutrition and brain neurotransmitters. *In:* Human Nutrition. Vol. I Nutrition, Pre and Postnatal Development (R. B. Alfin-Slater and D. Kritchevsky. Gen. Ed. M. Winick Special Ed) pp. 103-132 Plenum Press. Nueva York, 1979.

8. Cortés Bucio, A.- Somatometría en menores de Tlapa, Gro. Tesis de Postgrado. Hospital de Pediatría C.M.N./IMSS.México, 1982.

9. Crawford, M.H.; Leyshon, W.C.; Brown, K.; Lees, F. and Taylor, L.- Human Biology in Mexico. II-A comparison of blood group, serum and red cell enzymes frequencies and genetic distances of the indian population of Mexico *Am. J. Phys, Anthrop.* 41:251, 1974.

10. Czarnecki, S.K. and Kritchevsky, D.- Trace elements. In: Human Nutrition. vol. 39 Nutrition and the Adult Micronutrients (R.B. Alfin-Slater and D. Kritchevsky. Gen. Edit) pp. 319-350. Plenum Press. Nueva York, 1979.

11. Foster, G.H.- Social anthropology as related to the nutrition in the preschool child. *In:* Nat. Ac Scs/Nat. Res Counc. Internat. Conf. Prev. Malnut. in Preschool Child Washington D.C. 1964.

12. Gálvez de la Vega, M.A.- Niveles de L.H. y F.S,H. en adolescentes deprivados. Tesis de Postgrado. Hospital de Pediatría, C.M.N./IMSS. México, 1981.

13. Gómez, F.; Ramos Galván, R. y Cravioto, J.- Nutritional Recovery Syndrome (Preliminary report). *Pediatrics.* 10:513-526, 1952.

14. Gómez, F.; Ramos Galván, R.; Cravioto, J. y Frenk, S. Malnutrition and Kwarshiorkor. *Acta Paed. Stockolm.* 43: (Suppl 100):336, 1954.

15. Gómez, F.; Ramos Galván, R.; Cravioto, J. y Frenk, S. Malnutrition in infancy and childhood with special reference to Kwarshiorkor. *Advances in Pediatrics.* Vol. 7:131-169, 1955.

16. Gómez, F.; Ramos Gálvan, R.; Cravioto, J. and Frenk, S.- Prevention and treatment of chronic severe infantile malnutrition (Kwarshiorkor). *Ann. Nueva York. Acad. of Sci.* 69:969, 1958.

17. Habicht, J.P.; Martorell, R.; Yarbrough, C.; Malina, R.M. ans Klein, R.E.- Height and weight standards for preschool children. Are there really ethnic differences in growth potential? *Lancet* 1:611, 1974.

18. Hagen, W.- The secular acceleration of growth and the individual. *In:* Modern Problems in Pediatrics. VII.- The growth of the normal child during the first three years of life. pp. 8-12. S. Karger. Basel. 1962.

19. Hahn, P.- Nutrition and metabolic development in mammals. *In:* Human Nutrition, vol. I. Nutrition. Pre and Postnatal Development (R.B. Alfin-Slater and D. Kritchvsky, Gen. Edit. M. Winick. Special Ed). pp. 1-40 Plenum Press. Nueva York, 1979.

20. Jolliffe, N.- The pathogenesis of deficiency diseases. *In:* Clinical Nutrition (N. Jolliffe, F.F. Tisdall and P.H. Cannon Eds). pp. 3-38, Paul B. Hoeber Inc. Nueva York, 1950.

21. Lisker, R.- Genetic polymorphism in Mexican population. *In:* Salzano, F. (Ed). The ongoing evolution of Latin. American population. Ch. C. Thomas. Springfield. 1971.

22. Lisker, R.- Estructura genética de la población mexicana. Aspectos médicos y antropológicos. Salvat ed. México, 1980.

23. Martorell, R.; Valverde, V. and Delgado, H.- La antropometría en los sistemas de salud. *In:* Simposio sobre tecnología apropiada para la salud. Org. Panam Salud (Ed). Washington, D.C. 1980 (Spanish copy).

24. Martorell, R.; Lechtig, A.; Habicht, J.P.; Yarbrough C. and Klein, R.E.- Normas antropométricas de crecimiento físico para países en desarrollo: Nacionales o extranjeros. *Bol. Of. Sanit. Panm.* 79:524, 1975.

25. Massler, M. and Suher, T.- Calculation of normal weight. *Child Develop.* 16:111, 1945.

26. Matson, A. y Swanson, J.- Distribution of hereditary blood antigens among the Maya and Non Maya indians in Mexico and Guatemala. *Am. J. Phys. Anthrop.* 17:49, 1959.

27. Matson, A. and Swanson, J.- Distribution of hereditary blood antigens among indians in middle America: Tzotzil and other Maya, *Am. J. Phys. Antrop.* 21:1, 1963.

28. Parra, A.; Ramos Galván, R.; Cervantes, C.; Sánchez, M. and Gálvez de la Vega, M.A.- Plasma gonadotrophins profile in relation to body composition in underprivileged boys. *Acta Endocr.* 99:326, 1982.

29. Patton, R.G. and Gardner, L.I.- Influence of family environment of growth: The Syndrome of Maternal Deprivation. *Pediatrics.* 30:957, 1962.

30. Powell, G.F.; Brasel, J.A. and Blizzard, R.M.- Emotional deprivation and growth retardation simulating idiopathic hypopituitarism. I. Clinical evaluation of the syndrome. *N. Engl., J. Med.* 276:1271, 1967.

31. Powell, G.F.; Brasel, J.A.; Raite, S. and Blizzard, R.M.- Emotional Deprivation and Growth Retardation Simulating Idiopathic Hypopituitarism. II.- Endrocrinologic Evaluation of the Syndrome. *N. Engl. J. Med.* 276:1279, 1967.

32. Ramos Galván, R.- Desnutrición, un componente del síndrome de deprivación social. *Gaceta méd.* México, 96:929, 1966.

33. Ramos Galván, R.- Heomeorresis en la desnutrición humana. *In:* Segundo Congreso de la Ac. Nac. Med. (Ac. Nac. Med. eds). Vol. 1 pp. México, 1969.

34. Ramos Galván, R.- Desnutrición y crecimiento físico. Comentarios. *In:* Nuevos conceptos sobre viejos aspectos de la desnutrición (Ac. Mex. Ped. eds.) pp. 247-265 México, 1973.

35. Ramos Galván, R.- Somatometría pediátrica. *Arch. invest. méd.* México 6 (Suppl 1):83, 1975.

36. Ramos Galván, R.- Consecuencias de la desnutrición crónica en los grupos humanos. *Gaceta méd.* México, 111:297, 1976.

37. Ramos Galván, R.- La somatometría en el diagnóstico del esta de nutrición. *Gaceta méd.* México, 111:297, 1976.

38. Ramos Galván, R.- El significado de la talla. *Cuadernos de Nutrición.* 3:199, 1978.

39. Ramos Galván, R.- Dimorfismo sexual en la composición corporal. Un análisis somatométrico. *In:* Estudios de Antropología Biológica. (Villanueva, M. y Serrano, C. eds). pp. 433-460. UNAM. México, 1982.

40. Ramos Galván, R.- Estudio del crecimiento físico, un método clínico y de campo mal aprovechado. *Rev. méd. IMSS.* (Méx.), 21:5, 1983.

41. Ramos Galván, R. and Cravioto, J.- Desnutrición. Concepto y ensayo de sistematización. *Bol. méd. Hosp. Infantil* (Méx.), 15:763, 1958.

42. Ramos Galván, R.; Mariscal, A.C.; Pérez Ortiz, B.; Viniegra C.A.; Castro, A. and Alvarez Rincón, M.C.- Mortalidad preescolar y desnutrición. *Bol. méd. Hosp. Infantil* (Méx.), 25:269, 1968.

43. Ramos Galván, R.; Mariscal, A.C.; Viniegra, C.A. and Pérez Ortiz, B.- Desnutrición en el niño. Chapter IV Patogenia. (Hosp. Inf. Méx. eds) pp. 21-31, México. 1969.

44. Ramos Rodríguez, R.M.- Crecimiento físico, composición corporal y proporcionalidad. Estudio en un grupo de mujeres de 12 a 20 años. Tesis recepcional. pp. 49-60. ENAH-SEP. México, 1978.

45. Ramos Rodríguez, R.M.- El segmento superior en la evaluación del potencial genético de crecimiento en talla. Una hipótesis que considerar. II. Cong. Int. Auxología. Dic. 1979. La Habana, Cuba.

46. Ramos Rodríguez, R.M.- El significado del segmento superior. Una hipótesis por considerar. *Bol. méd. Hosp. Infantil* (Méx.) 38:583, 1981.

47. Reba, R.C.; Cheek, D.B. and Leitnaker, F.C.- Body potassium and lean body mass. In: Human growth. Body compsitium, cell growth, energy and intelligence (Check, D.B. ed). Lea Febiger Philadelphia, 1968.

48. Redfield, R.- La sociedad "folk" *Rev. Méx. Soc.* 4:4, 1942.

49. Rogouski, S.J. and Winick, M.- Nutrition and cellular growth. *In:* Human Nutrition. Vol. I Nutrition. Pre and Postnatal development (R.B. Alfin-Slater and D. Kritchevsky Gen. Edit; M. Winick. Special Ed.). pp. 61-102, Plenum Press. Nueva York, 1979.

50. Sánchez Aedo, L.R.- Análisis de la proporcionalidad corporal en 1500 estudiantes de la Universidad Ibero Americana. Depto. de Ciencias de la Nutrición y Alimentos. U.I.A. México, 1982.

51. Sánchez Suárez, B.A.- Somatometría en mujeres puérperas y sus productos. Estudio en Cadereyta, Qro. Tesis de Postgrado. Hospital de Pediatría, C.M.N.- IMSS. México, 1982.

52. Sandstead, H.H.- Methods for determining nutrient requeriments in pregnancy. *Am.J. Clin. Nut:* 34:697, 1981.

53. Shive, W. and Lansford, E.M.- Role of vitamins as coenzymes. *In:* Human Nutrition. vol. 3B — Nutrition and the Adult Micronutrients (R.B. Alfin-Slater and D. Kritchevsky Gen. Edit), pp. 1-72 Plenum Press. Nueva York, 1979.

54. Swadesh, M.- Indian linguistic groups of Mexico. I.N.A.H. México, 1959.

55. Tanner, J.M.- Fetus into man. Physical Growth from Conception to Maturity, pp. 78-88. Harvard Univ. Press. Cambridge Mass. 1978.

56. Viteri, F.E.; Torún, B.; Immink, M.D.C. and Flores, R.- Marginal malnutrition and working capacity. *In:* Nutrition in Health and disease and International Development. Symposia from the XII International Congress of Nutrition (A.E. Harper and G.K. Davis, Eds.), pp. 277-283. Alan R. Liss Inc. Nueva York, 1981.

57. Waterlow, J.C.; Buzina, R.; Keeler, W.; Lane, J.M.; Nichaman, N.Z. and Tanner, J.M.-The presentation and use of height and weight data for comparing the nutritional status of growth of children under the age of ten years. *Bull. W. H.O.* 55:489, 1977.

58. Zardain, I.C.; Mena, M.S. y Ramos Galván, R.- Estudio somatométrico en un grupo de preescolares y en sus progenitores. *Cuadernos de Nutrición* (Méx.) 1978, 3:263-275.

59. Zavala, C.; Alatorre, S. y Lisker. R.- Distancias génicas entre grupos indígenas mexicanos. En. Inst. de Invest. Antropológicas UNAM.- Estudios de Antropología biológica (Primer Coloquio Juan Comas). UNAM. Méx. 1982, pp. 141-154.

60. Zerfas, A.C.- Anthropometric field methods. *In:* Human Nutrition. Vol. 2 — Nutrition and Growth. (R.B. Alfin-Slater and D. Kritchevsky Gen. Ed. D.B. Jelliffe and E.F.P. Jelliffe Special Ed), pp. 339-364. Plenum Press. Nueva York. 1979.

APPENDIX 1

Height, lower and upper segments in cm. at different ages

Age (years)	Males Height	Lower segment	Upper segment	Females Height	Lower segment	Upper segment
5 years	107.58 ± 3.64	52.72 ± 2.4	54.86 ± 2.4	107.59 ± 4.27	53.16 ± 2.6	54.43 ± 2.0
5 3/12	109.19 3.71	53.57 2.5	55.62 2.4	109.09 4.27	53.96 2.6	55.13 2.0
5 6/12	110.70 2.79	54.76 2.5	56.04 2.5	110.59 4.26	54.93 2.6	55.66 2.0
5 9/12	112.20 3.87	55.64 2.6	56.66 2.5	112.19 4.30	55.89 2.6	56.30 2.0
6 years	113.68 3.96	56.59 2.6	57.09 2.6	113.59 4.32	57.01 2.7	56.58 2.0
6 3/12	115.18 4.03	57.59 2.7	57.59 2.6	114.99 4.40	57.82 2.7	57.17 2.0
6 6/12	116.59 4.12	58.60 2.7	55.99 2.6	116.50 4.49	58.94 2.7	57.56 2.0
6 9/12	117.99 4.20	59.50 2.8	58.49 2.7	117.99 4.68	59.98 2.7	58.01 2.0
7 years	119.49 4.30	60.50 2.8	58.99 2.7	119.49 4.90	61.03 2.7	58.46 2.0
7 3/12	121.18 4.40	61.50 2.9	59.68 2.7	120.90 5.02	62.07 2.7	58.83 2.0
7 6/12	122.69 4.49	62.50 2.9	60.19 2.8	122.18 5.13	62.98 2.8	59.20 2.0
7 9/12	123.91 4.59	63.50 3.0	60.58 2.8	123.39 5.22	63.92 2.8	59.47 2.0
8 years	125.49 4.68	64.40 3.0	61.08 2.8	124.99 5.31	64.83 2.8	60.16 2.0
8 3/12	126.87 4.77	65.40 3.1	61.47 2.8	126.49 5.33	65.72 2.9	60.77 2.1
8 6/12	127.99 4.86	66.30 3.1	61.69 2.9	127.69 5.32	66.60 2.9	61.09 2.1
8 9/12	128.67 4.95	67.20 3.1	61.67 2.9	128.99 5.37	67.40 2.9	61.59 2.1
9 years	130.39 5.02	68.10 3.2	62.29 2.9	130.09 5.41	68.21 3.0	61.88 2.2
9 3/12	131.69 5.14	68.89 3.2	62.80 2.9	131.29 5.53	69.14 3.0	62.15 2.3
9 6/12	132.99 5.27	69.69 3.2	63.30 3.0	132.69 5.65	70.09 3.1	62.60 2.3
9 9/12	134.19 5.37	70.50 3.3	63.69 3.0	134.29 5.81	71.11 3.1	63.18 2.4

APPENDIX 2

Percentage represented by height, upper and lower segments related to final height
(from birth to 18 years of age)

Ages in	Males			Females		
years	Height	Lower segment	Upper segment	Height	Lower segment	Upper segment
5 years	62.26	30.51	31.75	66.99	33.10	33.89
5 3/12	63.19	31.00	32.19	67.93	33.60	34.33
5 6/12	64.06	31.63	32.43	68.86	34.20	34.66
5 9/12	64.93	32.20	32.73	69.86	34.80	35.06
6 years	65.79	32.81	32.98	70.73	35.50	35.23
6 3/12	66.66	33.33	33.33	71.60	36.00	35.60
6 6/12	67.47	33.91	33.56	72.54	36.70	35.84
6 9/12	68.28	34.43	33.85	73.47	37.35	36.12
7 years	69.15	35.01	35.14	74.40	38.00	36.40
7 3/12	70.13	35.59	34.54	75.28	38.65	36.63
7 6/12	71.00	36.17	34.83	76.08	39.22	36.86
7 9/12	71.81	36.75	35.06	76.83	39.80	37.03
8 years	72.62	37.27	35.35	77.83	40.37	37.46
8 3/12	73.42	37.85	35.57	78.76	40.92	37.84
8 6/12	74.07	38.37	35.70	79.51	41.47	38.04
8 9/12	74.46	38.89	35.87	80.32	41.97	38.35
9 years	75.46	39.41	36.05	81.00	42.47	38.53
9 3/12	76.21	39.87	36.34	81.75	43.05	38.70
9 6/12	76.96	40.33	36.63	82.62	43.64	38.98
9 9/12	77.66	40.80	36.86	83.62	44.28	39.34
10 years	78.41	41.38	37.03	84.62	44.92	39.70
10 3/12	79.10	41.84	37.26	85.61	45.57	40.04
10 6/12	79.86	42.30	37.56	86.73	46.23	40.50
10 9/12	80.67	42.71	37.96	87.79	46.85	40.94
11 years	81.36	43.23	38.13	88.91	47.48	41.43
11 3/12	82.17	43.69	38.48	90.09	48.08	42.01
11 6/12	82.92	44.16	38.76	91.09	48.69	42.40
11 9/12	83.68	44.62	39.06	92.15	49.20	42.95

SOME DATA DERIVED FROM NUTRITION LONGITUDINAL STUDIES RELEVANT TO THE INTERPRETATION OF NUTRITION AND GENETIC INTERACTION[1]

Joaquín Cravioto

*Instituto Nacional de Ciencias y Tecnología
para la Salud del Niño DIF,
Mexico City, Mexico*

Studies in nutrition involve three main variables: level of nutrient intake, response of the organism, and time. When time becomes the main variable, we talk about longitudinal studies. A longitudinal study is the quantitation of the nutrient response along the time dimension. This can be both chronological or biological.

For the last three decades, longitudinal studies have focused mainly on the relation between malnutrition, growth, and development. Most studies have been performed on children because of the period of rapid growth and the vulnerability of the central nervous system. They have been concerned with size and performance. The study of mental functions provides information about the development of the underlying central nervous system.

For instance, differences can be observed when raising rat litters. The smallest rat in a large litter (8) shows delayed development compared to the smallest rat in a small litter (2). Restriction of the diet involves delayed information through the senses which have not been developed, and therefore of central nervous system functions. Differences persist even after animals are weaned and put on a complete diet.

Biochemical studies show that proteolytic activity of liver enzymes is abnormal in small rats of large litters, even after they are properly fed. The same pattern appears in purposefully malnourished rats.

Studies performed on children of rural communities in Mexico show small differences when height increments are considered. However, real differences appear when the time dimension is taken into account. Well-nourished children reach maximum growth in less time than malnourished children.

---

[1]*Summary prepared by Isabel Pérez-Montfort*

Biochemical studies performed on malnourished children show abnormal phenylalanine-tyrosine ratio. Malnutrition can thus mimic inborn errors of metabolism, at least temporarily.

Longitudinal studies involving weight of children show that there is high probability of remaining either well-nourished or malnourished, depending on initial weight. Environmental and genetic modulators influencing weight at birth are important both at birth and at least during the first year of life. The symmetry of various growth and development curves in normal children is lost when malnutrition sets in.

The importance of longitudinal studies lies in their capacity to determine major differences between malnourished and nourished children. Tools and methodology for research exist, but data on the interaction between nutrition and genetics are still scarce.

PART VI

PROSPECTIVES

FUTURE NEEDS AND DEVELOPMENTS

M. C. Nesheim

Cornell University,
Ithaca, N.Y.

The responsibility for summarizing and projecting future needs following a wide ranging conference such as this one is formidable and I will attempt only to summarize some impressions that have come to me as a nutritionist as this meeting has progressed.

When we began this meeting, Dr. Velázquez in his welcoming address told us that the goals of this workshop were to initiate development of an interface between nutrition and genetics, define questions that needed answers, understand methodological tools available to both fields, define priority research areas and develop personal contacts to stimulate international cooperation in the area of genectics and nutrition. I think all will agree that we have had an extremely wideranging discussion. We have covered nearly all aspects of the questions raised by Dr. Velázquez and Dr. Bourges in their original paper, but sorting out the answers to some of those questions from the discussion has been a real challenge. I will not try to summarize this meeting in the true sense of the word, but I will try to extract some themes and ideas of what we have been talking about.

First let me say that the last objective that was listed for this meeting has been fulfilled very well. The interaction between individuals within the disciplines has been a special feature of our time here. I certainly want to thank Dr. Velázquez and Dr. Bourges for giving us the opportunity to spend this time in rather intense formal and personal discussion. Meetings of this type have a particular camaraderie about them, and this has developed most successfully during our four days together.

The general theme that we have discussed in many contexts, has been metabolic variation. We have considered many of its aspects and we have discussed many of the genetic and environmental factors that may influence metabolic variation. I think we all understand that variations that we find in individuals and in populations is not always genetic variation, and that one of the challenges is to distinguish genetic variations from environmental ones.

417

Nutritionists generally are concerned with the degree of genetic variation in nutritional requirements. As our geneticist colleagues have observed in this meeting, nutritional requirements are not always a benign subject in the nutrition community. We always have considerable debate about criteria for establishing requirements, what a requirements actually is, and what we are really going to do with requirements when we have agreed on them. I suggest we must recognize that nutritional requirements, as we understand them, are important. We spend a lot of time considering requirements; we appoint expert committees, and we spend long hours haggling over what seems to be a few decimal points in requirement levels. Why, then, are requirements to important to us?

First, we use nutritional requirements as a means for assessing the adequacy of population dietary intakes. Dr. Payne and Dr. Beaton have discussed this use of nutritional requirements and have suggested that when considering nutritional requirements and deviations from nutritional requirements, we need to find a way of expressing probabilities of the health consequences that may ensue from deviations from nutritional requirements. This important concept is a part of a growing recognition in nutrition that we have to be able to establish the functional consequences of deviations from nutritional norms.

Economists and planners, when they begin to consider nutrition ask us "What do you mean by this requirement? What are the consequences of a 25% lower intake by a population? How can we do an economic analysis of the benefits of a nutrition program until we are able to have some perspective as to biological consequences of deviations from nutritional requirements?" So nutritional requirements are very important to the nutrition community, as are the consequences of deviations from them.

Nutritional requirements also serve as targets for dietary recommendations. We have to have some way of telling people about desirable dietary practices. In this context, variation among the nutritional requirements of individuals is quite important. For example, when recommendations for nutritional standards are made for populations, is the individual variation so great as to make these general recommendations relatively meaningless for certain individuals within the population? This is a crucial point when we try to deal with the issue of nutritional requirements, and is a major reason for investigating the question of genetic variation in nutritional requirements.

In this meeting, we have made relatively little progress in answering that question, but perhaps we have obtained some new perspectives. The discussions on inborn errors of metabolism have been particularly stimulating. Inborn errors are sometimes discussed as being special cases that need specific treatment apart from general population recommendations, and they are assumed to have relatively little significance when considering variation in nutrient metabolism in the vast majority of the population. This meeting has provided a different perspective on inborn errors.

The discussion on the phenylketonuric variants, for example, by Dr. Cederbaum was particularly enlightening. The observed variation, that has been detected in practically all of the regulatory sites in the conversion of phenylala-nine to tyrosine, is of particular interest. The consequences of variations in phenylalanine metabolism, i.e. the elevation of phenylalanine in body fluids, has some rather spectacular biological consequences and, therefore, the variation results in a particular disease that is the result of genetic variation. The consideration of the receptor defects in hyperlipidemias indicated that there are also multiple variants affecting lipoprotein receptors. The degree that other metabolic variants exist that cause less spectacular physiological effects in pathways that affect specific nutrients and their use deserves to be eluci-dated further. This concept should pervade the thinking of those who are try-ing to consider metabolic variations that affect nutritional needs.

Sutton and Wagner [1] have reviewed data indicating that an amino acid substitution resulting from variation in a gene for a particular enzyme can re-sult in functional effects that can range all the way from abolishing the detect-able activity of the enzyme to effecting only a slight change in affinity of the enzyme for its substrate. If this full range of effect on metabolism is expressed in human populations some important nutritional variation rather than stri-king metabolic disease may result.

Nutritional requirements in the usual sense are hard to assess for the genetic variation. I do not think that our concept of nutritional requirements is specific enough for a geneticist to do very good genetic analysis of variation that occurs within a population. Dr. Motulsky made this point in his presentation, and I think that we must be more specific as to what are the metabolic variations that may have some quantitative effect upon nutritional needs in the population. Perhaps if some of the steps that lead to variation in nutritional requirements can be isolated, the assessment of genetic effects will be somewhat more precise.

It also seems likely that the amount of genetic variation one finds in a meta-bolic step depends upon the biochemical complexity of that particular pathway. I was impressed when Dr. Rosenberg, in discussing the methylmalonate acidemias and the observed variations in B-12 metabolism, commented that it took a lot of genetic information to describe the pathway. He suggested that the amount of variation that might occur within that pathway was probably more than you might find in a somewhat simpler metabolic pathway. There are other examples of this in the literature.

I presented an example yesterday of a rather complex metabolic pathway in experimental animals [2] that was associated with considerable genetic varia-tion. We have done the same kind of studies with the conversion of tryptophan to nicotinic acid [3]. This is a rather complex metabolic pathway, and genetic selection experiments can readily be carried out showing that it is possible to change in experimental animals the efficiency of conversion of tryptophan to NAD.

We have not considered much data at this meeting that will help estimate ge-netic variation that human populations might show in nutritional requeri-ments. As a guess, from the little information I am aware of, I think it is likely that the variation in quantitative needs for specific nutrients that we find among individuals is probably not as variable as our discussions of potential metabolic variation might lead us to believe. My estimate would be that something between 25 to 50 percent variation in the amount of a nutrient needed to cause a specific biological result will encompass the vast majority of the population.

Several fold differences in requirement that more enthusiastic disciples of biochemical individuality have suggested as being present in populations, probably are very unusual and it seems likely that nutritional requirements that are generally known, have meaning to individuals over a relatively small range.

I think that some of the data presented here, Dr. Snyderman's observations, for example, were quite impressive in the relatively small variation in amino acid needs that she determined for a large number of infants. Dr. Scrimshaw discussed variations in relation to nitrogen requirements that were relatively low.

All of the variations observed are not necessarily due to genetic variation, however, and this must be better established by future research. The major nutritional deficiencies that we find in the world today, outside of the problems of protein energy malnutrition, are iodine deficiency, vitamin A deficiency and iron deficiency. There are vast numbers of people who are consuming relatively marginal or deficient levels of these particular nutrients [4]. I think the components of variation in the utilization of these nutrients probably can be assessed by the use of appropriate genetic epidemiological techniques. Such considerations may be incorporated in some nutrition surveys in an attempt to examine the genetic variations observed in utilization of these nutrients. Such studies would be a useful future collaboration between geneticists and nutritionists and might help to determine some of the genetic influences on nutrient deficiency diseases that we see in populations.

We discussed in some detail the problems with protein energy malnutrition and the overwhelming influence of environmental factors as opposed to genetic factors in variations among individuals. Some of these specific nutrient deficiencies might lend themselves to genetic analysis. Dr. Torún made a specific plea that we look at some of these genetic relationships related to iodine deficiency, and I think that is something we should take to heart.

I was also particularly impressed by Dr. Schull's presentation and his suggestion that we carry metabolic variations around with us that we do not know about that only show up when we expose ourselves to a somewhat different environment. Individuals who respond somewhat differently from the majority of the population, may turn out to be genetic variants that are expressed only in a very specific environment. Such individuals might be recognized when certain kinds of dietary changes occur in relation to drug metabolism, or in other situations where populations are suddenly confronted with environments that have changed.

It is typical of nutrition today that we seem to divide discussions of nutrition into the more traditional problems of undernutrition as being separate from the problems of overnutrition. The considerations of overnutrition, or some would say inappropriate dietary patterns, is a relatively new subject in nutrition. A great deal of controversy has been generated in nutrition in the last few years as to what is the relationship, not of individual nutrients, but of dietary patterns and the incidence of chronic disease in populations.

I thought it was interesting that this subject was introduced to this conference by Dr. Neel, a geneticist, rather than a nutritionist, and I think it shows the public health concern in many developed societies for the issues related to chronic disease that cross many discipline lines. Dr. Neel discussed what he termed multigenetic nutritional disorders and he considered mature-onset diabetes mellitus, essential hypertension and cancer of the colon, as examples of these multigenetic nutritional disorders. He considered the absence of these diseases in unacculturated primative populations and their high prevalence in modern developed societies as an indication of a widespread genetic susceptibility to environmental influences. He advocated mass measures, applied to the general population, that would decrease the likelihood of disease among the susceptible in the population. These measures in this case were to be related to excessive salt intake and exercise, and he indicated that we should take any steps that we could to control obesity. Dr. Neel suggested that it would be possible from a genetic point of view to identify high risk families, but he considered that the cost to our society would be too great, and that from a public health point of view, we would be better off to move toward mass measures applied to the population rather than to specific measures to individuals that were identified within the population. At another time in this meeting, coronary heart disease was discussed as a disease affected by environmental influences, and both Dr. Connor and Dr. Blackburn suggested that community-wide strategies of prevention are likely to be most effective in reducing population coronary heat disease risk. I am among those nutritionists that find these arguments quite persuasive.

However, Dr. Motulsky raised the possibility that further definition of population groups at risk may be possible, and I would hope that our geneticist colleagues would help to clarify this situation. Part of the debate within the nutrition community about this issue has been precisely whether we can identify individual at-risk groups within the population, and whether we can provide more effective counselling with individuals within at-risk groups than we can by educational measures applied to the general population. Therefore, I hope that collaboration with geneticists can continue in this particular area so that we can establish which conditions need to be dealt with on a mass basis and which have a greater possibility for more specific individual recommendations.

Dr. Payne raised as an ethical issue the strength of proof that is necessary before community-wide measures could be taken. He indicated that parhaps we should not interfere with people's lifestyles unless our evidence for benefit is strong. I think there is another side to that ethical issue; if we know and have evidence, but perhaps not complete evidence, that certain behavioral factors or lifestyle factors may contribute to disease in a population, then there is another ethical issue, involving what we have to do about informing people even before the absolute proof is established. We have not resolved this ethical balance in our meeting here, but the issue is an important one and probably the solution lies in the strength of measures that we take to deal with these issues in communities. Where the proof is particularly strong, the measures that one can take might be strong, and where the proof is not quite as strong, we should expend more effort on education and public understanding of the issues in helping people make individual choices.

We have not resolved the genetic and nutritional relationships dealing with energy balance and obesity. I think the conference as a whole skirted this issue because we really do not know quite how to come to grips with it. There were some excellent papers on obesity but the genetic-nutrition interaction here is not well understood. There certainly seem to be individual differences. Those working in the obesity area increasingly describe individual differences in response to energy intake and to other factors that affect the deposition of energy in the body. Recently, there have been some exciting new ideas in energy balance and these have rather specific metabolic components to them. The genetic understanding of this energy balance is going to become much easier once the components have been identified. Perhaps we will able to classify human genetic predisposition to obesity in the same way as Dr. Coleman has developed with the rodent models that he discussed with us so well in his presentation earlier. I believe that there has to be a lot of collaboration between our two disciplines in the area of obesity in the future because human obesity is not a simple, single entity and the record of success of treatment is pretty dismal.

We discussed many other exciting things during the past few days that I have not mentioned. From my own point of view, I have gained a greater understanding of how geneticists view problems that are of concern to nutritionists and I hope we all now have a base on which to build further collaboration.

REFERENCES

1. Sutton, H.E. and R.P. Wagner 1975 Mutation and enzyme function in humans. *Am. Rev. Genetics* 9:187-212.
2. Wang, Shu-heh, L.O. Crosby and M.C. Nesheim 1973 Effect of dietary excesses of lysine and arginine on the degradation of lysine by chicks. *J. Nutr.* 103:384-391.
3. Nesheim, M.C. 1972 Genetic variation in nicotinic acid requirement of chicks. *J. Heredity* 63:347-350.
4. FAO 1977 The Fourth World Food Survey. FAO, Rome.

FUTURE NEEDS AND DEVELOPMENTS:
A GENETICIST'S POINT OF VIEW

Luigi Cavalli-Sforza

Genetics Department
Stanford University Medical Center
Stanford, California

INTRODUCTION

New Genetics

The distinction between phenotype and genotype is at the root of genetics. Phenotype is "the observed": height, weight, skinfolds, or any other trait that intests us. Genotype, in classical genetics, is all that is transmitted from parent to child. In a given environment, genotype determines phenotype or more exactly, a statistical distribution of phenotypes.

"New genetics" permits us to replace this highly abstract concept, genotype, with a concrete molecular structure: DNA. Instead of inferring an individual's genotype from its ancestry or progeny, we can read directly from a sequence of DNA nucleotides. We replace earlier statements about genotypes, usually made in terms or probability, with the results of analytical chemical methods. These describe DNA structure in terms of the sequence of the four nucleotides A, G, C, and T (corresponding to the bases adenine, guanine, cytosine and thymine).

These advances are having, (and in the next decade they will have even more), gigantic effects on our biological thinking and technology.

We have known for a long time that each of us is unique; now we know precisely how incredibly unique we are. The DNA contained in a human gamete consists of approximately 3 billion pairs (3 million kb. or kilobases) of nucleotides aligned in the double helix. This DNA is distributed in the 23 chromosomes. In ordinary (non gametic) cells, chromosomes come in pairs. One member of each pair comes from the father, and one from the mother. Thus, a non-gametic cell contains 6 million kb. The information contained in a particular DNA segment of, for instance, the paternal chromosome, resembles that in the

423

corresponding or homologous segment in the maternal chromosome. Differences between them cause genetic variation and evolution. These changes, which arise from mutation, consist mostly of replacement of one nucleotide with another. Mutations are rare; they occur about once in every 100 to 1000 million gametes per generation per nucleotide. The average gamete, containing three million kilobases, might have 3 to 30 new mutations, randomly scattered throughout its DNA. Also, mutations that occurred in earlier generations may be transmitted from parent to child over many generations, and thus accumulate. Whether or not a mutation has a phenotypic effect, depends on the position of the nucleotide involved in the susbtitution and on the type of replacement. If the mutation has a phenotypic effect it may be subject to natural selection.

A new DNA type caused by mutation can be lost by chance or adverse selection against the particular phenotype it determines. Over the generations, this modified DNA can become more common than the nonmutated type. Through chance or natural selection, the new sometimes replaces the old.

If we choose a random segment of paternal DNA and compare it with its maternal homologue, we find that they differ, on the average, at one in every 500-1000 nucleotides. This measures, simply and directly genetic variation in a population. In a DNA segment of, say, 20 kb, we expect about 10 differences, on the average, between the paternal and the maternal segment. We would predict the same amount of variation between homologous segments taken from two individuals of the same population. For a whole chromosome set (3 million kilobases), we anticipate 6 million mutations.·

To find all the differences between two random chromosomes, we must determine the nucleotide sequence of two entire segments-a feasible, but prohibitively long, experiment. Another alternative approach will miss most mutants but will quickly detect enough to be useful for many purposes. This method uses restriction enzymes. They break DNA wherever a certain nucleotide sequence occurs. For instance, the restriction enzyme called SstI breaks the sequence GAGCTC. Any chromosome set can thus be broken into millions of fragments of variable length. Electrophoresis separates fragments by length. A specific fragment can be identified on the electrophorogram by its ability to specifically anneal ("hybridize") with a radioactive, partly homologous, fragment. The radioactive probe thus reveals, on an autoradiograph, the position of a desired DNA fragment and helps determine the lenght (in kb) of its homologous fragment or fragments in the genome.

Suppose a segment of DNA is fragmented at the arrows (the "restriction sites").

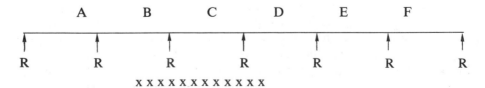

The radioactive probe is indicated with a row of x's: fragments that are homologous with the probe and therefore anneal with it appear on the autoradiograph as radioactive bands. All other fragments—millions—are invisible. In the example above, only the three fragments B, C, D, show. If a mutation has modified an existing restriction site, or generated a new one, the fragmentation pattern will change. Suppose the R site between fragments C and D has been lost through a mutation in a nucleotide of the corresponding restriction site sequence GAGCTC. The DNA does not break in that position. The probe reveals only two fragments, one of length B, the other C + D.

The probe essential for the procedure is obtained by cloning the relevant piece of human DNA. A fragment containing an interesting gene or region is put into the circular chromosome of the bacteriophage (a bacterial virus) or of a plasmid (a non-essential bacterial minichromosome which can be transmitted from cell to cell). This human DNA fragment, usually between 1 and 40 kb long, can be produced very cheaply in any quantity. Besides generating the probes necessary for restriction analysis, this process is also useful for sequencing DNA, and for bacterial production of proteins, one of the chief industrial applications of genetic engineering.

Many human genes have already been cloned, and many more will be in the near future. This makes the analysis of genetic variation much more precise than ever before. It raises the number of potentially known "genes" from the thousands to the millions now known; to all DNA. We have seen that the gene is a more complex structure than we thought. The part of DNA coding for a specific protein is, on the average, 1 kb long. It is only about one-tenth or one-twentieth of the DNA segment containing a protein-coding gene. We still know too little about many of the non-coding parts of DNA. Certainly at least some of them help regulate gene action.

Cloning the genes for lipoproteins, membrane receptors, enzymes, and other cell fractions of nutritional interest will generate an unprecedented mass of genetic information. The DNA sequence is extremely informative. For instance, it supplies knowledge of the amino acid sequence of a protein more easily than does sequencing of the protein. Human DNA regions best known today include those directing the synthesis of insulin, immunoglobulins, and the protein part of hemoglobins.

Present genetic technology is starting to fulfill the wildest dreams of geneticists, and developments in sight can lead to genetic therapy by gene replacement. But geneticists are also interested in understanding phenotypes. The analysis of gene products, from messenger, protein and enzyme products all the way to morphological, physiological and behavioral traits, is inevitably complex. Very few systems have been worked out, and only in a limited way. In general, situations in which a single gene difference is known and clear cut, as for instance in inborn errors of metabolism, lend themselves best to analysis in depth. Polygenic systems, in which many different genes each contribute a bit to a phenotypic trait, are most difficult to study. A very productive but demanding approach to the study of a polygenic trait is that of reconstructing the mosaic of participating polygenes by using genetic markers for each of them. An important beginning to this approach was made with the demonstration, that electophoretic variants of lipoproteins A and E are found in different parts of the overall distribution of serum cholesterol levels. This approach might account for an important part, perhaps even all, of the genetics variation in cholesterol levels. The necessary markers were provided by electrophoretic study of proteins. DNA restriction analysis can supplement it by supplying a wealth of other genetic markers of the chromosome segments involved. DNA markers are not confined to the structural variation which can be studied by protein analysis. They can also uncover variation in regulatory genetic units. Such an analysis has the greatest potential and will cover a ground today largely uncharted, for practically any genetic system.

The Norm of Reaction

At the end of the chain of events from gene to phenotype, the importance of environment, or "nurture", usually becomes overwhelming. Nutritionists are close to realizing a dream of geneticists: the adequate discription of the genotype-phenotype relation. This is greatly helped by resorting to a basic concept, the norm of reaction, introduced a long time ago in genetics and mentioned here by R. Ward [27]. It was never used in man except for sporadic, hypothetical cases: IQ and, in a slightly less hypothetical situation, skin color [7, 8, 16]. Nutritional studies give an excelent chance to use and amplify this very basic model, which substantially clarifies this complex issue.

One example is that of dietary cholesterol(x) versus serum cholesterol (y). Plotted on a graph, they form a norm-of-reaction curve. Different genotypes give different curves (Fig. 1).

To plot the curve for a single genotype, values from several genetically identical individuals are observed at various levels of dietary intake. Unfortunately, few people are genetically identical. To simplify the problem, we study one gene at a time. At least two alleles of it must be known and labelled by a protein of DNA marker (*e.g.,* lipoproteins E and A, or hyperlipidemias as reviewed by Motulsky, [21]. We can then group together individuals with the same allele (s). To have data for various input levels in the same individuals requires dietary experiments. The lower curve in Fig. 1 shows data from different cultures with known cholesterol intake (Blackburn, 17). This helps supply a first approximation for the reaction norm (lower curve, Fig. 1) of an average "normal" genotype (assuming this does not vary too much in the different ethnic groups). The upper (semi-hypothetical) curve is for familial hyperlipidemia. The dotted curves are norms of reaction of other hypothetical genotypes.

Blackburn [1] gave us expected cholesterol levels in three hypothetical genotypes on five diets. Plotting his data on a "norm of reaction" graph clarifies his model. The curves of his three genotypes are parallel, straight lines. This

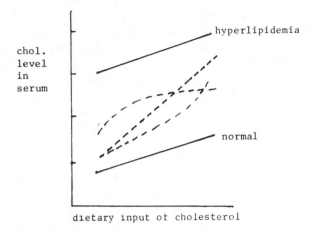

Figure 1. Data from different cultures with known cholesterol intake.

correspondes to an exactly additive interaction between genotype and environment. Adding a given amount of cholesterol to the diet changes serum cholesterol by the absolute amount for any genotype. Increasing dietary cholesterol by one step always raises cholesterol level by 25 mg/dl. Genotype changes only the baseline of the norm of reaction.

This is the additive model. It is the simplest mode of interaction between genotype and environment. Statisticians call this graph one of no interaction. It is certainly the first model to be tested. In Fig. 1, the norm of reaction of the heterozygotes for familial hyperlipidemia (upper solid line). The data suggest that these are approximately straight, parallel lines. Naturally, the "normal" population contains many genotypes.

Extending the concept of "norm of reaction" [7] helps us to understand components of variation better. How do we derive the total distribution of cholesterol in a population? We need information on the reaction norm plot for each genotype represented in the population. We also need to investigate sources of variation which are usually all classified as "environmental" and grouped together, but should be kept distinct.

1) Experimental error.

2) "Internal" variation. Or the expected differences between individuals of identical genotype in exactly the same environment. This is likely to be small, perhaps negligible for many characters. It arises through stochastic developmental processes, and might be tested in humans by comparing identical twins on the same diet.

3) Previous individual history. Sometimes external events that occurred prior to observation, irreversibly influence an individual's reaction. These events, a life history component, are partially confused with "internal" variation. We can evaluate their importance only on the basis of longitudinal data, along with knowledge of life history. Consequences of early deprivation: Cravioto [11], and Sukhatme and Margen's model [26] exemplify this. The observations on PKU (Cederbaum, 10) make it certain that life history, especially the early one, can be extremely important for some traits. "Critical periods" in development are known for any class of traits, but poorly studied in man.

4) Variation in the environmental parameter (s). This is on abscissa of Fig. 1, and is distinct for different individuals of the population. It is especially important, because a fraction, perhaps an important one, of the environment is transmitted over generations. In this case environmental variation is easily confused with genetic effects, as we shall discuss later.

5) When one analyzes only the genotypes formed by the alleles of one gene at a time, there may be an important residual genetic variation due to other genes affecting trait.

The diverse information required poses difficult problems for the experimenter. I have no sadistic motivation in adding that, to completely predict population behavior, one also needs the frequencies of the various genotypes in the population. We also have to know about possible genotype-environment GE correlations to be kept distinct from GE interaction. In the simplest case (as in Blackburn's model), GE interaction is additive, while more complex norm of reactions are not parallel (and this is synonymous with the existence of GE interaction).

By contrast, GE correlation is defined as the situation in which different genotypes of the same population have a different distribution of environments, i.e., of abscissa values. Medical advice may succeed in convincing individuals with "high" genotypes to considerably lower their cholesterol input. This can generate some negative GE correlation. By contrast, spontaneous behavior might induce a positive correlation. My personal experience suggests that "high" genotypes may spontaneously select high environments; my sample is limited, however, to one person: myself. My preference for food seems to be strictly proportional to its cholesterol content. However, I do not have very good information on my genotype for cholesterol.

We can extend the norm of reaction curve to more than one environmental parameter, for instance smoking and physical exercise for cholesterol HDL. We then have to struggle with three-dimensional representation. Figure 2 shows an approximate example derived from average population data (for lack of single genotype data) with the help of Henry Blackburn. The line in the 1-environmental parameter of Figure 1 becomes a surface. In a situation of additive interaction between the two environmental parameters of Figure 1 becomes a surface. In a situation of additive interaction between the two environmental parameters, the straight line in Figure 1 will become an even surface. Each genotype will have its own surface.

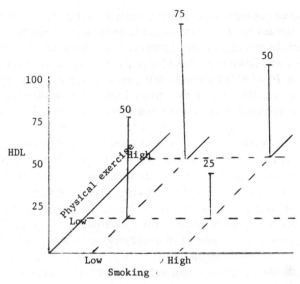

Figure 2. "Norm of reaction" surface. (A single genotype should be shown).

Individual history might be represented by a time dimension. A statisfactory description of all relevant facts is likely to require many dimensions. Before throwing up one's hands in despair, one should consider using some well known, powerful statistical techniques. They can reduce dimensionality, with minimum loss of information. The use of multiple regression methods, which are closely related, is already very familiar to students of cholesterol levels.

Cultural Transmission and Evolution

It is still widely believed by many geneticists and other scientists that similarities between parent and child, sib and sib, or identical twins, are proof and measurement of what Galton [14], who started this approach, called "natural inheritance". Similarities between relatives, evaluated by correlation coefficients, yield estimates of heritability. Heritability supposedly measures the fraction of total phenotypic variation due to genetic differences between individuals of a population.

I share Dr. Garby's lack of patience for heritabilities [15]. Correlations and derived heritability estimates merely indicate, sometimes only tentatively, that genetic variation affects a specific phenotype. We inherit both genes and much of our "culture" (including characteristics such as language, skills, behaviors, and tastes), from our parents. In genetic transmission, parents are the only factors. Cultural inheritance depends on parents and many other people-sibs, friends, teachers, social leaders and groups. Nevertheless, depending on traits and societies, parents can still be very influential. The simultaneous presence of genetic and cultural parent-child transmission makes it very difficult, however, to separate the effects of genes and culture. Kuru and hepatitis B are two diseases that entered human genetic literature due to *bona fide* genes. They left it when scientists discovered that both are chronic viral infections, which parents frequently transmit to their children [2, 5].

How can we distinguish between natural and cultural inheritance? We all accept evidence for genetic inheritance when the trait follows Mendelian patterns. Inborn errors of metabolism are the classic examples. Lactose malabsorption is a borderline case [18]. I tend to believe that lactose malabsorption is due to at least one gene difference, but some of my colleagues are less happy with this idea. This problem was examined on the basis of data collected in Italy by T. Cavalli-Sforza [9]. The experimental error of existing methods, unfortunately, is large. Its magnitude seems to justify, at least in part, the disagreement with the Mendelian model observed by Lisker. However, the gene's geographic distribution (Simoons, 24) agrees well with local history of milk consumption. Lactose absorption is probably the best documented case of genetic adaptation (by natural selection) in the field of nutrition.

Good evidence of a genetic background also comes from strong association of traits with *bona fide* genetic markers. The associations of HLA with several diseases provide solid examples (Bodmer & Bodmer, 3). For most other traits, especially those showing continuous variation, heritability estimates do not distinguish between the contributions of genetic and cultural components. Correlations of adopted children with biological and foster relatives supply some information. Unfortunately, good adoption data are rare.

Some other criteria can help support cultural inheritance. Migrant studies are especially interesting; differences in correlation with father and with mother are other criteria. Both were used by R. Ward [27] in his paper. A third method, twin studies, may sometimes be used to back up cultural, rather than genetic, inheritance. Political attitudes [6] *e.g.* preference of parent and child for the Republican or Democratic party, strongly agree with each other. Is this due to a political gene? Twin studies (Loehlin and Nichols, 17) show that there is also a strong correlation between members of a twin pair for traits concerning political attitudes, but it is of about the same strenght in identical and in fraternal twin pairs. This seems to dispose of the political gene. When, the correlation is higher for identical twins than for fraternal, however, one should be careful of concluding uncritically in favor of genetic transmission.

In a recent book [5], M. Feldman and I developed a formal treatment of cultural transmission and evolution. We tried to be as quantitative as possible. We drew from models of genetics and biological evolution, and from the mathematical theory of epidemics. We also experimented with new ones accounting for the numerous models of cultural transmission: from parent to child (vertical), between age-peers (horizontal), teacher to students, social leaders of all sorts to dependents, subordinates, or fans (a transmission called "from one towards many"), social group pressures ("many towards one") and so on. We evaluated the evolutionary consequences of these modes of transmission, particularly on the variation between groups and within groups, *i.e.,* between individuals of the same social group. Variance between groups is likely to be highest in the one-towards-many type of transmission, and lowest is the many-to-one transmission. Within groups it is highest in vertical transmission [5, 6].

Vertical cultural transmission is likely to be important in nutrition. For instance, tastes might be influenced, to some extent irreversibly, by the food available at a young age. There might also be genetic components to tastes; one, the capacity of tasting phenylthiourea is well known, but whether it influences food preference is less clear. Experimental evidence includes very special types of maternal and more complex transmission (Galef and Clark, 12). Weaned rats prefer food that their lactating mother ate (Galef and Henderson, 13). In kittens, food preferences transmitted by the mother may last until the adult state (Wywicka, 28).

Questions of palatability border on behavior. Many nutritional problems are truly behavioral. The area of food preferences seems one in which studies of transmission are of considerable practical importance.

Genetics was originally the study of variation and inheritance. Much of the variation that we observe in nutrition is really of cultural origin. It reflects cultural adaptations to potential food sources in different environmental and historical niches. I consider problems of variation and inheritance as pertaining to genetics, even if they have nothing to do with DNA, since concepts and methods similar to the ones in classical genetics help solve them. Such was the motivation to write the recent book [3], in collaboration with M. Feldman, on cultural transmission and evolution. In it we use ideas from genetics for treating problems of inheritance and variation, totally distinct from those of DNA genetics.

This approach is not to be confused with other recent attempts at considering relations between genes and culture. A widely publicized one, stemming from sociobiology, is based on the idea that genes hold culture on a leash, sometimes a very short leash (Lumsden and Wilson, 19). In nutrition, we have only a few examples of genetic adaptations to different foods. They are sufficient, however, to indicate that, on the contrary, culture may hold genes on a very short leash. The clearest case of a genetic, not only cultural or physiological, adaptation to certain foods is that of lactose absorption, believed to be due to cultural adaptation to adults' use of milk (Simoons, 24). Another possible candidate is the disapeareance of gluten intolerance (Simoons, 25) in populations that have used wheat and barley for long periods of time. Another interesting example is the relatively high frequency of sucrase deficiency in Eskimos, [20] who only recently started to consume sucrose. It is known that populations which do not use a given gene sometimes lose it.

Along the lines of genetic adaptations following cultural changes, I would like to plead for research on one problem. When exposed to a protein-poor diet, Pygmies, who are hunter-gatherers, have more kwashiorkor than do African farmers on the same diet. Indeed, this diet is standard diet for the farmer. Studies of the amino acid profile [22], show an increased phenylalanine-tyrosine ratio in normal adult Pygmies. This is not due to a genetic condition, since the abnormal ratio vanished on exposure to a balanced diet [23]. It does not exclude, however, the possibility of genetic differences in risk of kwashiorkor of other severe protein/ caloric malnutrition. Most hunter-gatherers, such as Pymies, Bushmen, and Eskimos, eat high-protein diets. Farmers from developing countries take in small amounts of protein. If protein-thrifty genotypes exist (or nitrogen-thrifty, or perhaps thrifty for more specific things), they are probably rare among hunter-gatherers. They would be more frequent among farmers, who are under the pressure of protein-poor diets. As with lactose malabsorption, selection might not yet have had time to completely eradicate non-thrifty genotypes. Therefore, these genotypes may still be present among farmers, though less commonly than among huntergatherers. Such genotypes may run the risk of kwashiorkor. However, this disease represents an extreme manifestation. With a probability of only, say, 10 % in the appropriate genotype (s) exposed to extreme environmental conditions, there would be little correlation between sibs. Parent-child correlations cannot be explored because affected children have died before becoming parents. Thus, evidence of genetic determination of kwashiorkor would be hard to obtain from correlations between first degree relatives. I suggest we study the N-balance of children who have recovered for kwashiorkor and compare it with that of suitable controls. Other analysis might be more suitable. One clue comes from our observation of a high phenylalanine/tyrosine ratio in malnourished Pygmies, which corresponds to Cravioto's observations in Central America [11]. The partial deficit of black pigment in the hair of kwashiorkor patients parallels that observed in PKU patients. This also points to inhibition of phenylalanine hydroxylase (or at least of that pathway) as one facet of kwashiorkor worth studying more closely. We should remember that more than one gene may be necessary for observing the kwashiorkor phenotype.

Students of the genetic variation that affects nutrition have many interesting discoveries ahead of them. Such studies are likely to be especially successful if centered around *specific* clear-cut metabolic changes and qualitative and quantitative variation of *specific* enzymes or proteins likely to be involved in metabolism or transport. Clear-cut, single-gene determined variation of biochemical significance will be a most promising field for the nutritional problemas under study. The search for quantitative variation and the estimation of heritabilities, are especially arduous for traits that are hard to measure accurately. Generally they are of little scientific or practical significance. The "holistic" approach, considering polygenic variation in toto, is less rewarding than the single gene approach.

Natural selection must have stabilized the genetic variation of food dependencies within narrow bounds. It must have been continuously selected for genotypes that would place the population well away from "danger zones" of the risk/environment diagrams discussed by the earlier speakers. Genetic variation may be relatively low for traits that have been strongly selected over a long period of time. However, it is more likely that a fraction of the population is now in the danger zone when environmental conditions have recently changed due to cultural or ecological shifts.

Neel has stressed the potential importance of some of these changes. Both genetic and cultural evolution will eventually remedy such situations. But genetic changes are slow, and some people might still be behind in the process of genetic adaptation. Here genetic research may be especially rewarding, as is happening, for instance, in the analysis of cholesterol levels. The transition from hunting-gathering to agriculture [4], which took place only recently (the last ten thousand years) revolutionized the nutritional environment. It also probably caused genetic adaptations besides those which we have already studied.

REFERENCES

1. Blackburn, II. Determinants of individual and population blood lipoprotein levels: Nutritional-genetics interactions (this symposium).
2. Bodmer, W.F. and Cavalli-Sforza, L.L. "Genetics, Evolution and Man", 782 pp. W.H. Freeman and Company, San Francisco. 1976.
3. Bodmer, W.F. and Bodmer, J.G. Evolution and function of the IILA system. *Br. Med. Bull.* 34: 309, 1978.
4. Cavalli-Sforza, L.L. Human evolution and nutrition. *In* "Food, Nutrition and Evolution" (D.N. Walcher and N. Kretchmer, eds.) pp. 1-7. Masson Publishing Company USA. 1981.
5. Cavalli-Sforza, L.L. and Feldman, M., "Cultural Transmission and Evolution: A Quantitative Approach". 388 pp. Princeton University Prees, Princeton, 1981.
6. Cavalli-Sforza, L.L., Feldman, M.W., Chen, K.H. and Dornbusch, S.M. Theory and observation in cultural transmission. *Science* (in press, October 1982).
7. Cavalli-Sforza, L.L. The rote of plasticity in biological and cultural evolution. *Annals of N.Y. Acad. of Sci.* 231: 43, 1974.
8. Cavalli-Sforza, L.L. and Feldman, M.W. Cultural versus biological inheritance: Phenotypic transmission from parent to children. *Am. J. Hum. Genet.* 25: 618, 1973.
9. Cavalli Sforza, T. and Menozzi, P. Observation on lactase deficiency in adults in Italy.
10. Cederbaum, S.D. Phenylketonuria (this symposium).
11. Cravioto, J. Longitudinal studies (this symposium).
12. Galef, B.G. and Clark, M.M. Mother's milk and adult presence + two factors determining initial dietary selection by weanling rats. *Jrnl. of Comp. and Physiol. Psych.* 78: 220, 1972.
13. Galef, B.G. and Henderson, P.W. Mother's milkk + A determinant of the feeding preferences of weaning rat pups. *Jrnl. of Comp. and Phys. Psych.* 78: 213, 1972.
14. Galton, F. "Natural Inheritance", 259 pp. McMillan, London and New York, 1889.
15. Garby, L. Energy balance and obesity (This symposium).
16. Gottesman, I.I. Genetic aspects of intelligent bahavior. In "The Hand book of Mental Deficiency + Psychological Theory and Research" (N. Ellis, eds.), pp. 253-296. McGraw-Hill, New York, 1963.
17. Loehlin, J.C. and Nichols, R.C. "Heredity, Environment and Personality", pp. Univ. of Texas Press, Austin, 1976.
18. Lisker, R. Lactase deficiency (this symposium).
19. Lumsden, C.J. and Wilson, E.O. "Genes Mind and Culture: The Geoevolutionary Process 428 pp. Harvard Univ. Press. Cambridge and London, 1981.

20. McNair, A., Gudman-Hoyer, E., Jarnum, S. *et/al.,* Sucrase malabsorption in Greenland. *Brit. Med. J.* 2: 19-21, 1972.
21. Motulsky, A. The Mendelian Hyperlipidemias (this symposium).
22. Paolucci, A.M., Spadoni, M.A., Pennetti, V. and Cavalli-Sforza, L.L. Serum free amino acid pattern in a Babinga Pygmy adult population. *Amer. J. Clin. Nutrition* 22: 1642, 1969.
23. Paolucci, A.M., Spadoni, M.A., and Pennetti, V. Modifications of serum-free amino acid patterns of Babinga adult pygmies after short-term feeding of a balanced diet. *Am. J. Clin. Nutr.* 26: 429, 1973.
24. Simmoons, F. The geographic hypothesis and lactose malabsorption. A weighing of the evidence. *Dig. Dis. Sci.* 23: 963, 1978.
25. Simoons, F. Celiac disease as a geographic problem. *In* "Food, Nutrition and Evolution" (D.N. Walcher and N. Kretchmer, eds.), pp. 179-199. Masson Publishing Company USA, New York, 1981.
26. Sukhatme, P.V. and Margen, S. Models for protein deficiency. *Amer, J. Clin. Nutr.* 31: 1237, 1978; and Autoregulatory hemeostatic nature of energy balance. *Am. J. Clin. Nutrit.* 35: 355, 1982.
27. Ward, R.H. Genetic epidemiology as a potential tool in nutritional research (this symposium).
28. Wyrwicka, W. Imitation of mother's inappropriate food preference in weanling kittens. *Pav. J. Biol, Sci.* 13: 55, 1978.

Index